NUTRITION AND DIET RESEARCH PROGRESS

FOOD ALLERGIES

SYMPTOMS, DIAGNOSIS, AND TREATMENT

NUTRITION AND DIET RESEARCH PROGRESS

Additional books in this series can be found on Nova's website under the Series tab.

Additional E-books in this series can be found on Nova's website under the E-books tab.

NUTRITION AND DIET RESEARCH PROGRESS

FOOD ALLERGIES

SYMPTOMS, DIAGNOSIS, AND TREATMENT

PATRICIA M. RODGERS
EDITOR

Nova Science Publishers, Inc.
New York

For permission to use material from this book please contact us:
Telephone 631-231-7269; Fax 631-231-8175
Web Site: http://www.novapublishers.com

Additional color graphics may be available in the e-book version of this book.

LIBRARY OF CONGRESS CATALOGING-IN-PUBLICATION DATA

Food allergies : symptoms, diagnosis, and treatment / editor, Patricia M. Rodgers.
p. ; cm.
Includes bibliographical references and index.
ISBN 978-1-61728-748-0 (hardcover)
1. Food allergy. I. Rodgers, Patricia M.
[DNLM: 1. Food Hypersensitivity--diagnosis. 2. Food Hypersensitivity--therapy. 3. Child. 4. Infant. WD 310 F6854 2010]
RC596.F65 2010
616.97'5--dc22

2010022740

Published by Nova Science Publishers, Inc. ✝ New York

CONTENTS

PREFACE

Food allergy is an adverse reactions resulting from an inappropriate immunological response to a food antigen. It usually presents as multi-system involvement with gastrointestinal symptoms, cutaneous symptoms, and respiratory symptoms occuring in 50 to 80%, 20 to 40%, and 4 to 25% of cases, respectively. This new book reviews research from around the globe in the study of food allergies including fish allergy diagnosis and detection; allergy mitigation by dietary components; the pathophysiology and mechanisms of food allergy; emergency department anaphylaxis management and management of children with food allergies.

Chapter 1 - Food allergy is an adverse reaction resulting from an inappropriate immunological response to a food antigen. It usually presents as multi-system involvement. Gastrointestinal symptoms, cutaneous symptoms, and respiratory symptoms occur in 50 to 80%, 20 to 40%, and 4 to 25% of cases, respectively. Gastrointestinal manifestations include oral allergy syndrome, gastrointestinal anaphylaxis, allergic eosinophilic esophagitis, allergic eosinophilic gastroenteropathy, food protein-induced enteropathy, food protein-induced enterocolitis syndrome, food protein-induced proctocolitis, gluten-sensitive enteropathy, infantile colic, irritable bowel syndrome, and constipation. Cutaneous manifestations are urticaria/angioedema, atopic dermatitis, contact dermatitis, and dermatitis herpetiformis. Finally, rhinitis/rhinoconjunctivitis, asthma, Heiner syndrome, and serous otitis media are the respiratory manifestations of food allergy. Other manifestations include systemic anaphylaxis, food-dependent exercise-induced anaphylaxis, migraine, epilepsy, diabetes mellitus, nephrotic syndrome, nocturnal enuresis, anemia, thrombocytopenia, vasculitis, and arthropathy/arthritis.

Skin-prick testing with food extracts is often used to screen patients with suspected IgE-mediated food allergies. Simultaneously, since many children with IgE-mediated food allergies have elevated serum IgE levels, serum IgE antibodies specific for allergens can be measured in vitro by RAST, ELISA, or FEIA techniques. However, the double-blind placebo-controlled food challenge is objective and is considered the "gold standard" for the diagnosis of a food allergy. Nonetheless, an open or single-blind food challenge is acceptable when the resulting symptoms can be objectively observed. Definitive treatment of food allergy is strict elimination of the offending food from the diet. Symptomatic reactivity to food allergens is generally very specific, and patients rarely react to more than one food in a botanical or animal species. If elimination diets are prescribed, care must be taken to ensure that they are palatable and nutritionally adequate. Patients must have a good knowledge of foods containing the allergen and must be taught to scrutinize the labels of all packaged food carefully. Emergency treatment of food-induced anaphylaxis centers on basic life support principles, and intramuscular injection of epinephrine. A fast-acting H_1 antihistamine should be considered for the child with progressive or generalized urticaria or disturbing pruritus. Pharmacological therapies such as mast cell stabilizers have little role in the treatment of food allergy.

Chapter 2 - Allergy to fish is one of the most common IgE-mediated food allergies, especially in geographical regions where fish is frequently consumed. Most fish-allergic patients are sensitized to β-parvalbumin, a highly stable protein of 11-12 kDa. Several isoforms of parvalbumins can be found in the same muscle tissue. These isoforms share conserved protein domains. Common IgE epitopes have been considered as an explanation for the extensive allergic cross-reactivity to different fish species. However, frequency and intensity of allergic reactions to fish are highly variable in sensitized patients.

The diagnosis of fish allergy has made progress over the last decade. New approaches have been investigated for component-resolved diagnosis. Parvalbumin molecules from different species are being produced as recombinant proteins and become available for use in allergen-specific serum IgE quantification. Component-resolved diagnosis provides also the opportunity to test IgE for fish allergens other than parvalbumin. The availability of well-characterized minor allergens in routine assays is important to improve the future clinical diagnosis of fish allergy. Diagnostic tools like the microarray system are being commercialized addressing the challenge of patient-specific allergy profiling.

To date, specific immunotherapy is not available for fish-allergic patients. A new EU project aims now to test a hypo-allergenic variant of recombinant parvalbumin in a clinical immunotherapy trial. For the time being, patients are advised to avoid any kind of fish and fish products, unless it was shown that some fish were tolerated by the individual. In the US and Europe, fish and fish-derived ingredients are included in the list of important food allergens. In order to protect fish-allergic consumers, regulatory food authorities require manufacturers to label fish and fishery products. Food monitoring and tracing became a legal issue. In the recent past, the need for reliable assays motivated research to develop analytical assays for fish allergen detection. Detection of fish allergens has been approached by a number of studies both on the protein level as well as on the DNA level, so that it can be expected that commercial assays will be available soon.

This chapter will provide a general overview of fish allergy and of the relevant molecular biology background. Recent developments in diagnosis of fish allergy and detection of fish allergens will be discussed.

Chapter 3 - Proper and well-balanced immune functioning is of pivotal importance to health and well-being. In the past decades, there has been an apparent decrease in the prevalence of classical infectious diseases, with a concomitant increase in immune-related disorders, including allergies. Causally, a relationship with changes in life-style-related factors, amongst which hygienic practice, is often laid.

Diet and nutrition can affect functioning of various immune parameters. This concept can be explored to prevent or mitigate allergic reactions via the development of targeted food products or ingredients. This review describes recent findings with respect to food products and ingredients that show potential in this respect, with special emphasis on pro- and prebiotics, ß-glucans, fungal immunomodulatory proteins and ω-3 polyunsaturated fatty acids. The micro-organism-related products appear to strengthen Th1-mediated immunity, thus possibly restoring defective immune maturation due to overly hygienic living conditions.

Also ω-3-PUFAs may hold promise to attenuate allergic symptoms, although this concept appears to function via mechanisms that are clearly distinct from the micro-organism derived compounds.

Chapter 4 - Food allergy, whose symptoms may vary widely from one patient to the other, has a wide prevalence, affecting 6% of children and 3 to 4% of adults (Benhamou, 2009; Simpson, 2008). It has a potential impact on family life and the accidental contact to food allergens is a latent risk for sudden and life-threatening reactions (Burks, 2008). To our knowledge, the best form of treatment is still food avoidance, which can further reduce quality of life for patients and their families. It is important for all health professionals working with these patients to gain understanding of the mechanisms of this disease, and thus diminish the difficulty in establishing the diagnosis.

In normal conditions, the physiological access of dietary macromolecules into the organism through the gut mucosa generally induces a phenomenon called oral tolerance (OT) in which the immunological reactions are mediated by regulatory lymphocytes in a non inflammatory milieu (Burks, 2008). On the other hand, the ingestion of food proteins may also result in abnormal responses, leading to immunological consequences such as food allergy and inflammatory gut reactions (Benhamou, 2009). Food allergies, characterized both by humoral and cellular mechanisms, are reactions initiated by immunological mechanisms and should be called food hypersensitivity. In many cases the immunological reaction is mediated by IgE - typified as a Th2 response - which accounts for most of the acute reactions that are not restricted to the gut. The cases in which the main mechanisms involve IgG and cellular reactions - typified as Th1 responses - the symptoms tend to be chronic and are frequently restricted to the gut (Eigenmann, 2009).

Accidental exposure remains a serious problem for individuals who are allergic to specific food allergens. Patients with severe forms of food allergy must not only be alert to situations in which exposure is possible but must also be prepared to treat reactions when they occur. This is particularly important when the individual has little control over their surroundings or cannot request medical attention (Comstock, 2008).

Food allergies have increased over the past decade and are an important problem in daily clinical practice. Adverse reactions to food may result in a large number of clinical signs involving skin, circulatory system, and the gastrointestinal tract. Food allergies can also lead to fatal final consequences such as hypotension an anaphylaxis. The diagnosis relies on a detailed history, an elimination diet, skin tests, laboratory tests, and food challenges. The basis of the food allergy treatment is the elimination diet.

Chapter 5 - Allergic disorders have been a rising health problem in Western Countries over the last three decades. The majority of allergic disorders are elicited by IgE-dependent activation of the immune system; therefore, monitoring of serum IgE is commonly used for diagnosis of allergic conditions. Importantly, a significant number of patients present with allergic symptoms in the absence of elevated serum IgE. Here, the authors propose that total-body IgE cannot be correctly assessed by looking at serum IgE alone. In the absence of elevated serum IgE, tissue-resident IgE or IgE bound to peripheral blood cells might be critically involved in the elicitation of allergic symptoms. In this comment, the authors discuss options to expand diagnostic measures to an assessment of total-body IgE rather than serum IgE levels alone. Such additional diagnostic approaches might be particularly useful for evaluating the allergic status of patients with low serum IgE.

Chapter 6 - Anaphylaxis is a serious allergic reaction that is rapid in onset and may cause death.[1] The management of anaphylactic reactions occurs most commonly in the emergency department.[2, 3] Furthermore, food-related allergic reactions have been shown to be the leading cause of anaphylactic reactions treated in the emergency department.[4] A systematic algorithm for the diagnosis and management of anaphylaxis, especially food-related reactions, would allow emergency medicine practitioners to better recognize and manage anaphylaxis in the emergency department.

Chapter 7 - Food allergy is defined as an adverse reaction because of an abnormal immunological response to food protein. The immune pathogenesis is, in the majority of cases, IgE-mediated although it may also be cell-mediated (non-IgE) or mixed IgE/cell-mediated. Food allergy affects as many as 2 to 8% of young children and the presentation can be highly variable. There is usually a clear temporal relationship between food exposure and the development of allergic symptoms. At times, symptoms may develop hours or days after food exposure making the diagnosis difficult.

Food allergy usually presents as multi-system involvement, most commonly gastrointestinal symptoms which occur with a frequency of 50 to 80% of cases. These are followed by cutaneous symptoms and respiratory symptoms, occurring in 20 to 40%, and 4 to 25% of cases, respectively. Gastrointestinal manifestations include oral allergy syndrome, gastrointestinal anaphylaxis, allergic eosinophilic esophagitis, allergic eosinophilic gastroenteropathy, food protein-induced enteropathy, food protein-induced enterocolitis syndrome, food protein-induced proctocolitis, gluten-sensitive enteropathy, infantile colic, irritable bowel syndrome, and constipation. Cutaneous manifestations are urticaria/angioedema, atopic dermatitis, contact dermatitis, and dermatitis herpetiformis. Rhinitis/rhinoconjunctivitis, asthma, Heiner syndrome, and serous otitis media are the respiratory manifestations of food allergy. Other manifestations include systemic anaphylaxis, food-dependent exercise-induced anaphylaxis, migraine, epilepsy, diabetes mellitus, nephrotic syndrome, nocturnal enuresis, anemia, thrombocytopenia, vasculitis, and arthropathy/arthritis. This chapter discusses the various clinical manifestations of food allergy.

Chapter 8 - The prevalence of cow's milk allergy (CMA) ranges from 0.5% to 7.5% in children in the first half year of life, although generally resolves by 3 years of age. However, it may be a precursor to other, and sometimes more serious, atopic diseases, asthma, and respiratory allergies. The prevention of cow's milk proteins sensitisation, early allergy and atopic dermatitis is therefore an important strategy in limiting atopic disease in later childhood and adulthood, and research efforts have been done into prevention strategies. Because infants may absorb more food allergen during their first year than later in life, the best strategy to prevent food sensitisation is to avoid the relevant allergenic proteins, with exclusive breast-feeding as a first option. The second option is the use of hypoallergenic (HA) hydrolysates based formulas during the first 6 months of life, mainly in none or partially breastfed infants from atopic families (at risk infants).

Since residual allergenicity has been reported in several commercial preparations developed from enzymatic hydrolysis of heat treated (HT) proteins, the use of high hydrostatic pressure (HHP) as an alternative to HT has generated increasing interest over the last decade, investigation widely developed by our group. The combined HHP and enzymatic treatments of proteins might be of interest to the dairy industry to produce new foods suitable for children having a milk allergy and also for those from atopic families (at risk infants).

The main objective of this review is to provide the reader with an up-to-date summary and analyse new trends which have emerged in the last few years in this developing area.

Chapter 9 - Food allergy, atopic dermatitis, rhinitis and allergic asthma are common atopic diseases in Western countries and their prevalence has been rising the past thirty years (1-3). Prevention of food allergy induced by the three major food allergens, hen's egg, cow's milk and peanut is considered important to prevent related diseases like atopic dermatitis, allergic rhinitis and allergic asthma later in life. There is a strong relation between food allergy and eczema in young children under the age of 1 year (4-6). The route of sensitization to food allergens is still not completely elucidated and might involve the skin or airways beside sensitization via the gastrointestinal tract. Breastfeeding is still considered the best way of preventing food sensitization. Prebiotic oligosaccharides and cytokines like IL10 and TGF_{β} which are abundantly present in human milk, might provide an immunological milieu that favors the induction of oral tolerance in the Th2 prone infant. However, if breastfeeding is not possible or sufficient, hydrolysed formulae are the second best option for children with a genetic predisposition to develop allergic diseases. Recent studies provide evidence that the induction of specific oral tolerance is preferred in preventing sensitization to food allergens early in life (7-10). For prevention of clinical symptoms in sensitized children, different approaches of specific immune modulation are currently investigated to desensitize or tolerize cow's milk allergic infants; subcutaneous immunotherapy (SIT), sublingual immunotherapy (SLIT) or oral immunotherapy (OIT). In the current chapter primary prevention of allergic disease or treatment strategies to prevent clinical symptoms in sensitized individuals are described. Furthermore, the use of animal models is discussed in relation to food allergy, atopic dermatitis and the predisposition to other allergies later in life (i.e. atopic march).

Chapter 10 - The definitive treatment of food allergy is strict elimination of the offending food from the diet. Symptomatic reactivity to food allergens is generally very specific, and patients rarely react to more than one food in a botanical or animal species. If elimination diets are prescribed, care must be taken to ensure that they are palatable and nutritionally adequate. Patients must have a good knowledge of food containing the allergen and must be taught to scrutinize the labels of all packaged food carefully.

Formula-fed infants with cow's milk allergy should be fed an elemental or extensively hydrolysed hypoallergenic formula. Soy formulas are inappropriate alternatives as a significant number of infants who are allergic to cow's milk are also allergic to soy. Most children outgrow their food hypersensitivity. As such, rechallenge testing for food allergy should be performed; the interval between rechallenges should be dictated by the specific food allergen in question, the age of the child, and the degree of difficulty in avoiding the food in question

Emergency treatment of food-induced anaphylaxis should follow the basic life support ABC principles, with the simultaneous intramuscular injection of adrenaline. A fast-acting H_1 antihistamine should be considered for the child with progressive or generalized urticaria or disturbing pruritus. Pharmacological therapies such as mast cell stabilizers have very little role to play in the treatment of gastrointestinal manifestations of food allergy.

In high-risk infants, exclusive breastfeeding with introduction of solid foods not earlier than 6 months of age may delay or possibly prevent the onset of food allergy in some children. Avoidance of allergenic foods by lactating mothers is often recommended. When breastfeeding is not possible, the use of a partially or extensively hydrolysed hypoallergenic formula is desirable. Prophylactic medications have not been shown to be consistently effective in the prevention of life-threatening reactions to food. Their use may mask a less severe reaction to a culprit food, knowledge of which might prevent a more severe reaction to that food in the future.

In: Food Allergies: Symptoms, Diagnosis, and Treatment
Editor: Patricia M. Rodgers
ISBN: 978-1-61728-748-0

Chapter 1

FOOD ALLERGY: AN OVERVIEW*

Alexander K. C. Leung [≠1] ***and James S. C. Leung*** [2]
[1]Department of Pediatrics, University of Calgary,
Alberta Children's Hospital, Calgary, Alberta, Canada
[2]Department of Pediatrics, University of Toronto,
Hospital for Sick Children, Toronto, Ontario, Canada

ABSTRACT

Food allergy is an adverse reaction resulting from an inappropriate immunological response to a food antigen. It usually presents as multi-system involvement. Gastrointestinal symptoms, cutaneous symptoms, and respiratory symptoms occur in 50 to 80%, 20 to 40%, and 4 to 25% of cases, respectively. Gastrointestinal manifestations include oral allergy syndrome, gastrointestinal anaphylaxis, allergic eosinophilic esophagitis, allergic eosinophilic gastroenteropathy, food protein-induced enteropathy, food protein-induced enterocolitis syndrome, food protein-induced proctocolitis, gluten-sensitive enteropathy, infantile colic, irritable bowel syndrome, and constipation. Cutaneous manifestations are urticaria/angioedema, atopic dermatitis, contact dermatitis, and dermatitis herpetiformis. Finally, rhinitis/rhinoconjunctivitis, asthma, Heiner syndrome, and serous otitis media are the respiratory manifestations of food allergy. Other manifestations include systemic anaphylaxis, food-dependent exercise-induced anaphylaxis, migraine, epilepsy, diabetes mellitus, nephrotic syndrome, nocturnal enuresis, anemia, thrombocytopenia, vasculitis, and arthropathy/arthritis.

Skin-prick testing with food extracts is often used to screen patients with suspected IgE-mediated food allergies. Simultaneously, since many children with IgE-mediated food allergies have elevated serum IgE levels, serum IgE antibodies specific for allergens can be measured in vitro by RAST, ELISA, or FEIA techniques. However, the double-blind placebo-controlled food challenge is objective and is considered the "gold standard" for the diagnosis of a food allergy. Nonetheless, an open or single-blind food

---

* Portions of this article appeared previously in Advances in Pediatrics [1] and Food Allergies: New Research [2,3], and have been used with permission from the publishers.

≠ Address correspondence to: Dr. Alexander K.C. Leung MBBS, FRCPC, FRCP (UK&Irel), FRCPCH, FAAP, Clinical Professor of Pediatrics, The University of Calgary, #200, 233 – 16th Avenue NW, Calgary, Alberta, Canada T2M 0H5, Telefax: (403) 230-3322, Telephone: (403) 230-3300, e-mail: aleung@ucalgary.ca challenge is acceptable when the resulting symptoms can be objectively observed. Definitive treatment of food allergy is strict elimination of the offending food from the diet. Symptomatic reactivity to food allergens is generally very specific, and patients rarely react to more than one food in a botanical or animal species. If elimination diets are prescribed, care must be taken to ensure that they are palatable and nutritionally adequate. Patients must have a good knowledge of foods containing the allergen and must be taught to scrutinize the labels of all packaged food carefully. Emergency treatment of food-induced anaphylaxis centers on basic life support principles, and intramuscular injection of epinephrine. A fast-acting H_1 antihistamine should be considered for the child with progressive or generalized urticaria or disturbing pruritus. Pharmacological therapies such as mast cell stabilizers have little role in the treatment of food allergy.

Introduction

Food allergy (food hypersensitivity) is an adverse reaction resulting from an inappropriate immunological response to an antigen contained in food or food additive [1-5]. The reaction occurs in susceptible patients, and may be independent of the quantity of the offending substance ingested. Food allergy should be distinguished from food intolerance (nonallergic food hypersensitivity), which is an adverse reaction to food resulting from unique physiologic characteristic of the host, such as a metabolic disorder (e.g., lactase deficiency) [6]. Food toxicity is a separate entity resulting from effects of toxic contaminant or ingredient in food that effect healthy individuals in sufficient doses [6].

Epidemiology

In the United States, up to 25% of adults self-report having a food allergy, and up to 25% of households report alteration of household dietary for individuals with perceived food allergies [7]. However, the prevalence of true, immunologically mediated food allergy is estimated to be 4 to 8% in children less than five years old in industrialized countries [5-7]. The prevalence decreases after 5 years of age, such that an estimated 1 to 4% of adults in industrialized countries have food allergies [7]. These data reflect the general tendency for children to develop immunologic or "oral" tolerance to their food allergens with advancing age [5]. Approximately 85% of children with IgE mediated food allergies lose their food hypersensitivity by 3 to 5 years of age [8]. However, this natural history will vary with the specific food allergen. For example, cow's milk protein allergy that develops within the first year of life, resolves spontaneously in 80% of cases by age five years [9]. This is contrasted with peanut allergies that develop in childhood but resolve in approximately 20% of cases by adulthood [10]. New onset food allergies during adulthood are rare [7].

In young children, the most frequently implicated foods include eggs, cow's milk, tree nut, peanut, soy, wheat, seafood, citrus fruits, and chocolate [7]. In comparison, shellfish, peanuts, fish and tree nut allergies are frequently seen in adults as they are rarely outgrown [7]. Although often suspected, wheat and soy allergies are traditionally difficult to prove [7]. Geographic clustering of particular food allergies with particular populations has been noted [7].

However, there is controversy regarding an increasing prevalence of specific food allergies in specific populations [7]. Although surveillance has increased in recent years, there is now clear evidence supporting and increased incidence of food allergy [11]. Evidence with peanuts is particularly compelling, with prospective studies from the United States and United Kingdom reporting a doubling in the prevalence of peanut allergies in young children over the last ten years [12,13]. Not surprisingly, this controversy has garnered significant media attention, and despite strong research initiatives, the precise etiology and rationale for these changes remains unclear [11].

PATHOGENESIS

In the majority of cases, food allergies result from an IgE-mediated immune response. However, non-IgE-mediated responses may also occur. IgE-mediated reactions are caused by inflammatory mediators and cytokines released when food-derived antigens that are absorbed into blood, bind onto specific IgE residing on the surface of mast cells and basophils as well as lymphocytes, platelets, eosinophils and macrophages [14]. This binding results in release of histamine, heparin, prostaglandins, tryptase and leukotrienes which when act systemically inducing vasodilatation, mucus secretion, smooth muscle dilation [15]. These reactions are associated with rapid development of symptoms, usually within minutes to 2 hours, although late phase reactions from IgE-mediated cytokines may occur [14].

On the other hand, non-IgE reactions develop over hours, days or even weeks after exposure to food allergen [16]. The pathogenesis of these reactions is far less understood, with insufficient evidence to support type III (immune complex mediated) or type IV (cell-mediated) as exclusive processes [5]. This lack of understanding is partly due to the delayed onset of symptoms combined with lack of efficiency in making diagnosis once suspected [16]. Non-IgE reactions primarily affect the gut, and are histologically characterized by intense eosinophilic infiltration of the specific organ involved and may lead to chronic disorders such as allergic eosinophilic gastroenteropathy [16]. These reactions cause significant morbidity, but rarely mortality in patients [16].

In recent years, studies have focused on understanding the molecular pathogenesis, natural history and the recent increase in prevalence of food allergies. Specifically, a number of studies have queried the predisposition of young children towards food allergy, followed by their subsequent resolution with age. Understanding these fundamental mechanisms is believed by many to be a key to developing novel therapies and addressing the increasing incidence of food allergy [11]. At present, it is believed that a complex interplay of factors including:

- An immature gut mucosa in infants permitting increased absorption of intact food antigens.
- An immature immune system, especially at the gut mucosal level in infants unable to differentiate between innocent food allergens/nutrients, symbiotic gut flora and virulent microbes. Aging allows immunologic tolerance to develop and hence resolution of symptoms with age.
- Specific food allergens that elicit greater immunologic response.

- Genetic polymorphisms in particular populations that react immunologically to particular food allergens.

Although the specific details and proposed molecular interactions with these hypotheses is beyond the scope of this clinically-oriented paper, excellent reviews on this topic were recently published by Cocharane et al and Jyonouchi [11,16].

TABLE 1. Clinical Manifestations of Food Allergy

Generalized manifestations
Systemic anaphylaxis
Food-dependent exercise-induced anaphylaxis
Gastrointestinal manifestations
Oral allergy syndrome
Gastrointestinal anaphylaxis
Allergic eosinophilic esophagitis
Allergic eosinophilic gastroenteropathy
Food protein-induced enteropathy
Food protein-induced enterocolitis syndrome
Food protein-induced proctocolitis
Gluten-sensitive enteropathy
Infantile colic
Irritable bowel syndrome
Recurrent abdominal pain
Constipation
Cutaneous manifestations
Urticaria/angioedema
Atopic dermatitis
Contact dermatitis
Dermatitis herpetiformis
Respiratory manifestations
Rhinitis/rhinoconjunctivitis
Chronic sinusitis
Asthma
Heiner syndrome
Serous otitis media
Ménière's disease
Neurologic manifestations
Migraine
Epilepsy
Endocrine manifestation
Diabetes mellitus
Renal manifestations
Nephrotic syndrome
Hematologic manifestations
Anemia
Thrombocytopenia
Rheumatic manifestation
Vasculitis
Arthropathy/arthritis

Clinical Manifestations

Food allergies typically present with multi-system involvement. From a clinical and diagnostic perspective, it is helpful to subdivide clinical manifestations according to the predominant organ system(s) involved. Gastrointestinal symptoms occur most commonly with a frequency between 50 and 80% of cases, followed by cutaneous symptoms occurring in 20 to 40% and respiratory symptoms occurring in 4 to 25% of cases, respectively [14]. Symptoms may be mild or severe and most often occur within one to two hours after the offending food has been eaten. Occasionally, the onset of symptoms may be delayed for 48 to 72 hours.

Generalized Manifestations

Systemic Anaphylaxis

Systemic anaphylaxis secondary to ingestion of food allergen is potentially fatal, and the most common cause of anaphylaxis treated in emergency departments [6]. However, overall, systemic anaphylaxis is an uncommon manifestation of food allergy [17]. Systemic anaphylaxis usually occurs within minutes, but occasionally hours after the ingestion of an offending food [18]. Peanuts, nuts, eggs, and seafood are responsible for the majority of these reactions [19]. Early symptoms may include pruritis, "metallic" taste in the mouth, sensation of tightness in the throat, flushing, urticaria, dizziness, nausea, vomiting, abdominal pain, angioedema, and wheezing [20]. This may rapidly progress to laryngeal edema, dyspnea, stridor, diaphoresis, cyanosis, chest pain, hypotension, cardiac dysrhythmias, and shock [21,22]. The degree of anaphylactic reactions varies and may be manifested in a partial form. In general, the more rapidly anaphylaxis occurs after exposure to an offending agent, the more likely the anaphylactic reaction is to be severe and potentially life-threatening [19]. Anaphylactic reactions to foods can be biphasic with an early and late phase separated by one to eight hours or there may be multiple recurrences separated by asymptomatic periods lasting for hours [14,23]. Some very severe anaphylactic reactions are protracted and last continuously for many hours without remission [14]. Risk factors for severe anaphylactic reactions include history of a previous anaphylactic reaction, history of poorly controlled asthma, allergy to peanuts, nuts and shellfish, and use of ß-blockers or acetycholinesterase inhibitors [4,24]. Low levels of serum platelet-activating factor acetylhydrolase may be a marker for more severe food-induced anaphylaxis [24].

Food-Dependent Exercise-Induced Anaphylaxis

Anaphylaxis has been reported after the ingestion of foods in association with exercise [25-27]. Food-dependent exercise-induced anaphylaxis represents 7 to 9% of anaphylactic reactions [28]. The condition is twice as common in females and 60% of cases occur in individuals under the age of 30 years [24,28]. There is often a history of atopy [28]. One subset of patients may develop anaphylaxis in temporal proximity to ingestion of any type of food [20,29]. The other subset may develop anaphylaxis with exercise in conjunction with ingestion of a specific food [20]. The latter subset is more common than the former subset [20]. Foods associated with food-specific exercise-induced anaphylaxis include crustaceans, celery, grapes, tomato, wheat, buckwheat, chicken, and dairy products [29,30]. Rarely, two foods have to be eaten together to provoke an anaphylactic attack [31]. When each food is taken separately, food-dependent exercise-induced anaphylaxis does not occur [31]. Typical symptoms include urticaria, angioedema, dyspnea, and abdominal pain [32]. These may progress to hypotension and shock. Loss of consciousness is seen in approximately 30% of cases [32].

Although various exercises may lead to anaphylaxis in susceptible individuals, jogging is the exercise most frequently reported, followed by aerobics and walking [28,29,33]. Anaphylaxis usually occurs when exercise takes place within two to four hours of food ingestion [20]. Unlike exercise-induced anaphylaxis, anaphylactic symptoms develop only in the presence of both food ingestion and exercise [34]. Food-dependent exercise-induced anaphylaxis often presents with scalp pruritis prior to systemic symptoms [20].

The exact mechanism of food-dependent exercise-induced anaphylaxis is not known. There is evidence of IgE-mediated sensitization to the food allergen [28]. Skin testing may show an immediate flare-and-wheal reaction to the implicated food [27]. Blood flow differences to the gut, increased food allergen absorption, increased spontaneous leukocyte histamine release, lowered mast cell releasability threshold, and enhanced mast cell responsiveness to physical stimuli may have a role in the pathogenesis of this condition [27,29,33].

Gastrointestinal Manifestations

Oral Allergy Syndrome

Oral allergy syndrome (pollen-food allergy syndrome) is a complex of symptoms induced by exposure of the oral and pharyngeal mucosa to plant protein allergens [35,36]. Patients are usually sensitized to an aeroallergen initially [35]. The IgE antibodies to the aeroallergen cause the oral allergy syndrome [37]. Botanical cross-reactivity as a result of shared epitopes between pollen and causative fruits and vegetables has been suggested as a possible mechanism of local mast cell activation [38]. The oral allergy syndrome is considered a form of contact urticaria that is confined mainly to the oropharynx [5]. Symptoms include rapid onset of itching, tingling, burning, and/or angioedema of the lips, tongue, palate, and throat within minutes of ingestion of fresh fruit and vegetable [36]. Symptoms usually resolve rapidly. Occasionally, the clinical course is more dramatic with potentially fatal pharyngeal swelling or progression towards a generalized anaphylactic reaction [14,39]. The syndrome generally occurs in patients with inhalant allergy to birch, mugwort, or ragweed pollen and is associated with the ingestion of various fresh fruits (e.g., apples, bananas, melons, citrus fruits) and raw vegetables (e.g. carrots, tomatoes, celery) [40-43]. It is uncommon to have several fruits and vegetables that cause the oral allergy syndrome in one patient [44]. However, cross-reactivity with different fruits processing homologous protein segments has been described [45]. Oral allergy syndrome is more prevalent in adults than in children [46].

Most patients have some degree of allergic conjunctivitis or allergic rhinitis because the IgE antibodies to an aeroallergen cross-react with the fruit or vegetable proteins [35,47]. It is interesting to note that if the offending fruit or vegetable is cooked, then the patient does not usually experience any symptom as the food allergens are generally destroyed by heating [35]. Patients who remain sensitive to cooked fruit or vegetable may be sensitive to proteins that do not cross-react with pollens and do not actually have oral allergy syndrome [42,48]. Although these patients react to food typically associated with oral allergy syndrome, the absence of pollenosis and presence of symptoms beyond the oropharynx suggest conventional food allergy rather than oral allergy syndrome [42].

Gastrointestinal Anaphylaxis

Gastrointestinal anaphylaxis is an IgE-mediated gastrointestinal hypersensitivity that often accompanies other systemic manifestations of food allergy [49]. This may be manifested as nausea, vomiting, abdominal pain, flatulence, abdominal distension, or diarrhea [5]. The reaction usually occurs within minutes to 2 hours of food ingestion [50]. Repeated ingestion of a food allergen may induce partial desensitization of mast cells in the gastrointestinal tract resulting in milder symptoms [5,39].

Allergic Eosinophilic Esophagitis

Allergic eosinophilic esophagitis is characterized by intense eosinophilic infiltration of the esophageal mucosa (>20 eosinophils per high-power field) and severe basal cell hyperplasia [51-54]. However, First International Gastrointestinal Eosinophil Research Symposium Subcommittees (FIGERS) recently suggested that the presence of 15 eosinophils in esophageal mucosa is sufficient to establish the diagnosis of eosinophilic esophagitis [55].

The condition is usually T-cell-mediated rather than IgE-mediated, and caused by allergens in the diet and, less commonly, in the air [52,54,56-58]. Allergic eosinophilic esophagitis occurs mainly in children and young adults [59-60]. This condition is being more frequently diagnosed over the past decade. The condition is more common in males and those with a family or personal history of atopy or proven food allergy [53,61]. Allergic eosinophilic esophagitis may present with irritability, sleep disturbance, food refusal, vomiting/ regurgitation, dysphagia, abdominal pain, substernal chest pain, occult blood loss, anemia, and failure to thrive [41,51,54,55]. Dauer et al retrospectively reviewed the records of 71 children with biopsy-proven allergic eosinophilic esophagitis and found that the most common symptom was dysphagia, being present in 36 (51%) patients [51]. Eighteen (50%) of the 36 patients with dysphagia experienced at least one episode of food impaction. Other common symptoms include vomiting (31%) and abdominal pain (24%). The symptoms of recurrent vomiting /regurgitation may mimic those of gastroesophageal reflux but are refractory to anti-reflux treatment [55,62,63]. These symptoms respond to dietary avoidance of food allergens [63].

Allergic Eosinophilic Gastroenteropathy

Allergic eosinophilic gastroenteritis is characterized by infiltration of the gastrointestinal tract with eosinophils, peripheral eosinophilia, and absence of vasculitis [64,65]. The eosinophilic infiltrates may be quite patchy and may involve the mucosa, muscular layer, or serosal layer of the stomach or small intestine [29,45].

Although allergic eosinophilic gastroenteropathy may affect all ages, the disease is more common in individuals in the third through fifth decades [64]. Patients with mucosal involvement usually have postprandial nausea, vomiting, abdominal pain, watery diarrhea with or without blood, iron deficiency anemia, occasionally steatorrhea, and weight loss in adults or failure to thrive in children [21,29,66]. Patients with muscular involvement may have symptoms and signs of gastric outlet or intestinal obstruction, depending on the site of bowel involvement [45]. The serosal form is characterized by ascites, abdominal pain, and abdominal distension and is extremely rare in children [45,67].

Food Protein-Induced Enteropathy

Food protein-induced enteropathy is characterized by protracted diarrhea and vomiting with onset usually in infancy. This may result in malabsorption, protein-losing enteropathy, and failure to thrive [42,50]. The disorder is caused by a T-cell-mediated response most commonly to cow's milk protein [45]. Intestinal biopsy typically reveals a patchy villous atrophy, increased crypt length, and prominent mononuclear round cell infiltrates [68].

Food Protein-Induced Enterocolitis Syndrome

Food protein-induced enterocolitis syndrome is a cell-mediated hypersensitivity disease that occurs mainly in infants under 3 months of age [69]. The condition usually resolves by 2 years of age but may, rarely, persist into late childhood [46]. Cow's milk and soy protein are most often responsible [41,53,67], other food antigens have occasionally been implicated [7]. Classic symptoms are protracted vomiting and diarrhea [29,50,70]. Additional signs and symptoms include irritability, lethargy, anemia, transient methemoglobinemia, abdominal distension, protein-losing enteropathy, and failure to thrive [42,45,70-72]. Stools generally contain occult blood, polymorphonuclear neutrophils, eosinophils, and Charcot-Leyden crystals [5]. Presumably, stimulation of T-cells by food allergens with secretion of tumor necrosis factor-α may play a role in the pathophysiology of this disorder [50,70,73]. A relative lack of expression of transforming growth factor-β may also have a role to play [70,73]. Skin tests for the offending antigen are usually negative [46]. Radioallergosorbent (RAST) assay, which detects specific IgE antibody, may also be negative in these patients. Jejunal biopsy specimens usually reveal villus atrophy and increased numbers of lymphocytes, eosinophils, and mast cells [29,74]. Colonoscopy and biopsy show inflammatory colitis and eosinophilic infiltration [75]. Symptoms usually resolve in 72 hours after the offending food substance has been removed from the diet.

Food Protein-Induced Proctocolitis

As with food protein-induced enterocolitis syndrome, food protein-induced proctocolitis is a T-cell mediated disorder. The disorder usually occurs in the first few months of life and is most often secondary to milk protein or soy protein hypersensitivity [67,74]. Unlike food protein-induced enterocolitis syndrome, infants with food protein-induced proctocolitis generally appear healthy and have normal weight gain. These infants usually have occult or gross blood and occasionally mucus in their stools but classically, do not have diarrhea [50,76,77]. In breastfed infants, elimination of food-allergen from the maternal diet may result in resolution of hematochezia. In general, hematochezia resolves within 72 hours of appropriate food-allergen avoidance [50]. Colonic biopsy samples reveal mucosal edema, erythema, friability, ulceration, nodular lymphoid hyperplasia and eosinophilic infiltration [29,78]. However, colonic biopsy findings are often nonspecific and unhelpful as the disease of focal in nature and require sampling from the appropriate sites [79]. The diagnosis is primarily clinical as laboratory tests are generally unreliable [79]. Food challenges are also helpful [79].

Gluten-Sensitive Enteropathy

Gluten-sensitive enteropathy (celiac disease) is a disorder in which small-bowel mucosal damage is the result of a permanent sensitivity to gliadin, the alcohol-soluble portion of gluten, present in wheat, barley, and rye. Patients with gluten-sensitive enteropathy typically present with diarrhea/steatorrhea, abdominal distension, muscle wasting, and failure to thrive [4]. Other clinical manifestations include irritability, anorexia, vomiting, abdominal pain, oral ulcers, digital clubbing, delayed puberty, and infertility [80,81]. Occasionally, patients with gluten-sensitive enteropathy may be asymptomatic [81]. The presence of anti-gliadin, anti-endomysial, and anti-tissue transglutaminase of the IgA isotype and anti-gliadin of the IgG isotype support the diagnosis [42]. However, anti-gliadin antibody of IgG subtype has been known to be positive in conditions such as cow's milk protein allergy, inflammatory bowel disease, and cystic fibrosis and therefore has poor specificity. In addition, patients with IgA deficiency may not have antibodies of IgA subtype in spite of suffering from gluten-sensitive enteropathy. It is recommended that the diagnosis of gluten-sensitive enteropathy be confirmed by intestinal biopsy before instituting dietary changes. Characteristically, biopsy of the jejunum shows villus atrophy, marked increase in crypt-villous ratio, and extensive cellular infiltrates [29]. Both cellular and complement-mediated cytotoxicity and lymphokine-induced damage have been implicated in the pathogenesis of the condition [63]. There is a genetic predisposition to the disease. There is a predominance of certain HLA types (B8, DQ2, DW3) in patients with gluten-sensitive enteropathy [4,5]. Environmental factors may influence expression of the genetic predisposition

Infantile Colic

There is increasing evidence that cow's milk proteins may play a role in infantile colic [82-88]. Approximately 25% of infants with moderate or severe colic have allergy to cow's milk protein [89,90]. Lothe and Lindberg showed that colic disappeared in 24 of 27 infants when they were given a cow's milk-free diet [86]. These infants were entered into a double-blind placebo-controlled crossover trial of whey protein. Eighteen infants receiving the whey protein capsules reacted with colic, two infants received placebo reacted with colic, and four infants did not react at all.

Iacono et al put 70 cow's milk formula-fed infants with severe colic on soy-milk formula [84]. In 50 infants, there was a remission of symptoms when cow's milk protein was eliminated from their diet. Two successive challenges caused the return of symptoms in all these 50 infants. Follow-ups, after an average period of 18 months, showed that in 22 of 50 (44%) of the infants who had cow's milk protein-related colic and 1 of 20 (5%) of those with non-cow's milk protein-related colic developed an overt form of alimentary intolerance. Lucassen et al randomly selected 43 healthy infants with colic to receive whey hydrolysate formula or standard formula [87]. They found a decrease in the duration of crying in those infants fed with whey hydrolysate formula.

Jakobsson et al studied the effectiveness of 2 formulae with extensively hydrolysed casein in 22 infants with severe colic [91]. One infant was considered as treatment failure and six infants as protocol failures. The remaining 15 infants showed a significant decrease in the lengths of time they cried as well as a decrease in the intensity of their crying on both formulae. When the infants were challenged in a double-blind design, 11 infants reacted with an increase in crying time to cow's milk protein or bovine whey protein.

Hill et al studied the effect of diet change in 38 bottle-fed and 77 breast-fed colicky infants in a double-blind, randomized, placebo-controlled trial [83]. Bottle-fed infants were assigned to either casein hydrolysate or cow's milk formula. All mothers of breast-fed infants were started on an artificial color-free, preservative-free, additive-free diet and were randomized to receive either an active low allergen (milk free) diet or a control diet. Hill et al showed that infants on the active diet had their distress reduced by 39% compared with 16% for those on the control diet.

Jakobsson and Lindberg put 66 mothers of 66 breast-fed infants with infantile colic on a cow's milk-free diet [92]. The colic disappeared in 35 infants; it reappeared after reintroduction of cow's milk into the mother's diet in 23 of the 35 infants. A double-blind crossover trial with cow's milk whey protein was performed in 16 of these 23 mothers and infants. Six infants had to be taken out of the study for various reasons. Of the remaining 10 infants, nine displayed signs of colic after their mothers had taken the whey-filled capsules.

Maternal ingestion of eggs, chocolate, citrus fruits, nuts, as well as certain seafood whilst breastfeeding may result in infantile colic [85,93,94]. Hill et al randomized mothers of 107 term breastfed infants younger than 6 weeks of age with colic to follow a low-allergen diet with elimination of dairy products, soy, wheat, eggs, peanuts, tree nuts, and fish (n=53) and a control group (n=54) whose diet contained the known allergen [95]. Forty seven mothers in the treatment group and 43 mothers in the control group completed the study. Infants were identified as responders if there was at least 25% reduction in duration of crying/fussing on days 8 and 9. The authors showed that 74% of infants in the treatment group versus 37% of infants in the control group were responders (p=<0.001).

Irritable Bowel Syndrome

The pathogenesis of irritable colon syndrome is likely heterogeneous. Food allergy has been implicated in the pathogenesis of a subset of patients with irritable bowel syndrome [96,97]. The association of irritable bowel syndrome with specific IL-10 genotypes supports involvement of the immune system in its pathogenesis [71,98,99]. Patients with irritable bowel syndrome have a greater area of intestinal mucosa occupied by mast cells than do healthy control individuals [100]. A study of dietary eliminations in patients with irritable bowel syndrome found a significant reduction in symptom score in those patients whose exclusions were guided by raised IgG antibodies to dietary antigens than did patients on a sham diet based on irrelevant antigens [101]. Reintroduction of eliminated foods resulted in aggravation of symptoms in patients whose dietary exclusions were guided by raised IgG antibodies to dietary antigens. Irritable bowel syndrome might result from an interplay between immunological dysfunction, impaired gut barrier functions, susceptible genes and other environmental factors [102]. It has been hypothesized that food antigens induce mast cells to secrete mediators that regulate gastrointestinal motility and pain perception through gastrointestinal neural system [96].

Recurrent Abdominal Pain

Recurrent abdominal pain is usually defined as three or more bouts of abdominal pain, severe enough to interfere with a child's normal activities, occurring over a period of not less than three months during the year preceding the examination [103,104]. Onset often occurs between five and 10 years of age. Typically, the pain is vague, poorly localized or periumbilical and may be crampy or sharp. Episodes of pain tend to cluster, alternating with pain-free periods of variable length [104]. Most episodes last for less than an hour. On cessation of the pain, the child is up and about as if nothing had happened. In the majority of cases, the cause is functional [104,105]. Organic causes account for 5 to 10% of cases [103,104]. Kokkonen et al studied 84 children with recurrent abdominal pain [105]. Food allergy was diagnosed in 28 (33%) children based on an open elimination challenge test. However, the study was criticized because a formal diagnosis would require a double-blind placebo-controlled food challenge [106]. Further studies using double-blind placebo-controlled food challenges are necessary before food allergy can be established as a cause of recurrent abdominal pain in children.

Constipation

The vast majority of constipation in children is functional [107,108]. Constipation resulting from IgE sensitization to cow's milk has been described [108]. Loening-Baucke reviewed the records of 4157 children between 0 to 24 months of age seen in general pediatric clinics for health maintenance and acute care visits [108]. Of the 185 children with constipation, food allergy was responsible for constipation in only 2 (1%) of these children [108]. In contrast, Iacono et al studied 27 consecutive infants with chronic "idiopathic" constipation and noted improvement or resolution of symptoms in 21(78%) of these infants after a 4-week period of a cow's milk-free diet [109]. These infants had a relapse of symptoms on cow's milk challenge. Iacono et al subsequently performed a randomized cross-over trial of a cow's milk-based diet versus a soy milk-based diet in 65 children with chronic constipation [110]. Forty-four (68%) of the 65 children had increased bowel movements and improvement of fecal score while receiving the soy milk. None of the children who received cow's milk had a response. In all 44 children with a response, the response was confirmed with a double-blind challenge with cow's milk. Daher et al studied 25 children with chronic constipation [111]. In seven (28%) patients, the constipation disappeared while they were following a diet free of cow's milk protein and reappeared within 48 to 72 hours after challenge with cow's milk. In two patients, a rectal biopsy revealed allergic colitis with eosinophilic infiltration and they therefore did not undergo the challenge. High serum levels of total IgE were observed in five (71%) of the seven patients who showed a clinical improvement. Two (29%) patients had a positive skin test and two (29%) had detectable levels of specific IgE. Carroccio et al treated 52 children with chronic constipation unresponsive to common treatment by exclusion of milk alone, or by an extensive oligoallergenic diet if unresponsive [112]. Twenty four patients were found to be suffering from cow's milk intolerance and six from multiple food intolerance. These patients had a normal stool frequency on elimination diet with recurrence of constipation on food challenge. These patients showed a significantly higher frequency of mucosal erosions, number of intraepithelial lymphocytes and eosinophils, and number of eosinophils in the lamina propria. The remaining 22 patients did not respond to the elimination diet. Murch identified 30 children with constipation who responded to the exclusion diet with resolution of symptom; six of these children were allergic to multiple antigens [71]. Rectal biopsy of the affected patients showed eosinophilic proctitis [71]. Carroccio et al performed a Medline search for articles published between 1970 and June 2006, using the key words "chronic constipation or constipation" and "food intolerance or allergy". The authors identified 33 papers but only 19 of them were related to the topic. Analysis of these papers showed a relationship between constipation and food allergy in a subgroup of pediatric patients with "idiopathic" constipation unresponsive to laxative treatment. Additional studies are necessary to substantiate the specific associations and to clarify the pathogenic mechanisms involved.

Cutaneous Manifestations

Urticaria/Angioedema

Acute urticaria and, to a lesser extent, angioedema are among the most common manifestations of food allergic reactions in children [21,29]. They tend to occur more commonly in younger patients and in atopic patients, in association with other systemic features [113]. Symptoms result from activation of IgE-bearing cells by circulating food allergens absorbed through the gastrointestinal tract. The foods most commonly incriminated include eggs, milk, peanuts, and nuts [114]. In several studies, urticaria/angioedema occurred in 10 to 15% of infants with challenge-proven milk allergy [115,116]. In a classic study of 554 adults with urticaria, food allergy was demonstrated as the cause in only 1.4% of cases [117].

Physical contact with foods may also cause acute urticaria [116,118,119]. Allergic contact urticaria can be seen in children who are sensitized to environmental allergens such as food or classically, latex allergy [120]. There is a potential for cross-reactivity with various foods in individuals with latex allergy [120]. Food allergy is rarely the cause of chronic urticaria, unless the offending food is eaten almost every day [21,29,49,113].

Atopic Dermatitis

Atopic dermatitis is a multifactorial disease, and food allergy is associated with 30 to 50% of young children who had moderate to severe atopic dermatitis [121-123]. Burks et al evaluated 46 patients who had atopic dermatitis from food hypersensitivity substantiated with double-blind placebo-controlled food challenges [124]. Sixty five food challenges were performed; 27 (42%) were interpreted as positive in 15 (33%) patients. Sampson et al studied 350 patients with severe atopic dermatitis for possible food hypersensitivity [49,125,126]. Food allergy was diagnosed by double-blind placebo-controlled food challenges. Cutaneous reactions developed in 75% of the positive challenges within minutes to two hours, but only 30% of the positive responses were isolated cutaneous symptoms alone [49]. Most of the skin manifestations consisted of a markedly pruritic, erythematous rash that developed in sites with a predilection for atopic dermatitis.

In a prospective study of 113 patients with atopic dermatitis, marked improvement was noted in those who were maintained on an allergen elimination diet when compared with a similar group of patients who did not have food allergy or who did not adhere to the elimination diet [125]. Breuer et al performed 106 double-blind placebo-controlled food challenges to cow's milk, egg, wheat, and soy on 64 children who had atopic dermatitis [127]. Twenty-eight (57%) of the 49 positive reactions resulted in late eczematous reactions, either as isolated events or in combination with immediate reactions. Hill et al evaluated 487 infants who had skin prick tests to cow's milk, egg, and peanut, and who had a family history of atopic dermatitis, asthma, or immediate food allergy in a parent or sibling [128]. One hundred and forty-one (28.9%) of these infants had atopic dermatitis by the age of 12 months. These authors found that as the severity of atopic dermatitis increased, so did the prevalence of IgE-mediated food allergy and also the frequency of adverse food allergy reactions. The relative risk of an infant who had atopic dermatitis to develop an IgE-mediated food allergy was 5.9 for the most severely affected group.

The pathogenesis of atopic dermatitis likely involves both immediate and late-phase effects of IgE-mediated food hypersensitivity reactions as well as cell-mediated reactions [21,49,118]. The immediate or early phase of the reaction results from IgE-mediated cutaneous mast cell activation [126]. The late phase is characterized by a mixed cellular infiltrate (eosinophils, neutrophils, lymphocytes, and basophils) at six to eight hours and thereafter by a mononuclear round cell infiltrate indistinguishable from that seen in eczematous skin [125,129,130]. The pattern of cytokine expression is predominantly that of the Th2 type, namely, interleukin-4, -5 and -13 [113,114]. A single ingestion of food allergen may not provoke an eczematous lesion, but chronic ingestion of a food allergen can result in the classic changes of atopic dermatitis [121]. Children who have atopic dermatitis and documented food allergy may develop typical eczematous lesions while the disease is active, but may develop urticaria with ingestion of a food allergen when the atopic dermatitis is in remission [123]. On the other hand, atopic dermatitis is also seen in patients with X-linked agammaglobulinemia, suggesting that, at least in some cases, atopic dermatitis is not IgE-mediated [131]. Testing for cow's milk allergy, Hill et al identified a delayed eczematous reaction in 17 of 135 children with atopic dermatitis [132]. Ten of the 17 children had negative prick test to cow's milk allergen, suggesting a non-IgE mediated pathogenesis. Lio suggests that there are at least two types of "food allergy" in patients with atopic dermatitis: the IgE-mediated immediate reactions and the cell-mediated eczematous reactions [131].

Contact Dermatitis

Contact dermatitis may be related to an immune-mediated reaction to food or a direct toxic effect of the food coming into contact with the skin [114,133]. Food-induced contact dermatitis is often seen among food handlers, especially those who handle raw shellfish and eggs [6,102,134]. Allergic contact cheilitis has been reported from the chewing of garlic [135] and from the contact of geraniol, a food additive contained in certain foods [136].

Dermatitis Herpetiformis

Gluten-sensitive enteropathy is found in 75 to 95% of patients with dermatitis herpetiformis [118,137]. Dermatitis herpetiformis is a cutaneous cell-mediated response to gliadin that is present in wheat, rye, and barley [29,114]. The disorder is characterized by a chronic, intensely pruritic, papulovesicular rash, symmetrically distributed over the extensor surfaces of the extremities and buttocks [68,114]. Approximately 80 to 90% of patients have the HLA-B8 haplotype, and more than 90% have the HLA-Dw3 haplotype [138]. Skin biopsy generally reveals granular and linear deposits of IgA, C3, as well as infiltrates with polymorphonuclear leukocytes. Immunoglobulin A deposits may activate complement through the alternative pathway and cause inflammation. An IgE-mediated hypersensitivity reaction does not contribute to the pathogenesis. IgA antibodies to smooth muscle endomysium and jejunum have been reported in patients with dermatitis herpetiformis-associated gluten-sensitive enteropathy [118]. Also, antibodies to tissue transglutaminase and epidermal transglutaminase are present in patients with dermatitis herpetiformis, suggesting that epidermal transglutaminase is the autoantigen in dermatitis herpetiformis [114].

Respiratory Manifestations

Rhinitis/ Rhinoconjunctivitis

Food-induced allergic rhinitis/rhinoconjunctivitis is more frequently observed in children than in adults [122,139]. Rhinitis/rhinoconjunctivitis following inhalation of food dusts or vapor is not uncommon in patients with food allergy [14]. Rhinitis/rhinoconjunctivitis typically occurs in association with other clinical manifestations such as cutaneous and/or gastrointestinal symptoms during acute allergic reactions to foods [40,140]. Rhinitis/

rhinoconjunctivitis as the sole manifestation of food allergy is quite uncommon [49,67,135,139]. Allergic rhinitis may be manifested as nasal congestion, sneezing, and rhinorrhea [141]. Allergic conjunctivitis is characterized by periocular erythema, ocular injection, pruritis, and tearing. It seems likely that ingested allergens can activate nasal mast cells in addition to mast cells elsewhere in the body [141].

Chronic Sinusitis

Allergy to food allergens has been suggested to be a rare cause of chronic sinusitis [142]. Food allergy should be suspected in refractory cases of chronic sinusitis in which no apparent cause can be found, especially in atopic individuals with perennial symptoms [120,142].

Asthma (Bronchospasm)

Asthma from food allergy is a mixed IgE- and cell-mediated response due to the involvement of IgE antibodies, mast cells, eosinophils, and T-lymphocytes [42]. The condition occurs more often in children than in adults [143,144]. In several studies, 2 to 6% of children with asthma were found to have wheezing provoked by blinded food challenges [139,143-146]. Asthmatic children have a 14-fold higher risk of developing a severe allergic reaction to food compared with children without asthma [144,147].

In some children, food allergy may increase airway reactivity so that other triggers or environmental factors can more readily precipitate an asthmatic attack [148,149]. Vapors containing proteins emitted from cooking food can induce asthmatic attacks [6,143,150,151]. Inhalational exposures to foods, particular in the workplace, account for approximately 1% of asthmatic attacks in the adult population [6,149]. "Baker's asthma" caused by inhalation of flour or mold-derived enzymes used as flour additives are one such example [29]. Affected individuals have asthmatic attacks in association with exposure to aerosolized wheat proteins and have positive skin prick tests or serum specific IgE to wheat proteins [146,149]. Likewise, peanut dust in airplanes can provoke allergic reactions in susceptible individuals [152]. Allergenic proteins may also reach the respiratory tract via the circulation or they may act via inflammatory mediators released from the skin or gastrointestinal tract [149].

Food allergy in early infancy increases the risk for developing asthma in later life [144,153,154]. This applies also to children who have outgrown their food allergies [155].

Heiner Syndrome

Primary pulmonary hemosiderosis with hypersensitivity to cow's milk (Heiner syndrome) is a rare condition that usually occurs in young children. The syndrome is characterized by chronic cough, wheezing, hemoptysis, pulmonary infiltrates, hemosiderosis, gastrointestinal blood loss, iron deficiency anemia, and failure to thrive [139,156]. Presumably, the syndrome results from aspiration of milk into the lungs with subsequent development of IgG cow's milk antibodies and an immune complex Arthus-type reaction in the alveoli [157]. If the vasculitis is severe, alveolar bleeding and pulmonary hemosiderosis may result [157]. Affected children have usually high titers of precipitins to multiple constituents of cow's milk and positive results on intradermal skin tests to various cow's milk proteins [156]. Dietary elimination of cow's milk results in symptomatic improvement, and reintroduction of cow's milk results in recurrence of symptoms. It has been postulated that antigen-antibody complexes and cell-mediated hypersensitivity play a pathogenic role in this syndrome based on the presence of elevated serum levels of milk-specific IgG antibodies and the in vitro proliferative response of the patient's lymphocytes to milk antigen [141].

Serous Otitis Media

Serous otitis media, defined as non-purulent collection of fluid in the middle ear, is a multifactorial disease [158]. Food allergy may play a role in the pathogenesis in a subgroup of children with serous otitis media [159-161]. It has been hypothesized that allergic inflammation in the nasal mucosa may cause Eustachian tube dysfunction that may result in serous otitis media [140,160]. IgG complexes with cow's milk protein might also contribute to the middle ear inflammation [162]. In the study by Aydoğan et al, food allergy was detected in 25 (44.6%) of 56 patients with serous otitis media [158]. In patients with food allergy, serous otitis media was detected in 7 (25%) of 28 patients. In the control group of 28 patients, food allergy was diagnosed in 5 (18%) patients and serous otitis media in one (3%) patient. The incidence of food allergy in serous otitis media group was statistically significant when compared to the normal group. The risk of otitis media in children having food allergy was 3.7 times higher than the control. Bernstein et al evaluated 100 patients aged 2 to18 years with recurrent serous otitis media for IgE-mediated hypersensitivity [159]. Thirty five of these patients had allergic rhinitis. Total IgE was increased in the middle ear fluid in 16 of the 35 patients with allergic rhinitis and in only 2 of the 65 patients in the non-allergic group. In 8 of these 16 patients (23% of the allergic group), levels of IgE per milligram of protein were higher in the middle ear effusion than in the corresponding serum, thus suggesting local production of IgE by the middle ear mucosa in these patients. In a subset of infants with recurrent serous otitis media, IgG complexes with food antigen may contribute to middle ear inflammation and serous otitis media [150,162]. Nsouli et al evaluated 104 unselected children with recurrent serous otitis media for food allergy [161]. There was a significant statistical association, by chi-square analysis, between food allergy and recurrent serous otitis media in 81 (78%) of the 104 patients. An elimination diet led to a significant amelioration of serous otitis media in 70 (86%) of 81 patients. An open challenge diet with the suspected offending food(s) provoked a recurrence of serous otitis media in 66 (94%) of 70 patients. Further studies with double-blind placebo-controlled food challenge are necessary to confirm these findings.

Ménière's Disease

Ménière's disease is characterized by recurrent vertigo, fluctuating hearing loss, aural fullness or pressure, and tinnitus [163,164]. Derebery et al did a mail-survey on 1490 patients with Ménière's disease [163]. Of 734 respondents with Ménière's disease, 296 (40.3%) had or suspected food allergies and 272 (37%) had confirmatory skin or in vitro tests for allergy.

These prevalence rates were significantly higher than those found in the control group of patients (n=172) with otologic problems other than Ménière's disease, of which 43 (25%) had or suspected food allergies and 38 (22.2%) had confirmatory skin or in vitro tests for allergy. Keleş et al studied 46 patients aged between 26 and 68 years and 46 aged-matched controls. The authors found that total serum IgE levels were above the normal levels in 19 (41.3%) of the patients with Ménière's disease and 9 (19.5%) of the controls [164]. A history of allergy was found in 31 (67.3%) of the patients with Ménière's disease and 16 (34.7%) of the controls. When the specific IgE levels were measured (all seasons, tree, fungus, fruit, egg white, cow's milk, wheat flour, corn flour, beef, and rice), the number of patients having all the panels negative was eight (17.9%) in patients with Ménière's disease and 31 (67.3%) in the controls. Cow's milk allergy was the most common identifiable cause of Ménière's disease. It has been hypothesized that immune complexes circulating in the blood might hinder the filtering ability of the endolymphatic sac [164].

Neurologic Manifestations

Migraine

Medical consensus is that food allergy does not play a significant role in migraine [122]. Several double-blind studies have shown that some patients with migraine had adverse reactions to certain foods, as shown by dietary exclusion and subsequent challenge [165-167]. However, there was no clearly proven immunologic effect of food components in many of these patients [168]. Foods rich in tyramine, tryptamine, serotonin, and histamine can trigger migraine, and this is based mainly on pharmacologic rather than immunologic effects [169,170]. According to the revised nomenclature for allergy published by the European Academy of Allergy and Clinical Immunology, these kinds of adverse reactions are classified as toxic reactions rather than food hypersensitivity [171].

Epilepsy

Associations between epilepsy and food allergies are controversial at best. Several authors have proposed a possible role of food allergy in a subset of children with epilepsy [172-174]. However a great deal of additional research must be performed. Frediani et al have noted a significantly higher proportion of allergic disorders in 72 epileptic patients versus 202 aged-matched controls [173]. Using skin prick tests, the percentage of epileptic children who tested positive for cow's milk protein (24/72), lactalbumin (16/72) and β-lactoglobulin (10/72) was significantly higher than the percentage of controls who tested positive for the same allergens: 7/202 for cow's milk protein, 4/202 for lactalbumin, and 2/202 for β-lactoglobulin. In patients with allergic disorders, there is an increase in the proportion of electroencephalographic anomalies, often in the form of occipital dysrhythmias [173]. Crayton et al reported on a patient whose epileptic fits were triggered and increased in frequency by double-blind food challenges [172]. Frediani et al reported on a nine-year-old boy whose epileptic symptoms disappeared as a result of an allergen-free diet with no anticonvulsant therapy [174].

Endocrine Manifestation

Diabetes Mellitus

Cow's milk has been implicated as a possible trigger of an autoimmune response destroying pancreatic ß-cells in genetically susceptible individuals, thereby leading to diabetes mellitus [175-177]. Karjalainen et al measured IgG antibovine serum albumin antibodies in the serum of 142 children with newly diagnosed insulin-dependent diabetes mellitus [177]. These children had elevated serum concentrations of IgG antibovine serum albumin antibodies that declined after diagnosis and reached normal levels in most patients within one to two years. These authors speculate that patients with insulin-dependent diabetes mellitus have immunity to cow's milk albumin, with antibodies to an albumin peptide that are capable of reacting with a β-cell-specific surface protein. Such antibodies could participate in the development of islet cell dysfunction. Cavallo et al measured the in vitro peripheral T-lymphocyte response to β-casein in 47 patients with recent-onset insulin-dependent diabetes mellitus [175]. Twenty four of 47 (51.1%) patients with insulin-dependent diabetes mellitus versus 0 of 10 patients with autoimmune thyroid disease and 1 of 36 (2.8%) healthy people had a positive response to ß-casein. A positive response was defined as a stimulation index above the mean value plus 2 SD of healthy people. These authors suggest that exposure to cow's milk triggers a cellular and humoral anti- ß-casein immune response that may cross-react with a β-cell antigen and lead to destruction of the β-cell. A subsequent study, however, showed a lack of association between early exposure to cow's milk and β-cell autoimmunity [178]. Norris et al screened 253 children aged nine months to seven years with first-degree relatives who had insulin-dependent diabetes mellitus for β-cell autoimmunity [178]. Eighteen cases of β-cell autoimmunity were detected at baseline. These children were compared with 153 unrelated autoantibody-negative children selected from the cohort as controls. There were no differences in the proportion of cases and controls that were exposed to cow's milk or foods containing cow's milk by 3 months or 6 months of age. Further studies are necessary to clarity this important issue.

Renal Manifestation

Nephrotic Syndrome

Food allergy may play a role in the pathogenesis of nephrotic syndrome in a selected group of children [179-182]. Sandberg et al reported 6 children with steroid-responsive nephrotic syndrome [179]. In the relapse period, a milk-free diet led to remission without steroid therapy. In the remission period, challenge with cow's milk resulted in a relapse in 4 patients. Sieniawska et al evaluated the role of cow's milk in 17 children with steroid-resistant nephrotic syndrome [182]. Cow's milk was excluded from the diet for at least 14 days without changing the previously ineffective prednisone dosage. Six patients went into remission three to eight days after the elimination of cow's milk. After a period of two to three weeks of remission, cow's milk challenge was positive in three of the six patients. The group of responders to a milk-free diet was characterized by young age, feeding with cow's milk or unmodified powdered milk formulas in the neonatal period, and coexistence of allergic symptoms. The authors suggest that cellular mechanisms may play a role in cow's milk-induced steroid-resistant nephrotic syndrome as evidenced by the late-onset reaction to cow's milk challenge, positive leukocyte migration inhibition tests, absence of specific IgE antibodies, and negative skin test results. These studies, however, contain some design flaws and better objective studies are needed to prove the association between milk ingestion and nephrotic syndrome.

Hematologic Manifestations

Anemia

Iron deficiency anemia may develop in children with cow's milk allergy secondary to gastrointestinal blood loss. This may be caused by milk-induced enterocolitis syndrome, milk-induced colitis, and allergic eosinophilic gastroenteropathy, and Heiner syndrome.

Thrombocytopenia

A few anecdotal reports suggest that thrombocytopenia may be caused by food allergy [183-185]. Whitefield and Barr reported a girl with the syndrome of thrombocytopenia and absent radius who showed marked gastrointestinal disturbance with clinical evidence of cow's milk allergy and in whom there appeared to be a direct correlation between cow's milk exposure, gastrointestinal upset, and thrombocytopenia [183]. Jones reported a newborn male infant with idiopathic thrombocytopenic purpura in whom withdrawal of a milk formula produced an improvement in the platelet count and reintroduction of the milk formula led to hematologic relapse on two occasions [184]. It has been suggested that a type II cytotoxic reaction may account for the thrombocytopenia seen after the ingestion of milk [185].

Rheumatic Manifestations

Vasculitis

Food-induced vasculitis has been described [186,187]. In the majority of cases, it is mediated by type III immunologic reaction in which the antigen combines with its specific IgG and complement to form circulating complexes [186]. The circulating complexes deposit in the small blood vessels and initiate vasculitis. Occasionally, food-induced vasculitis may be IgE-mediated. Businco et al reported two patients with leucocytoclastic vasculitis confirmed by skin biopsy [186]. The first patient had cutaneous vasculitis with large joint involvement, caused by cow's milk and egg as confirmed by blind food challenge. The second patient had cutaneous and mucous membrane vasculitis with large joint involvement caused by chocolate. Lunardi et al described five patients with allergy and cutaneous vasculitis of 1 to 13 years' duration [187]. Double-blind food challenges identified the offending agent to be a food in two patients, an additive in another two patients, and both food and additive in the fifth patient.

Arthropathy/Arthritis

A few anecdotal reports suggest that arthropathy/arthritis may be the result of food hypersensitivity [188-190]. Parke et al described a 38-year-old woman who had progressive rheumatoid arthritis for 11 years [191]. Her rheumatoid arthritis improved within three weeks of changing to a milk-free diet and deteriorated within 24 hours with a milk challenge. Golding reported three patients with food-induced synovitis [192]. van de Larr et al described six patients with rheumatoid arthritis that responded to a diet limited to an elemental formula [193]. Double-blind placebo-controlled trial confirmed a relationship with specific food in four of the six patients. Long-term benefit from avoidance of the specific foods, however, was noted only in two patients. Panush monitored 97 patients with inflammatory arthritis and found that no more than 5% of the patients with rheumatic disease had immunologic sensitivity to foods [190]. Denman et al have not been able to detect any consistent correlation between controlled dietary challenges and exacerbations of inflammatory arthritis [194]. In those cases in which inflammatory arthritis responds to dietary manipulation, it is possible that dietary restriction non-specifically moderates the inflammatory manifestations of the disease or the placebo effect may be responsible [194]. Karatay et al have shown that individualized diet challenges consisting of allergenic foods may regulate tumor necrosis factor-α and interleukin-1β levels in selected patients with rheumatoid arthritis [195]. Tumor necrosis factor-α and interleukin-1β are cytokines that promote inflammation and may play an important role in the development of rheumatoid arthritis [195].

Clinical Evaluation

History and physical examination are the cornerstones for the diagnostic workup of any food allergy [6]. However, their value can fluctuate depending on dietary history recall, and timing of presentation from reaction. In this light, accurate diet diaries are invaluable tools for clinicians. Key points to document include foods consumed, route of exposure, descriptions of symptoms, timing on symptom onset and resolution, consistency of symptoms with food consumption, treatments attempted and response [5-7].

Diagnostic Studies

A number of diagnostic studies are indicated based on clinical impression. Several, similar diagnostic algorithms have been proposed, but no one algorithm is universally accepted [6]. Regardless, the results of these studies should be interpreted in light of history and physical examination [6]. In this light, referral to allergy specialists for testing is prudent [7]. In addition, further testing may be required to evaluate specific clinical presentations, such as endoscopy for suspected allergic eosinophilic esophagitis and biopsy for celiac disease. A detailed discussion of these numerous confirmatory tests for clinical presentations is beyond the scope of this review.

ELIMINATION DIETS

Elimination diets are frequently suggested as an initial investigation for food allergy. These diets involve the complete elimination of suspected food allergens for at least two weeks with close follow-up monitoring for resolution of clinical symptoms [6]. However, despite being fundamentally simple and cost-effective means of assessing food allergies, they are rarely diagnostic [7]. In practice, these diets are difficult to implement and require correct allergen identification, complete avoidance of the suspected allergen and the lack of other confounding factors occurring the testing period [5-7]. They are especially difficult to interpret in patients with other chronic conditions such as atopic dermatitis that may occur in isolation or as part of a constellation of symptoms with food allergy [5].

SKIN PRICK TESTING

Skin prick testing with food extracts is often used to screen patients with suspected IgE-mediated food allergies [7]. It is rapid and useful in demonstrating clinical response to allergen exposure [5]. Fundamentally, testing determines the presence of allergen-specific IgE antibodies. Patients are exposed to commercially or freshly prepared food allergens mixed with glycerin (1:10 or 1:20 ratio), as well as a positive control (generally histamine) and negative control (saline) in the form of small drops applied to the surface of the skin [5]. A "prick" is then used to break the skin barrier. By convention, a food allergen producing a wheal with a diameter 3 mm greater than the negative control is considered "positive" [5]. Because of the small risk of systemic anaphylaxis, the test should be performed in settings capable of managing this adverse event.

This test is reproducible and generally has a sensitivity of 90% but a specificity of 50% [7,196]. These values vary with age of patient, food allergen utilized. In general, commercially prepared reagents are labile and less allergenic than freshly prepared reagents with suspected fruit and vegetable allergies [6,43]. The positive predictive value and negative predictive value are 50% and 95%, respectively [197]. As such, skin prick testing is useful for ruling out IgE-mediated food allergies when results are negative, but only suggestive of possible food allergy if positive [7]. Two important exceptions include systemic anaphylaxis initiated by exposure to a single allergen which is diagnostic of food allergy and children less than one year old which may have food allergy diagnosed in the presence of a negative result [6]. Nonetheless, indiscriminate testing of multiple food allergens without clinical suspicion is not recommended as there is a fairly high potential for false positives [6].

In Vitro Tests for Total and Specific IgE

Many children with IgE-mediated food allergies have elevated serum IgE levels. Serum IgE antibodies specific for allergens can be measured in vitro by qualitative techniques such as RAST (Radio absorbant serum test), and ELISA (Enzyme-linked immunosorbant assay). In practical terms, these tests have similar sensitivity and specificity as skin-prick tests and are used in a similar fashion to screen and rule-out IgE mediated food allergies [6].

However, newer, quantitative techniques such as CAP FEIA® (Fluorenzyme immunoassay) (CAP Systems FEIA, Pharmacia-Upjohn Diagnostics) are now favored over qualitative techniques due to their greater specificity and positive predictive values [198]. Currently, for a number of foods, there are known IgE levels with a 95% positive predictive of food allergy [6]. By convention, patients with IgE levels greater than these standardized thresholds can be diagnosed with food allergy [6]. Likelihood ratio data are also available to account for varying prevalence with specific allergies in specific populations [7]. These assays are most useful when milk, egg, peanut and possibly soy, wheat and fish allergies are suspected as they are the most studied [6].

Food Challenge

An open or single-blind food challenge is practical in a clinic setting and acceptable when the resulting symptoms can be objectively observed [6]. The main disadvantage is the increased incidence of false-positive results, primarily because of biased interpretation by the patient, parents, and physician. However, the double-blind placebo-controlled food challenge has long been considered the "gold standard" for the diagnosis of food allergy. This method can be applied to both suspected IgE and non-IgE mediated food reactions [5]. This type of food challenge is objective and should be used if a positive open challenge yields only a subjective response on the part of the patient, if the symptoms are vague or ill defined, or if there is a psychological component to the reaction. However, the test can be time-consuming in a clinic setting, and carries a risk of systemic anaphylaxis and therefore is impractical for screening purposes. If IgE-mediated reactions are suspected, blinded food challenges are often initiated after a skin-prick and in vitro test has been completed. For patients being evaluated for resolution of food allergy, a food challenge will often be initiated after skin-prick and in vitro tests convert to negative.

Although no specific protocol has been widely accepted, the general principles of the food challenge are common. To begin, all foods and medications suspected of causing adverse reactions or complicating the interpretation of results are eliminated for 10 to 14 days. This allows for previous symptoms to resolve before the food challenge takes place and exaggerate any response during the food challenge [6]. The suspected food is administered in a gradual fashion, starting with a small quantity, and the dose is doubled appropriately at 15 to 20 minute intervals until symptoms occur or a reasonable serving size has been ingested. In a single blind challenge, the suspected food is hidden in some neutral, tolerated food or in capsules and the patient is unaware of the ingested food. In a double blind challenge, both the physician and patient are unaware and a neutral third party is involved. Following, patients may be observed for up to three days for symptoms, especially if a non-IgE mediated reaction is suspected [6]. Afterwards, the specific foods consumed are revealed. Extreme caution, with appropriate supports and close observation is recommended for children with previous severe systemic anaphylaxis. If the blind challenge is negative, the food should then be consumed openly in the usual quantities under observation to rule out the rare false-negative challenge.

MANAGEMENT

The key to the management of food allergy is avoidance of foods known to or suspected of having caused a reaction [29]. Other approaches include pharmacotherapy, education of patients, and dietary manipulations for the prevention of food allergy in high-risk individuals. Currently, there is no effective and safe immunotherapy in the management of patients with food allergy. Referral to an allergist is generally recommended.

AVOIDANCE OF FOOD ALLERGENS

The definitive treatment of food allergy is strict elimination of the offending food from the diet [5]. It is unusual for a child to be allergic to more than one food. Bock studied 480 children with probable food hypersensitivity and found that allergic reaction to more than two foods occurred in only 10 (2.1%) of the 480 children [199]. Symptomatic reactivity to food allergens is generally very specific, and patients rarely react to more than one food in a botanical or animal species [5,49,67]. However, in pollen-related food allergy, cross-reactions can occur between phylogenetically distantly related species such as birch and kiwi or soy [200],

Although the fundamental concept is simple, avoiding an offending food antigen is often difficult in practice, especially if the offending food is ubiquitous. In particular, accidental exposure is a major obstacle. Approximately 50% of affected individuals experience accidental exposure and reactions every 3 to 5 years [201]. In addition, cross-contamination of food with the offending antigen, leading to inadvertent ingestion, is commonly described [202]. Accidents frequently occur in daycare centers, schools, and restaurants [202]. Of the 32 food-related fatalities reported by Bock et al, at least 87% of patients had a previous history of reaction to the responsible food allergen [203]. Avoidance of skin contact and inhalation of offending food allergen is also necessary [204-206].

On the other hand, the indiscriminate application of elimination diets without a firm diagnosis is a widespread malpractice and may lead to psychological dependence on an unsound diet, as well as vitamin deficiencies, malnutrition, and failure to thrive if multiple foods are inadvertently avoided [5,207-209]. Venter et al followed a birth cohort of 966 infants on the Island of Wight, United Kingdom born between September 2001 and August 2002 to the age of one year [210]. Cumulative incidence of parentally reported food hypersensitivity was 25.8%. Open or double-blind, placebo-controlled food challenges were used to confirm suspected reactions. Only 2.2% of those tested were confirmed to have food allergy, indicating the need to evaluate suspected food allergy to avoid needless dietary restriction.

In some children ingesting inappropriate elimination diets, eating disorders may develop. If elimination diets are prescribed, care must be taken to ensure that they are palatable and nutritionally adequate. Patients should be provided with information on what alternative foods are available so that good variety in the diet can be maintained [211]. A formal dietetic evaluation is recommended.

Patients and other caregivers must have a good knowledge of foods containing the allergen and must be taught to scrutinize the labels of all packaged food carefully [212]. Careful label reading is a cornerstone of food avoidance [213]. In one study, only 4 (7%) of 60 parents were able to identify milk protein in 14 sample labels [214]. Incorrect or ambiguous labeling of foods may result in accidental ingestion of the offending food [202]. Also, some of the terms used do not clearly indicate the presence of a food allergen. The United States Food and Drug Administration (FDA) now requires food manufacturers to declare and clear label all functional ingredients on food labels [215]. The Food Allergen Labeling and Consumer Protection Act (FALCPA) effective in January 2006 requires simple terms to indicate the presence of major food allergens [216]. FALCPA requires food manufacturers to state explicitly the presence of eight major food allergens, namely, milk, egg, wheat, soybean, peanut, tree nuts, fish, and shellfish. New EU labeling laws require the presence of the following food allergens at any level to be stated on the label: celery, cereals containing gluten (wheat, barley, rye and oats), crustaceans, eggs, fish, milk, mustard, tree nuts, peanuts, sesame seeds, soybeans, SO_2 and sulfites (at level >10 mg/kg or >10 mg/L) [216]. It is mandatory to list all sub-ingredients and specify the source of ingredients previously listed as "natural flavor". However, foods that are not prepackaged are not covered by this legislation [211]. Patients and/or their caregivers should be cautioned about the presence of the offending food as a "hidden" ingredient in processed foods [217,218]. In addition, at restaurants, it is important that patients learn to communicate with staff regarding their food allergies [15].

Overall, food avoidance diets in children are generally required on a transient basis as most outgrow their food allergies. As noted before, the loss of hypersensitivity is especially likely to occur in infants and young children, although older children and adults may also lose their hypersensitivity [219]. The degree of compliance with allergen avoidance and the allergen responsible may influence the outcome [220]. Consequently, rechallenge testing for food allergy should be performed; the interval between rechallenges should be dictated by the specific food allergen in question, the age of the child, and the degree of difficulty in avoiding the food in question.

Environmental Management

Patients should be aware of high-risk environments. High-risk areas include common eating places such as childcare centers, school cafeterias, restaurants, and ice cream shops [29]. School and childcare centers should have policies facilitating food allergen avoidance such as prohibition of sharing of food or utensil and increased staff supervision during meal times [29]. Patients with reactions to airborne antigens (such as steamed fish, flour additives in Baker's asthma, peanut dust on airplanes) are at particular risk [29].

PHARMACOTHERAPY

Patients with a history of anaphylactic reaction over the age of seven years as well as caregivers should be taught how to self-administer epinephrine and should have an epinephrine autoinjector such as Anapen/Anapen Jr® (Lincoln Medical Ltd, Wiltshire, United Kingdom), EpiPen/EpiPen Jr® (Dey Pharma, L.P. of Napa, California), or Twinjet/Twinjet Jr® (Shionogi Pharma, Inc, Georgia) and antihistamine available at all times [7,200]. It is suggested that patients at risk for anaphylaxis should always carry two doses of self-injectable epinephrine [221,222]. An identification necklace or bracelet such as MedicAlert® (MedicAlert Canada, Ontario, Canada) stating the patient's sensitivity is also advised [218]. The physician should take appropriate steps to ensure that the patients and their caregivers understand the indications and use of the device thoroughly. These individuals should also be provided with a written anaphylaxis action plan. The instructions should be clear, simple, and age appropriate. Rehearsal of the procedure is important.

Patients and/or their caregivers must be educated about early recognition of allergic symptoms and early management of an anaphylactic reaction [6]. Schools should be equipped to treat anaphylaxis in allergic students and physicians should help instruct school personnel about these issues [200]. Referral to an allergist is also recommended [223].

Epinephrine helps to block severe allergic reactions and anaphylaxis by suppressing leukotriene and histamine release [224,225]. Epinephrine reverses vasodilatation, increases blood pressure, dilates airways, reduces laryngeal edema and angioedema, and increases myocardial contractility [224,225]. For the treatment of anaphylaxis, the recommended dose of epinephrine 1:1000 (1mg/ml) is 0.01 mg/kg intramuscularly, up to a maximum of 0.3 mg (0.3 ml) in children and 0.5 mg (0.5 ml) in adults [224,226]. Peak concentrations are reached within 10 minutes of intramuscular administration [225,227]. As Anapen Jr®, EpiPen Jr®, and Twinjet Jr® contain 0.15 mg of epinephrine and Anapen®, EpiPen®, and Twinjet® contain 0.3 mg of epinephrine, it would be desirable to have a wider range of auto-injector doses [202,224]. The subcutaneous route is no longer recommended as the systemic levels of epinephrine are highly unpredictable from this mode of administration [202]. In addition intramuscular injections into the thigh result in more rapid absorption and higher plasma epinephrine levels than intramuscular injections into the arm [212,221,226,228-229]. Epinephrine works best when given early [202,224].

After first aid treatment, the patient should be transferred to the nearest emergency department for monitoring and additional treatment as required. Anaphylactic patients should continue being observed in hospital for at least 4 to 12 hours after epinephrine administration, even if they are apparently well, because of the possibility of a biphasic reaction [7]. Biphasic reactions occur in 6% of anaphylaxis with the second "peak" occurring within 4 to 12 hours in 96% of cases [7]. If necessary, epinephrine may be repeated at 5 minutes intervals [224,221]. In one study, 16% of patients presenting to the emergency department with food-induced anaphylaxis required an average of two doses of epinephrine [221].

In patients with severe anaphylaxis unresponsive to intramuscular epinephrine or with cardiovascular collapse, epinephrine should be given intravenously and transferred to intensive care with blood pressure and continuous cardiac monitoring [225,226].

Many patients also require volume support, oxygen, nebulized bronchodilators, parenteral diphenhydramine, ranitidine, and glucocorticosteroids [6,7,212,226]. Should this be the case, the patient should be placed in a recumbent position with lower limbs elevated, as tolerated symptomatically [212,226,228]. This may prevent orthostatic hypotension.

For the child with progressive or generalized urticaria or distressing pruritis, the administration of a fast-acting oral H_1 antihistamine such as hydroxyzine or diphenhydramine should be considered [67,224,226,230]. H_2 receptor blockers such as ranitidine are less helpful as only a small number of H_2 receptors are found in the skin [230]. It is critical to note that unlike epinephrine, antihistamines do not block systemic reactions in anaphylaxis [6]. They are mainly useful in relieving symptomatic pruritus [6].

The use of drugs such as disodium cromoglycate, ketotifen, and prostaglandin synthetase inhibitors in the treatment of food allergy has generally been disappointing, either because of minimal efficacy or unacceptable adverse effects [5,200]. Systemic corticosteroids are rarely used in the treatment of food allergy, except in severe anaphylaxis, allergic eosinophilic esophagitis, allergic eosinophilic gastroenteropathy, and dietary-induced enteropathy [6,231]. The side effects of long-term systemic corticosteroid therapy are unacceptable.

Currently, oral administration of activated charcoal is not considered a practical first-aid treatment for food anaphylaxis. Prophylactic medications have not been shown to be consistently effective in the prevention of severe life-threatening reactions to foods [29]. Their use may mask a less severe allergic reaction to a culprit food, the knowledge of which might prevent a more severe allergic reaction to that food in the future [29]. The use of prophylactic medications is therefore discouraged.

Probiotics and Prebiotics

The use of probiotics and prebiotics in the management of food allergy is controversial [232]. It has been hypothesized that the increased sensitization to food allergens might result from reduced infection or exposure to microbial products such as endotoxin in early childhood [233]. Prospective studies have found that infants who are prone to develop atopic dermatitis have lower numbers of *Bifidobacterium* in their intestinal microflora [234-236]. Evidence also suggests that probiotics may reverse the increased intestinal permeability characteristic of children with food allergy and enhance specific IgA responses frequently defective in children with food allergy [237]. *In vitro* studies show that allergic patients induce less IL-10 production and more proinflammatory cytokine production than those nonallergic individuals [238,239]. Presumably, probiotics act on the intestinal mucosa and stimulate T-cell differentiation in favor of Th1 over Th2, with resultant decreased production of IgE and increased production of IgA [238,240]. Probiotics might also correct aberrations in gut permeability [241,242]. Prebiotics work by selectively stimulating the growth or activity of a limited number of bacterial strains in the intestinal flora.

Much work has been done on the use of probiotics and, to a lesser extent, prebiotics in the management of atopic dermatitis. Several randomized controlled trials failed to show the beneficial effects of probiotics in the prevention of atopic dermatitis [243]. Other studies yielded different results [243-248]. Kalliomäki et al randomized 159 mothers and their respective infants with a family history of atopy to receive either a placebo or 10^{10} CFU of *Lactobacillus* GG for 2 to 4 weeks before delivery and for 6 months after delivery, respectively [244]. Twenty three percent of the children in the probiotic group versus 46% of children in the control group were found to have atopic dermatitis at two years of age (RR: 0.51; 95% confidence interval: 0.32-0.84) [244]. The effect was still observed two years later: 26% of children in the treatment group versus 46% of children in the placebo group had atopic dermatitis (RR: 0.57; 95% confidence interval: 0.33-0.97) [245].

Viljanen et al randomized 230 infants who had suspected cow's milk allergy in a double-blinded study to receive *L. rhamnosus* GG (n=80), a mixture of four probiotic strains (n=76), or a placebo (n=74), given twice daily with food for four weeks [248]. The authors found that *L. rhamnosus* GG was an effective therapy for atopic dermatitis in IgE-sensitized infants but not in non-IgE-sensitized infants.

In a double-blind, placebo-controlled trial, Tamura et al randomized 109 adult patients with allergic rhinitis to drink fermented milk containing *Lactobacilli casei* strain Shirota (n=55) or placebo (n=54) for 8 weeks [249]. The authors found no significant difference between the two groups during the ingestion period. In the subgroup of patients with moderate to severe nasal symptom scores before starting ingestion of test samples, supplementation with the probiotic tended to reduce nasal symptom-medication scores.

In a double-blind placebo-controlled trial, Taylor et al randomized 226 newborn infants of atopic mothers to receive either 3 x 10^9 CFU of *Lactobacillus acidophilus* (n=115) or placebo (n=111) daily for 6 months [250]. A total of 178 infants (89 in each group) completed the study. The authors found that the rates of atopic dermatitis were similar in the two groups at 6 months and 12 months of follow-up. At 12 months, the rate of sensitization was significantly higher in the probiotic group (p=0.03). These findings challenge the use of probiotics in the prevention of allergy.

Kukkonen et al randomized 1,223 pregnant women carrying high risk infants at increased risk for allergy to receive a probiotic (n=610) or a placebo (n=613) for 2 to 4 weeks before delivery [251]. Their infants received the same probiotic plus galacto-oligosaccharides (n=461) or a placebo (n=464) for 6 months. These children were evaluated at 2 years of age for cumulative incidence of allergic diseases (food allergy, eczema, asthma, and allergic rhinitis) and IgE sensitization (positive skin prick test response or serum antigen-specific IgE level). The authors found that probiotic and prebiotic treatment, compared with placebo, had no effect on the cumulative incidence of allergic diseases but tended to reduce IgE-associated atopic diseases (odds ratio: 0.71; 95% confidence interval: 0.5 to 1; p=0.052). Probiotic and prebiotic treatment did reduce eczema (odds ratio: 0.74; 95% confidence interval: 0.55 to 0.98; p=0.35) and atopic eczema (odds ratio: 0.66; 95% confidence interval: 0.46 to 0.95; p=0.025).

In a double-blind placebo-controlled trial, Weston et al randomized 56 children aged 6 to 18 months who had moderate to severe atopic dermatitis to receive *L. fementum* VRI-033 PCC (n=28) or placebo (n=28) twice daily for eight weeks [252]. Fifty children completed the study. The authors found that the reduction in the SCORAD index was significant in the probiotic group (p=0.03) but not in the placebo group. In a double-blind study, Passeron et al randomized 48 children to receive either *L. rhamnosus* Lcr 35 plus a prebiotic preparation (n=28) or an identically appearing probiotic preparation alone three times a day for three months [253]. In the symbiotic group, the mean total SCORAD score was 39.1 before treatment versus 20.7 after three months of treatment (p< 0.0001). In the probiotic group, the mean SCORAD score was 39.3 before treatment versus 24 after three months of treatment (p<0.0001). The authors concluded that symbiotics and prebiotics used alone were effective in the treatment of atopic dermatitis.

Probiotics and prebiotics are included in some infant formulas with the aim of inducing the development of a *Bifidobacterium*-dominated intestinal flora. At present, probiotics or prebiotics are not established treatment modalities for atopic dermatitis [232,238]. They are ineffective in the prevention and treatment of reactive airway disease [238]. The routine use of probiotics and prebiotics in food allergy management requires further study

DIETARY MANIPULATION IN THE PREVENTION OF FOOD ALLERGY IN THE GENERAL POPULATION

Recently, perspectives on dietary manipulation and food allergies have dramatically changed. According to a recent landmark clinical report (intended to replace previous position statements) by the Committee on Nutrition and Section on Allergy and Immunology of the American Academy of Pediatrics, there is now limited evidence to support dietary manipulation in preventing food allergies in the general, low-risk population [254].

Although evidence for prevention of atopic dermatitis and wheezing in early life is conflicting, there is insufficient evidence that exclusively breastfeeding prevents food allergy [7,254]. Long-term, randomized, control trials have shown no significant difference in risk of food allergy at 7-years of age in children exclusively breastfed from mothers on allergen-elimination diets [255, 256]. Nonetheless, breastfeeding is still recommended for its other well-described benefits in children.

Furthermore, because small amounts of food antigens ingested by the mother are excreted in breast milk [219], previous position statements by the AAP recommended avoidance of allergenic foods by lactating mothers [217,257,258]. However, this theoretical risk has not been observed. As summarized in a Cochrane review, there is inefficient evidence supporting maternal avoidance of common food allergens during breastfeeding in order to prevent food allergies in their children [254,259]. Currently, no specific dietary modification is recommended by lactating mothers. This position represents a change from previous statements.

Perhaps most dramatic, is the controversial shift in perspective with tapered introduction of solid foods to a child's diet. Traditionally, it was believed that the delayed introduction of common food allergens such as dairy, eggs, peanuts and tree nuts past 6 months chronological age would prevent food allergies [7]. However, despite being adopted into widespread clinical practice, there is little clinical evidence to support the efficacy of delayed solid introduction in preventing food allergies. In a recent major prospective birth cohort study (n=2073) by the Influences of Lifestyle-Related Factors on the Immune System and the Development of Allergies in Childhood (LISA) study group, no evidence was found to support the delayed introduction of solids in preventing food allergy [260]. In fact, some studies have shown that delayed introduction of food allergens actually confers a higher risk for future food allergy [261,262]. Given these findings, a joint-consensus document by the Adverse Reactions to Foods Committee, American College of Allergy, Asthma and Immunology currently states that the introduction of solids into an infant's diet should be individualized, and that egg, peanut, tree nuts, fish and seafood may be introduced, with caution, at six months age [263]. The American Academy of Pediatrics's recent clinical report acknowledges this lack of evidence but does not comment on clinical practice recommendations [254].

It has been suggested that supplementation with long-chain polyunsaturated fatty acids might reduce the incidence of atopic diseases [264-266]. A Cochrane systematic review showed no consistent beneficial effect on marine fatty acids (fish oil) supplementation in asthma prevention [267]. A meta-analysis showed that supplementation with fish oil did not improve the severity of atopic dermatitis [268].

Dietary Manipulation in the Prevention of Food Allergy in High-Risk Individuals

Evidence supporting the reduction of food allergy by dietary manipulation mainly applies to high-risk populations, defined by the American Academy of Pediatrics as infants with at least one first-degree relative with allergic disease [254]. Consequently, recommendations in high-risk individuals remain largely unchanged from previous position statements [254].

In high-risk infants, there is limited evidence that exclusive breastfeeding and delaying of solids until six months of age, breastfeeding might delay, or possibly prevent, the onset of food allergy [269]. A number of potential mechanisms have been proposed for the potential protective effects of breastfeeding. Colostrum may provide a protective coating to the gut that prevents the entrance of large foreign proteins and minimizing the possibility of an allergic response. Breastfeeding reduces the amount of foreign protein in the gastrointestinal tract and passively transfers maternal IgA to the infant, which minimizes the risk for absorption of antigens from the gastrointestinal tract. Transfer of cell-mediated immunity from mother to infant stimulates IgA synthesis in the infant [257]. Epidermal growth factor present in human milk hastens maturation of intestinal mucosa and epithelium, and strengthens the mucosal barrier to antigen. Several studies have shown that respiratory and gastrointestinal infections can predispose to the development of allergic diseases [257]. The allergy-preventive effect of breastfeeding might be secondary to a reduction in the number of infections in the infant.

Although evidence for food allergies is limited, partially hydrolysed formulas are often used for the prevention of atopy when breastfeeding is not possible in infants with a strong family history of allergy or elevated cord IgE levels to reduce possible food allergy symptoms [270]. These formulas have been developed with the aim of minimizing the number of sensitizing epitopes within milk proteins, while at the same time retaining peptides of sufficient size and immunogenicity to stimulate the induction of oral tolerance. Compared with extensively hydrolysed formulas, partially hydrolysed formulas are less expensive and more palatable [220]. Prospective controlled trials examining the use of extensively hydrolysed formulas and partially hydrolysed formulas for allergy prevention among high-risk infants show significant reductions in the cumulative incidence of atopic disease through the first five years of life compared with those fed with cow's milk formulas [270]. In the meta-analysis performed by Osborn et al, infants fed extensively hydrolysed formulas versus partially hydrolysed formulas had a significant reduction in food allergy (two studies, 341 infants; typical risk ratio: 0.43; 95%confidence interval: 0.19 to 0.99), but there was no significant difference in all allergy or any other specific allergy incidence [122].

Soy protein is immunogenic and allergenic, although less than cow's milk [272]. A meta-analysis of two studies (n=283) found no significant differences in childhood allergy cumulative incidence from the use of a soy formula compared to a cow's milk formula (typical risk ratio: 0.67; 95% confidence interval: 0.18 to 2.46) [273]. As there is no evidence of benefit, the use of a soy formula for prevention of food allergy cannot be recommended [254,273,274].

There is also evidence suggesting that early introduction of solid food may increase the risk of food allergy in high-risk individuals [274-277]. The existing literature suggests that the optimal developmental time for the introduction of selected supplemental food should be six months. For infants at risk, dairy products should not be introduced before 12 months, eggs 24 months, and peanut, tree nuts, fish, and seafood at least 36 months of age [278]. It is recommended that foods should be introduced one at a time and gradually [278]. Cooked, homogenized foods should be preferred to their fresh counterparts when a reduction of allergenicity has been clinically demonstrated for that processed food [278].

Marini et al prospectively studied 279 infants with high atopic risk who were put on an allergy prevention program and 80 infants with similar atopic risk but no intervention [279]. The intervention program included dietary measures (exclusive and prolonged milk feeding followed by a hypoallergenic weaning diet) and environmental measures such as avoidance of parental smoking in the presence of the babies. The incidence of allergic manifestations was much lower in the intervention group than in the nonintervention group at 1 year (11.5% vs. 54.4%), 2 years (14.9% vs. 65.6%), and 3 years (20.6% vs. 74.1%). Atopic dermatitis and recurrent wheezing were found in both the intervention group and the nonintervention group from birth to the second year of life, whereas urticaria and gastrointestinal disorders were only present in the nonintervention group in the first year of life. Halken et al studied 105 "high-risk" infants who were breast-fed and/or receiving a hypoallergenic formula combined with avoidance of solid foods during the first 6 months of life [280]. This prevention group was compared with a control group consisting of 54 identically defined "high-risk" infants who were on an unrestricted diet. The cumulative prevalence of atopic symptoms was significantly lower at 18 months in the prevention group (32%) than in the control group (74%) ($p < 0.01$) because of a reduced prevalence of recurrent wheezing (13% vs. 37%; $p < 0.01$), atopic dermatitis (14% vs. 31%; $p < 0.01$), vomiting/diarrhea (5% vs. 28%; $p < 0.01$), and infantile colic (9% vs. 24%; $p < 0.01$). The cumulative prevalence of food allergy was significantly lower in the prevention group (6% vs. 17%; $p < 0.05$). The authors concluded that feeding high-risk infants with breast milk and/or hypoallergenic formula, combined with the avoidance of solid foods during the first 6 months of life, has a protective effect on the risk of atopic dermatitis developing during the first 18 months of life.

Miscellaneous Aspects

Infants with cow's milk protein allergy should avoid cow's milk or formulas containing intact cow's milk proteins [281]. It has been estimated that 15 to 25% of infants who have IgE-mediated cow's milk allergy are also allergic to soy, but the rate of tolerance is only 50% for those with non-IgE-mediated cow's milk allergy [45,282]. Soy proteins have been identified that cross-react with cow's milk caseins [283]. A Cochrane analysis of studies comparing soy to hydrolysed cow's milk formulas found no significant difference in infant and childhood allergy and atopic disease [273]. As such, soy formula is not recommended for the prevention of allergy, or for food intolerance [284]. In addition, goat's milk is not recommended in infants with cow's milk allergy as goat's milk also shares some allergenic protein fractions with cow's milk [284,285]. Infants with cow's milk or soy hypersensitivity should be fed a hypoallergenic formula [286]. Extensively hydrolysed casein formulas such as Nutramigen® (Mead Johnson Nutrition [Canada] Co., Ottawa, Canada), Pregestimil® (Mead Johnson Nutrition [Canada] Co., Ottawa, Canada), and Alimentum® (Abbott Laboratories, Limited, Saint-Laurent, Quebec, Canada) have also been used successfully in this regard [286,287]. These formulas are hypoallergenic and well tolerated by children [288]. These formulas, however, are expensive and unpalatable. The partially hydrolyzed whey hydrolysate formulas such as Good Start® (Nestle Canada, Ontario, Canada) is less expensive and have a better taste [220]. However, it contains slightly larger peptides and significantly more immunologically identifiable cow's milk protein, and therefore not suitable for the treatment of cow's milk allergy [283]. Formulas whose protein source is free amino acids are available and are considered as nonallergenic. These formulas should be tried in infants who are very sensitive to cow's milk protein and cannot tolerate even extensively hydrolysed formulas. However, they are also very expensive. Amino acid-based formulas are also useful in the treatment of allergic eosinophilic esophagitis and allergic eosinophilic gastroenteropathy [289-291].

Patients with oral allergy syndrome generally do not experience symptoms when their offending fruit or vegetable is cooked, as proteinacious antigens are generally denatured by heat [35]. Thus, patients with this presentation can consumed cooked food antigen, but should avoid uncooked food antigens.

FUTURE THERAPEUTIC OPTIONS

There is currently no effective and safe specific immunotherapy for food allergens. The study of injectable specific immune therapy using peanuts was suspended because of the high rate of adverse reactions [292]. Traditional injection immunotherapy for other food allergies is not recommended either because of the risk of serious systemic reactions associated with such therapy [293]. Sublingual immunotherapy to food allergens is better tolerated and preliminary results are encouraging [289,294,295]. Long-term efficiency of sublingual immunotherapy, however, remains to be determined.

Vaccines for immunotherapy specially for food-induced anaphylaxis that are being developed include humanized anti-IgE monoclonal antibody therapy, sublingual immunotherapy, peptide immunotherapy, mutated protein immunotherapy, plasmid DNA immunotherapy, engineered recombinant protein immunotherapy, immunostimulatory sequence-modulated immunotherapy, cytokine-modulated immunotherapy, bacterial-encapsulated allergen immunotherapy, and homologous protein immunotherapy [5,202,295-298]. Allergen-specific immunotherapy should be considered for patients who have specific IgE antibodies to clinically relevant allergens and whose allergic symptoms are severe enough to warrant the time and risk of allergen immunotherapy [295].

Preliminary studies showed the potential use of humanized monoclonal anti-IgE antibody in food-allergic subjects [299,300]. Humanized monoclonal anti-IgE antibody binds to the third domain of the Fc region of the IgE molecule and prevents its binding to the high affinity receptor on mast cells and basophils [301]. The anti-IgE also down regulates the expression of the high affinity receptor on mast cells and decreases the release of histamine from basophils [302]. In a randomized, double-blind, placebo-controlled trial in 84 patients with a history of peanut allergy, Leung et al showed an increased threshold of tolerance in patients with severe peanut allergy on oral food challenge after being given every 4 weeks subcutaneous injection of TNX-901 for four doses [296]. TNX-901 is a humanized IgG_1 monoclonal antibody against IgE that binds with high affinity to an epitope in the CH_3 domain [296]. The effect was highly significant at the 450 mg dose level. However, even at the highest dose of TNX-901, approximately 25% of patients were not protected. The treatment was well tolerated with no systemic adverse events. Unfortunately, anti-IgE therapy is expensive and such therapy has to be administered on a regular basis so as to maintain its protective effect [6,15]. Currently, another anti-IgE humanized IgG_1 antibody (omalizumab) is being tested in subjects older than 6 years of age with peanut anaphylaxis [206]. Stern et al treated four adults with eosinophilic esophagitis with a human monoclonal IgG_1 antibody against interleukin-5 (mepolizumab) given by infusion on a monthly basis [303]. After three months of treatment (750 mg monthly), the mean and maximal esophageal eosinophilic count fell from 46 to 6 and from 153 to 28 per high-power field, respectively. The patients also reported improvement of clinical symptoms and quality of life.

Oral immunotherapy seems to represent an interesting and promising approach for the management of food allergy [295]. Enrique et al randomized in a double-blind, placebo-controlled fashion 23 patients with hazelnut allergy to receive either a standardized hazelnut extract or placebo using a sublingual-spit rush protocol over four days [304]. They then received maintenance sublingual immunotherapy for approximately three months. On repeat double-blind, placebo-controlled food challenge, patients in the treatment group had a mean quantity of hazelnut provoking objective symptoms and increased tolerance to hazelnuts from 2.29 gm to 11.59 gm (p=0.02) while patients in the placebo group had a non-significant increase from 3.49 gm to 4.14 gm.

Peptide immunotherapy utilizes peptide fragments containing T-cell-reactive epitopes rather complete protein molecules [293]. Apparently, this kind of therapy would induce T-cell unresponsiveness and production of interferon-γ in a concentration-dependent manner [206]. Peptide immunotherapy allows for formulation of vaccines against any target in which major allergenic proteins are known because IgE binding sites for each major allergen do not have to be mapped [206]. It is hoped that such therapy would render T-cells unresponsive to subsequent allergen exposure. Peptide immunotherapy might play a role in the future therapy of food allergy.

Mutated protein immunotherapy is based on the modification of the primary amino acid sequences of IgE-binding allergenic epitopes of the major allergens present in food, with the aim of reducing allergen potential thereby eliminating activation of mast cells and basophils [206,293]. Mutation of the IgE-binding sites leaves the T-cell response unaffected [305]. The large numbers of allergens present in each food hampers such therapy.

Plasmid DNA immunotherapy results in transcription and translation of encoded genes and elicits an antibody response in the host, thereby preferentially induces a Th1 immune response and suppression of IgE [201,306] Plasmid DNA requires immunostimulatory sequences for optimal immunogenicity [306].

Engineered recombinant protein technology makes room for the development of hypoallergenic derivatives of natural allergens, which would minimize the adverse effect of immunotherapy. Such allergens should not be able to activate cells via cross-linking of IgE antibodies, but should preserve T-cell epitopes and activate B-cells to induce blocking IgG antibodies [201].

Immunostimulatory sequence-modulated immunotherapy using CpG has been shown to be effective in reversing IgE-mediated sensitization in patients with ragweed allergy [307,308]. Likewise, immunostimulatory sequence-conjugated Ara h 2 has been shown to be beneficial in the treatment allergy in a murine model [6].

In animal studies, various Chinese herbs have been shown to block anaphylactic reactions resulting from food allergy [309-311]. The therapeutic effect was associated with immunoregulatory effects on Th1-Th-2 responses and reductions in IgE levels [310]. The exact mechanism is not known and further studies are required.

VACCINATIONS AND FOOD ALLERGIES

Although measles-German measles-mumps (MMR) vaccine is cultured from chick embryos, MMR vaccination is not contraindicated in children allergic to eggs [224,312]. The vaccine should, however, be administered in a supervised setting. On the other hand, the vaccine is contraindicated in children with known systemic allergic reaction to neomycin or gelatin as most reported drug allergies are due to these vaccine components [313].

According to the American Academy of Pediatrics, the influenza and yellow fever vaccines, which are cultured in chick embryo and contain small amounts of egg protein, should be avoided in those with severe anaphylactic reactions [314]. For those with non-anaphylactoid reactions, skin prick testing with the vaccine should be performed. Those with positive results should receive their vaccine in divided graded doses with close supervision after administration [314]. The recommended schedule is 0.05 ml of 1:10 dilution, followed by 0.05 mL, 0.10 mL, 0.15 mL and 0.20 mL of full strength vaccine, with doses spaced 15 to 20 minutes apart [314].

CONCLUSION

Food allergy is an inappropriate immunological response to exposed food. This immunological response is primarily IgE-mediated, but can also occur through other, non-IgE-mediated mechanisms. Food allergy primarily affects infants, with a natural history tending towards resolution by adulthood. In recent years, food allergy has clearly been shown to be increasing in prevalence. Although much remains unknown about this phenomenon, recent studies regarding the precise pathogenic mechanisms have begun to shed light on the matter.

Clinically, food allergy can present in an extraordinarily diverse manner. Typically, food allergy affects multiple organs, with the gastrointestinal, dermatological/integument and respiratory systems most commonly involved. Given this diversity, there is often a tendency for patients to over-report food allergy. Hence diagnosis can be a challenge. Skin prick tests, as well as in vitro testing have been applied with success for screening, but the gold standard for diagnosis remains a double blinded placebo control food trial. The slightly more practical, single blinded placebo controlled food trial can also be administered under the right circumstances.

Of the various clinical presentations of food allergy, systemic anaphylaxis is potentially the most important to recognize as it is potentially fatal and requires immediate management. Prompt airway management and intramuscular epinephrine injection are the cornerstones of management. In terms of long-term management, allergenic avoidance remains the mainstay of therapy, although other interventions such as dietary modification to prevent food allergy have been attempted with mixed results. In recent years, policies on dietary modification to prevent food allergy have changed considerably, with modification now recommended for those with higher risk of food allergy, rather than the general population as previously suggested. Therapies on the horizon include vaccination and immunotherapy.

References

[1] Leung, AK. Food allergy: a clinical approach. *Adv. Pediatr.* 1998;45:145-177.

[2] Leung, AK; Kamat, D. Clinical manifestations of food allergy. In: Chesterton, CM, (ed). *Food Allergies: New Research.* New York: Nova Science Publishers, Inc., 2008, pp.91-120.

[3] Leung, AK; Hon, KL. Management of the child with food allergy. In: Chesterton CM, (ed). *Food Allergies: New Research.* New York: Nova Science Publishers, Inc., 2008, pp.135-156.

[4] Burks, W; Ballmer-Weber, BK. Food allergy. *Mol. Nutr. Food Res.* 2006;50:595-603.

[5] Scurlock, AM; Lee, LA; Burks, AW. Food allergy in children. *Immunol. Allergy Clin. North Am.* 2005;25:369-388.

[6] Sampson, HA. Update on food allergy. *J. Allergy Clin. Immunol.* 2004;113:805-819.

[7] Lack, G. Food allergy. *N. Engl. J. Med.* 2008;359:1252-1260.

[8] Thong, BY; Hourihane, JO. Monitoring of IgE-mediated food allergy in childhood. *Acta Paediatr.* 2004;93:759-764.

[9] Bock, SA. Prospective appraisal of complaints of adverse reactions to foods in children during the first 3 years of life. *Pediatrics.* 1987;79: 683-688.

[10] Skolnick, HS; Conover-Walker, MK; Koerner, CB; et al. The natural history of peanut allergy. *J. Allergy Clin. Immunol.* 2001;107:367-374

[11] Cocharane, S; Beyer, K; Clausen, M; et al. Factor influencing the incidence and prevalence of food allergy. *Allergy.* 2009;64:1246-1255.

[12] Grundy, J; Bateman, BJ; Gantm, C; et al. Peanut allergy in three year old children - a population based study. *J. Allergy Clin. Immunol.* 2001;107(suppl):S231.

[13] Sicherer, SH; Munoz-Furlong, A; Sampson, HA. Prevalence of peanut and tree nut allergy in the United States determined by means of a random digit dial telephone survey: a 5-year follow-up study. *J. Allergy Clin. Immunol.* 2003;112:1203-1207.

[14] Asero, R; Ballmer-Weber, BK; Beyer, K; et al. IgE-mediated food allergy diagnosis: current status and new perspectives. *Mol. Nutr. Food Res.* 2007;51:135-147.

[15] Keet, CA; Wood RA. Food allergy and anaphylaxis. *Immunol. Allergy Clin. North Am.* 2007;27:193-212.

[16] Jyonouchi H. Non-IgE medited food allergy. *Inflamm. Allergy Drug Targets.* 2008;7(3):173-180.
[17] Sampson, HA. The immunopathogenic role of food hypersensitivity in atopic dermatitis. *Acta Derm. Venereol.* 1992;176:S34-S37.
[18] Golbert, TM; Patterson, R; Pruzansky, JJ. Systemic allergic reactions to ingested antigens. *J. Allergy.* 1969;44:96-107.
[19] Joint Task Force on Practice Parameters; American Academy of Allergy, Asthma and Immunology; American College of Allergy, Asthma and Immunology; Joint Council of Allergy, Asthma and Immunology. The diagnosis and management of anaphylaxis: an updated practice parameter. *J. Allergy Clin. Immunol.* 2005;115:S483-S523.
[20] Sampson, HA. Anaphylaxis and emergency treatment. *Pediatrics.* 2003;111: 1601-1608.
[21] Brigino, E; Bahna, SL. Clinical features of food allergy in infants. *Clin. Rev. Allergy Immunol.* 1995;13:329-345.
[22] Brown, SG. Cardiovascular aspects of anaphylaxis: implications for treatment and diagnosis. *Curr. Opin. Allergy Clin. Immunol.* 2005;5:359-364.
[23] Anderson, JA. Food allergy and intolerance. In: Lieberman, P; Anderson, JA. (eds). *Current Clinical Practice: Allergic Diseases: Diagnosis and Treatment.* 3rd edition. Totowa: Humana Press, 2007, pp. 271-294.
[24] Wang, J; Sampson, HA. Food anaphylaxis. *Clin. Exp. Allergy.* 2007;37:651-660.
[25] Maulitz, RM; Pratt, DS; Schocket, AL. Exercise-induced anaphylactic reactions to shellfish. *J. Allergy Clin. Immunol.* 1979;63:433-434.
[26] Sheffer, AL; Austen, KF. Exercise-induced anaphylaxis. *J. Allergy Clin. Immunol.* 1980;66:106-111.
[27] Kidd, JM III; Cohen, SH; Sosman, AJ; et al. Food-dependent exercise-induced anaphylaxis. *J. Allergy Clin. Immunol.* 1983;71:407-411.
[28] Beaudouin, E; Renaudin, JM; Morisset, M; et al. Food-dependent exercise-induced anaphylaxis – update and current data. *Eur. Ann. Allergy Clin. Immunol.* 2006;38:45-51.
[29] American College of Allergy, Asthma, & Immunology. Food allergy: a practice parameter. *Ann. Allergy Asthma Immunol.* 2006;96(Suppl 2):S1-S68.
[30] Noma, T; Yoshizawa, I; Ogawa, N; et al. Fatal buckwheat dependent exercise induced anaphylaxis. *Asian Pacific J. Allergy Immunol.* 2001;19:283-286.
[31] Dohi, M; Suko, M; Sugiyama, H; et al. 3 cases of food-dependent exercise-induced anaphylaxis in which aspirin intake exacerbated anaphylactic symptoms. *Arerugi.* 1990;39:1598-1604.
[32] Morita, E; Kunie, K; Matsuo, H. Food-dependent exercise-induced anaphylaxis. *J. Dermatol. Sci.* 2007;47:109-117.
[33] Anderson, JA. The clinical spectrum of food allergy in adults. *Clin. Exp. Allergy.* 1991;21:S304-S315.
[34] Silverstein, SR; Frommer, DA; Dobozin, B; et al. Celery-dependent exercise-induced anaphylaxis. *J. Emerg. Med.* 1986;4:195-199.
[35] Nash, S; Burks, AW. Oral allergy syndrome. *Curr. Allergy Asthma Rep.* 2007;7:1-2.
[36] Sugita, K; Kabashima, K; Nakashima, D; et al. Oral allergy syndrome caused by raw fish in a Japanese sushi bar worker. *Contact dermatitis.* 2007;56:369-370.

[37] Purohit-Sheth, TS; Carr, WW. Oral allergy syndrome (pollen-food allergy syndrome). *Allergy Asthma Proc*. 2005;26:229-230.

[38] Seidman, E. Food allergic disorders of the gastrointestinal tract. In: Roy, CC; Silverman, A; Allagille, D. (eds). *Pediatric Clinical Gastroenterology*. St Louis: Mosby. 1995; pp. 374-384.

[39] Sampson, HA. Food allergy – accurately identifying clinical reactivity. *Allergy*. 2005;60:19-24.

[40] Aiuti, F ; Paganelli, R. Food allergy and gastrointestinal diseases. *Ann. Allergy*. 1983;51:275-280.

[41] Amlot, PL; Kemeny, DM; Zachary, C; et al. Oral allergy syndrome: symptoms of IgE mediated hypersensitivity to foods. *Clin. Allergy*. 1987;17:33-42.

[42] Lee, LA; Buirks, AW. Food allergies: prevalence, molecular characterization, and treatment/prevention strategies. *Annu. Rev. Nutr*. 2006;26;539-565.

[43] Ortolani, C; Ispano, M; Pastorello, EA; et al. Comparison of results of skin prick tests (with fresh foods and commercial food extracts) and RAST in 100 patients with oral allergy syndrome. *J. Allergy Clin. Immunol.* 1989;83:683-690.

[44] Hallett, R; Teuber, SS. Food allergies and sensitivities. *Nutr. Clin. Care*. 2004;7:122-129.

[45] Garcia-Careaga, M; Kerner, JA, Jr. Gastrointestinal manifestations of food allergies in pediatric patients. *Nutr. Clin. Pract*. 2005;20:526-535.

[46] Spergel, JM; Pawlowski, NA. Food allergy: mechanisms, diagnosis, and management in children. *Pediatr. Clin. North Am*. 2002;49:73-96.

[47] Strobel, S; Hourihane, OB. Gastrointestinal allergy: clinical symptoms and immunological mechanisms. *Pediatr. Allergy Immunol*. 2001;12(Suppl 14):43-46.

[48] Pastorello, EA; Robino, AM. Clinical role of lipid transfer proteins in food allergy. *Mol. Nutr. Food Res*. 2004;48:356-362.

[49] Hoffman, KM; Sampson, HA. Evaluation and management of patients with adverse food reactions. In: Bierman, CW; Pearlman, DS; Shapiro, GG; et al. (eds). *Allergy, Asthma, and Immunology from Infancy to Adulthood*. Philadelphia: WB Saunders. 1996; pp. 665-686.

[50] Sicherer, SH. Clinical aspects of gastrointestinal food allergy in childhood. *Pediatrics*. 2003;111:1609-1616.

[51] Dauer, EH, Freese, DK; El-Youssef, M; et al. Clinical characteristics of eosinophilic esophagitis in children. *Ann. Otol. Rhinol. Laryngol*. 2005;114:827-833.

[52] Furuta, GT; Straumann, A. Review article: the pathogensis and management of eosinophilic oesophagitis. *Aliment. Pharmacol. Ther*. 2006;24:173-182.

[53] Heine, RG. Pathophysiology, diagnosis and treatment of food protein-induced gastrointestinal diseases. *Curr. Opin. Allergy Clin. Immunol*. 2004;4:221-229.

[54] Spergel, JM. Eosinophilic esophagitis in adults and children: evidence for a food allergy component in many patients. *Curr. Opin. Allergy Clin. Immunol*. 2007;7:274-278.

[55] Furuta, T; Liacouras CA; Collins, MH; et al. Eosinophilic esophagitis in children and adults: a systemic review and consensus recommendations for diagnosis and treatment. *Gastroenterology*. 2007;133:1342-1363.

[56] Noel, RJ; Rothenberg, ME. Eosinophilic esophagitis. *Curr. Opin. Pediatr*. 2005;17:690-694.

[57] Martin-Muńoz, MF; Lucendo, AJ; Navarro, M, et al. Food allergies and eosinophilic esophagitis – two case studies. *Digestion*. 2006;74:49-54
[58] Pentiuk, SP; Miller, CK; Kaul, A. Eosinophilic esophagitis in infants and toddlers. *Dysphagia*. 2007;22:44-48.
[59] Cheung, KM; Oliver, MR; Cameron, DJ, et al. Esophageal eosinophilia in children with dysphagia. *J. Pediatr. Gastroenterol. Nutr*. 2003;37:498-503.
[60] Croese, J; Fairley, SK; Masson, JW; et al. Clinical and endoscopic features of eosinophilic esophagitis in adults. *Gastrointest. Endosc*. 2003;58:516-522.
[61] Liacouras, CA. Eosinophilic esophagitis in children and adults. *J. Pediatr. Gastroenterol. Nutr*. 2003;37:S23-S28.
[62] Kaczmarski, SJ. Gastroesophageal reflux in children and adolescents. Clinical aspects with special respect to food hypersensitivity. *Adv. Med. Sci*. 2006;51:327-335.
[63] Kelly, KJ; Lazenby, AJ; Rowe, PC; et al. Eosinophilic esophagitis attributed to gastroesophageal reflux: improvement with an amino acid-based formula. *Gastroenterology*. 1995;109:1503-1512.
[64] Gonsalves, N. Food allergies and eosinophilic gastrointestinal illness. *Gastroenterol. Clin. North Am*. 2007;36:75-91.
[65] Klein, NC; Hargrove, RI; Sleisenger, MH; et al. Eosinophilic gastroenteritis. *Medicine (Baltimore)*. 1970;49:299-319
[66] Proujansky, R; Winter, HS; Walker, WA. Gastrointestinal syndromes associated with food sensitivity. *Adv. Pediatr*. 1988;35:219-238.
[67] Bock, SA; Sampson, HA. Food allergy in infancy. *Pediatr. Clin. North Am*. 1994;41:1047-1067.
[68] Mansueto, P; Montalto, G; Pacor, ML; et al. Food allergy in gastroenterologic diseases: review of literature. *World J. Gastroenterol*. 2006;12:7744-7752.
[69] Pirson, F. Food allergy: a challenge for the clinician. *Acta Gastroenterol. Belg*. 2006;69:38-42.
[70] Nowak-Wegrzyn, A; Sampson, HA; Wood, RA; et al. Food protein-induced enterocolitis syndrome caused by solid food proteins. *Pediatrics*. 2003;111:829-835.
[71] Murch, S. Allergy and intestinal dysmotility – evidence of genuine causal linkage? *Curr. Opin. Gastroenterol*. 2006;22:664-668.
[72] Yimyaem, P; Chongsrisawat, V; Vivatvakin, B, et al. Gastrointestinal manifestations of cow's milk protein allergy during the first year of life. *J. Med. Assoc. Thai*. 2003;86:116-123.
[73] Hojsak, I; Kljaić-Turkalj, M; Mišak. Z; et al. Rice protein-induced enterocolitis syndrome. *Clin. Nutr*. 2006;25:533-536.
[74] Sampson, HA. Food allergies. In: Oski, FA; DeAngelis, CD; Feigin, RD. (eds). *Principles and Practice of Pediatrics*. Philadelphia: JB Lippincott. 1994; pp. 227-232.
[75] Lake, AM. Dietary protein enterocolitis. *Curr. Allergy Rep*. 2001;1:76-79.
[76] Hirose, R; Yamada, T; Hayashida, Y. Massive bloody stools in two neonates caused by cow's milk allergy. *Pediatr. Surg. Int*. 2006;22:935-938.
[77] Swart, JF; Ultee, K. Rectal bleeding in a preterm infant as a symptom of allergic colitis. *Eur. J. Pediatr*. 2003;162:55-56.
[78] Proujansky, R; Winter, HS; Walker, WA. Gastrointestinal syndromes associated with food sensitivity. *Adv. Pediatr*. 1988;35:219-238.

[79] Troncone, R; Discepolo, V. Colon in food allergy. *J Pediatr Gastroentrol Nutr.* 2009;48 (Suppl 2):S89-91.

[80] Troncone, R; Bhatnagar, S; Butzner, D; et al. Celiac disease and other immunologically mediated disorders of the gastrointestinal tract: Working Group Report of the Second World Congress of Pediatric Gastroenterology, Hepatology, and Nutrition. *J. Pediatr. Gastroenterol. Nutr.* 2004;39:S601-S610.

[81] Dewar, DH; Ciclitira, PJ. Clinical features and diagnosis of celiac disease. *Gastroenterology.* 2005;128:S19-S24.

[82] Estep, DC; Kulczycki, A, Jr. Treatment of infant colic with amino acid-based infant formula: a preliminary study. *Acta Paediatr.* 2000;89:22-27.

[83] Hill, DJ; Hudson, IL; Sheffield, LJ; et al. A low allergen diet is a significant intervention in infantile colic: results of a community-based study. *J. Allergy Clin. Immunol.* 1995;96:886-892.

[84] Iacono, G; Carroccio, A; Montalto, G; et al. Severe infantile colic and food intolerance: a long-term prospective study. *J. Pediatr. Gastroenterol. Nutr.* 1991;12:332-335.

[85] Leung, AK; Lemay, JF. Infantile colic: a review. *J. R. Soc. Health.* 2004;124:162-166.

[86] Lothe, L; Lindberg, T. Cow's milk whey protein elicits symptoms of infantile colic in colicky formula-fed infants: a double-blind crossover study. *Pediatrics.* 1989;83:262-266.

[87] Lucassen, PL; Assendelft, WJ; Gubbels, JW; et al. Infantile colic: crying time reduction with a whey hydrolysate: a double-blind, randomized, placebo-controlled trial. *Pediatrics.* 2000;106:1349-1354.

[88] Savino, F. Focus on infantile colic. *Acta Paediatr.* 2007;96:1259-1264.

[89] Hill, DJ; Hosking, CS. Infantile colic and food hypersensitivity. *J. Pediatr. Gastroenterol. Nutr.* 2000;30:S67-S76.

[90] Kalliomäki, M; Lappala, P; Korvenranta, H; et al. Extent of fussing and colic type crying preceding atopic disease. *Arch. Dis. Child.* 2001;84:349-350.

[91] Jakobsson, I; Lothe, L; Ley, D; et al. Effectiveness of casein hydrolysate feedings in infants with colic. *Acta Paediatr.* 2000; 89:18-21.

[92] Jakobbson, I; Lindberg, T. Cow's milk proteins cause infantile colic in breast-fed infants: a double-blind crossover study. *Pediatrics.* 1983;71:268-271.

[93] Hewson, P; Oberklaid, F; Menahem, S. Infant colic, distress, and crying. *Clin. Pediatr.* 1987;26:69-73.

[94] Nutrition Committee, Canadian Paediatric Society. Dietary manipulations for infantile colic. *Paediatr. Child Health.* 2003;8:449-452.

[95] Hill, DJ; Roy, N; Heine, RG; et al. Effect of a low-allergen maternal diet on colic among breastfed infants: a randomized, controlled trial. *Pediatrics.* 2005;116:e709-e715.

[96] Kalliomäki, MA. Food allergy and irritable bowel syndrome. *Curr. Opin. Gastroenterol.* 2005;21:708-711.

[97] Park, MI; Camilleri, M. Is there a role of food allergy in irritable bowel syndrome and functional dyspepsia? A systemic review. *Neurogastroenterol. Motil.* 2006;18:595-607.

[98] Gonsalkorale, WM; Perrey, C; Pravica, V; et al. Interleukin 10 genotypes in irritable bowel syndrome: evidence for an inflammatory component? *Gut.* 2003;52:91-93.

[99] van der Veek, PP; van den Berg, M; de Kroon, YE; et al. Role of tumor necrosis factor-α and interleukin-10 gene polymorphisms in irritable bowel syndrome. *Am. J. Gastroenterol.* 2005;100:2510-2516.

[100] Barbara, G; Stanghellini, V; de Giorgio, R; et al. Activated mast cells in proximity to colonic nerves correlate with abdominal pain in irritable bowel syndrome. *Gastroenterology.* 2004;126:693-702.

[101] Atkinson, W; Sheldon, TA; Shaath, N; et al. Food elimination based on IgG antibodies in irritable bowel syndrome: a randomized controlled trial. *Gut.* 2004;53:1459-1464.

[102] Isolauri, E; Rautava, S; Kalliomäki, M. Food allergy in irritable bowel syndrome: new facts and old fallacies. *Gut.* 2004;53:1391-1393.

[103] Leung, AK; Wong, BE; Cho, HY, et al. Recurrent abdominal pain in childhood. *Singapore Pediatr. J.* 1996;38:44-48.

[104] Leung, AK; Lemay, JF; Barker, C. Recurrent abdominal pain in children. *Can. J. Diagn.* 2002;19(5):68-80.

[105] Kokkonen, J; Ruuska, T; Karttunen, T; et al. Mucosal pathology of the foregut associating with food allergy and recurrent abdominal pains in children. *Acta Paediatr.* 2001;90:16-21.

[106] Husby, S; Host, A. Recurrent abdominal pain, food allergy and endoscopy. *Acta Paediatr.* 2001;90:3-4.

[107] Leung, AK; Chan, PY; Cho, HY. Constipation in children. *Am. Fam. Physician.* 1996;54:611-627.

[108] Loening-Baucke, V. Prevalence, symptoms and outcome of constipation in infants and toddlers. *J. Pediatr.* 2005;146:359-363.

[109] Iacono, G; Carroccio, A; Cavataio, F; et al. Chronic constipation as a symptom of cow milk allergy. *J. Pediatr.* 1995;126:34-39.

[110] Iacono, G; Cavataio, F; Montalto,G; et al. Intolerance of cow's milk and chronic constipation in children. *N. Engl. J. Med.* 1998;339:1100-1104.

[111] Daher, S; Tahan, S; Solé, D; et al. Cow's milk protein intolerance and chronic constipation in children. *Pediatr. Allergy Immunol.* 2001;1:339-342.

[112] Carroccio, A; Scalici, C; Maresi, E; et al. Chronic constipation and food intolerance: a model of proctitis causing constipation. *Scand. J. Gastroenterol.* 2005;40:33-42.

[113] Burks, W. Skin manifestations of food allergy. *Pediatrics.* 2003;111:1617-1624.

[114] Fasano, MB. Dermatologic food allergy. *Pediatr. Ann.* 2006;35:727-731.

[115] Host, A; Halken, S. A prospective study of cow milk allergy in Danish infants during the first 3 years of life. *Allergy.* 1990;45:587-596.

[116] Hill, DJ; Firer, MA; Shelton, MJ; et al. Manifestations of milk allergy in infants: clinical and immunologic findings. *J. Pediatr.* 1986;109:270-276.

[117] Champion, RH; Roberts, SO; Carpenter RG; et al: Urticaria and angioedema: a review of 554 patients. *Br. J. Dermatol.* 1969;81:588-597.

[118] Lemanske, RF Jr.; Sampson, HA. Adverse reactions to foods and their relationships to skin diseases in children. *Adv. Pediatr.* 1988;35: 89-218.

[119] Winston, GB; Lewis, CW. Contact dermatitis. *Int. J. Dermatol.* 1982;21:573-578.

[120] Pastar, Z; Lipozencic, J. Adverse reactions to food and clinical expressions of food allergy. *SKINmed.* 2006;5:119-125.

[121] Sampson, HA. The immunopathogenic role of food hypersensitivity in atopic dermatitis. *Acta Derm. Venereol.* 1992;176:S34-S37.

[122] Gontzes, P; Bahna, SL. Food allergy for the primary care physician. *Primary Care.* 1987;14:547-558.
[123] Leung, AK; Hon, KL; Robson, WL. Atopic dermatitis. *Adv. Pediatr.* 2007;54:241-273.
[124] Burks, AW; Mallroy, SB; Williams, LW; et al. Atopic dermatitis: clinical relevance of food hypersensitivity reactions. *J. Pediatr.* 1988;113:447-451.
[125] Sampson, HA; McCaskill, CC. Food hypersensitivity and atopic dermatitis: evaluation of 113 patients. *J. Pediatr.* 1985;107:669-675.
[126] Sampson, HA; Mendelson, L; Rosen, JP. Fatal and near-fatal anaphylactic reactions to food in children and adolescents. *N. Engl. J. Med.* 1992;327:380-384.
[127] Breuer, K; Heratizadeh, A; Wulf, A; et al. Late eczematous reactions to food in children with atopic dermatitis. *Clin. Exp. Allergy.* 2004;34:817-824.
[128] Hill, DJ; Hosking, CS. Food allergy and atopic dermatitis in infancy: an epidemiology study. *Pediatr. Allergy Immunol.* 2004;15:421-427.
[129] Dolovich, J; Hargreave, FE; Chalmers, R; et al. Late cutaneous allergic responses in isolated IgE-dependent reactions. *J. Allergy Clin. Immunol.* 1973;52:38-46.
[130] Solley, GO; Gleich, GJ; Jordan, RE; et al. The late phase of the immediate wheal and flare skin reactions: its dependence on IgE antibodies. *J. Clin. Invest.* 1976;58:408-420.
[131] Lio, PA. Atopic dermatitis and food allergies: true, true and related? *Arch. Dis. Child. Educ. Pract. Ed.* 2007;92:ep56-ep60.
[132] Hill, DJ; Duke, AM; Hosking, CS; et al. Clinical manifestations of cow's milk allergy in childhood. II. The diagnostic value of skin tests and RAST. *Clin. Allergy.* 1988;18:481-490.
[133] Brancaccio, RR; Alvarez, MS. Contact allergy to food. *Dermatol. Ther.* 2004;17:302-313.
[134] Judd, L. A descriptive study of occupational skin disease. *N. Z. Med. J.* 1994;107:147-149.
[135] Ekeowa-Anderson, AL. Allergic contact cheilitis to garlic. *Contact Dermatitis.* 2007;56:174-175.
[136] Tamagawa-Mineoka, R; Katoh, N; Kishimoto, S. Allergic contact cheilitis due to geraniol in food. *Contact Dermatitis.* 2007;56:242-243.
[137] Hall, RP. Dermatitis herpetiformis. *J. Invest. Dermatol.* 1992;99:873-881.
[138] Solheim, BG; Ek, J; Thune, PO; et al. HLA antigens in dermatitis herpetiformis and coeliac disease. *Tissue Antigens.* 1976;7:57-59.
[139] El-Gamal, YM; Hossny, EM. Respiratory food allergy. *Pediatr. Ann.* 2006;35:733-740.
[140] James, JM. Respiratory manifestations of food allergy. *Pediatrics.* 2003;111:1625-1630.
[141] Burks, AW; Sampson, H. Food allergies in children. *Curr. Probl. Pediatr.* 1993;23:230-252.
[142] Ortolani, C. Atlas on mechanisms in adverse reactions to food. *Allergy.* 1995;50:5-81.
[143] James, JM; Crespo, JF. Allergic reactions to foods by inhalation. *Curr. Allergy Asthma Rep.* 2007;7:167-174.
[144] Ozol, D; Mete, E. Asthma and food allergy. *Curr. Opin. Pulm. Med.* 2008;14:9-12.
[145] Onorato, J; Merland, N; Terral, C; et al: Placebo-controlled double-blind food challenge in asthma. *J. Allergy Clin. Immunol.* 1986;78:1139-1146.
[146] Roberts, G; Lack, G. Food allergy and asthma – what is the link? *Paediatr. Respir. Rev.* 2003;4:205-212.

[147] Rance, F; Micheau, P; Marchac, V; et al. Food allergy and asthma in children. *Rev. Pneumol. Clin.* 2003;59:109-113
[148] James, JM; Eggleston, PA; Sampson, HA. Food allergy increases airway reactivity. *Am. J. Crit. Care Respir. Med.* 1994;149:59-64.
[149] Roberts, G; Lack, G. Relevance of inhalational exposure to food allergens. *Curr. Opin. Allergy Clin. Immunol.* 2003;3:211-215.
[150] Crespo, JF; Pascual, C; Dominguez, C; et al. Allergic reactions associated with airborne fish particles in IgE-mediated fish hypersensitive patients. *Allergy.* 1995;50:257-261.
[151] Roberts, G; Golder, N; Lack, G. Bronchial challenges with aerosolized food in asthmatic, food-allergic children. *Allergy.* 2002;57:713-717.
[152] Sicherer, SH; Furlong, TJ; DeSimone, J; et al. Self-reported allergic reactions to peanuts on commercial airlines. *J. Allergy Clin. Immunol.* 1999;104:186-189.
[153] Gustafsson, D; Sjöberg, O; Foucard, T. Sensitization to food and airborne allergens in children with atopic dermatitis followed up to 7 years of age. *Pediatr. Allergy Immunol.* 2003;14:448-452.
[154] Kotaniemi-Syrjanen, A; Reijonen, T; Romppanen, J. Allergen-specific immunoglobulin E antibodies in wheezing infants: the risk for asthma in later childhood. *Pediatrics.* 2003;111:e255-e261.
[155] Simpson, AB; Glutting, J; Yousef, E. Food allergy and asthma morbidity in children. *Pediatr. Pulmonol.* 2007;42:489-495.
[156] Heiner, DC; Sears, JW. Chronic respiratory disease associated with multiple circulating precipitins to cow's milk. *Am. J. Dis. Child.* 1960;100:500-502.
[157] Bahna, SL. Adverse food reactions by skin contact. *Allergy.* 2004;59(Suppl 78):66-70.
[158] Aydoğan, B; Kiroğlu, M; Altintas, D; et al. The role of food allergy in otitis media with effusion. *Otolaryngol. Head Neck Surg.* 2004;130:747-750.
[159] Bernstein, JM; Lee, J; Conboy, K; et al. Further observations on the role of IgE-mediated hypersensitivity in recurrent otitis media with effusion. *Otolaryngol. Head Neck Surg.* 1985;93:611-615.
[160] Luyasu, S; Morisset, M; Guenard, L; et al. Acute recurrent otalgia and food allergy: a case report and review of the literature. *Eur. Ann. Allergy Clin. Immunol.* 2005;37:60-62.
[161] Nsouli, TM; Nsouli, SM; Linde, RE; et al. Role of food allergy in serous otitis media. *Ann. Allergy.* 1994;73:215-219.
[162] Juntti, H; Tikkanen, S; Kokkonen, J; et al. Cow's milk allergy is associated with recurrent otitis media during childhood. *Acta Otolaryngol.* 1999;119:867-873.
[163] Derebery, MJ; Berliner, KI. Prevalence of allergy in Meniere's disease. *Otolaryngol. Head Neck Surg.* 2000;123:69-75.
[164] Keleş, E; Gödekmerdan, A; Kalidağ, T; et al. Ménière's disease and allergy: allergens and cytokines. *J. Laryngol. Otol.* 2004;118:688-693.
[165] Monro, J; Carini, C; Brostoff, J. Migraine is a food-allergic disease. *Lancet.* 1984;1:719-721.
[166] Mansfield, LE; Vaughan, TR; Waller, SF; et al. Food allergy and adult migraine: double-blind and mediator confirmation of an allergic etiology. *Ann. Allergy.* 1985;55:126-129.
[167] Egger, J; Carter, CM; Soothill, JF; et al. Oligoantigenic diet treatment of children with epilepsy and migraine. *J. Pediatr.* 1989;114:51-58.

[168] Stern, M. Allergic enteropathy. In: Walker, WA; Durie, PR; Hamilton, JR; et al. (eds). *Pediatric Gastrointestinal Disease*. St Louis: Mosby. 1996; pp. 677-692.

[169] Fotherby, KJ; Hunter, JO. Symptoms of food allergy. *Clin. Gastroenterol.* 1985;14:615-629.

[170] Pearson, DJ; McKee, A. Food allergy. *Adv. Nutr. Res.* 1985;7:1-37.

[171] Johansson, SG; Hourihane, JO; Bousquet, J; et al. A revised nomenclature for allergy. An EAACI position statement from the EAACI nomenclature task force. *Allergy.* 2001;56:813-824.

[172] Crayton, JW; Stone, T; Stein, G. Epilepsy precipitated by food sensitivity: report of a case with double-blind placebo-controlled assessment. *Clin. Electroencephalographol.* 1981;12:192-198.

[173] Frediani, T; Lucarelli, S; Pelliccia, A; et al. Allergy and childhood epilepsy: a close relationship? *Acta Neurol. Scand.* 2001;104:349-352.

[174] Frediani, T; Pelliccia, A; Aprile, A; et al. Partial idiopathic epilepsy: recovery after allergen-free diet. *Pediatr. Med. Chir.* 2004;26:196-197.

[175] Cavallo, MG; Fava, D; Monetini, L; et al. Cell-mediated immune response to ß casein in recent-onset insulin-dependent diabetes: implications for disease pathogenesis. *Lancet.* 1996;348:926-928.

[176] Harrison, LC. Cow's milk and IDDM. *Lancet.* 1996;348:905-906.

[177] Karjalainen, J; Martin, JM; Knip, M; et al. A bovine albumin peptide as a possible trigger of insulin-dependent diabetes mellitus. *N. Engl. J. Med.* 1992;327:302-307.

[178] Norris, JM; Beaty, B; Klingensmith, G; et al. Lack of association between early exposure to cow's milk protein and ß-cell autoimmunity: diabetes autoimmunity study in the young (DAISY). *JAMA.* 1996;276:609-614.

[179] Sandberg, DH; McIntosh, RM; Bernstein, CW; et al. Severe steroid-responsive nephrosis associated with hypersensitivity. *Lancet.* 1997;1:388-391.

[180] Genova, R; Sanfilippo, M; Rossi, ME; et al. Food allergy in steroid-resistant nephrotic syndrome. *Lancet.* 1987;1:1315-1316.

[181] Laurent, J; Rostoker, G; Robera, R; et al. Is adult idiopathic nephrotic syndrome food allergy? Value of oligoantigenic diets. *Nephron.* 1987;47:7-11.

[182] Sieniawska, M; Szymanik-Grzelak, H; Kowalewska, M; et al. The role of cow's milk protein intolerance in steroid-resistant nephrotic syndrome. *Acta Paediatr.* 1992;81:1007-1012.

[183] Whitefield, MF; Barr, DGD. Cow's milk allergy in the syndrome of thrombocytopenia with absent radius. *Arch. Dis. Child.* 1976;51:337-343.

[184] Jones, RHT. Congenital thrombocytopenia and milk allergy. *Arch. Dis. Child.* 1977;52:744-745.

[185] Caffrey, EA; Sladen, GE; Isaacs, PET; et al: Thrombocytopenia caused by cow's milk. *Lancet.* 1981;2:316.

[186] Businco, L; Falconieri, P; Bellioni-Businco, B; et al. Severe food-induced vasculitis in two children. *Pediatr. Allergy Immunol.* 2002;12:68-71.

[187] Lunardi, C; Bambara, LM; Biasi, D; et al. Elimination diet in the treatment of selected patients with hypersensitivity vasculitis. *Clin. Exp .Rheum.* 1992;10:131-135.

[188] Panush, RS; Carter, RL; Katz, P; et al. Diet therapy for rheumatoid arthritis. *Arthritis Rheum.* 1983;26:462-471.

[189] Panush, RS; Stroud, RM; Webster, EM. Food-induced (allergic) arthritis: Inflammatory arthritis exacerbated by milk. *Arthritis Rheum.* 1986;29:220-226.

[190] Panush, RS. Food induced ("allergic") arthritis: clinical and serologic studies. *J. Rheumatol.* 1990;17:291-294.

[191] Parke, AL; Hughes, GR. Rheumatoid arthritis and food: a case study. *Br. Med. J.* 1981;282:2027-2029.

[192] Golding, DN. Is there an allergic synovitis? *J. R. Soc. Med.* 1990;83:312-314.

[193] van der Laar, MA; van der Korst, JK. Food intolerance in rheumatoid arthritis. I. A double blind, controlled trial of the clinical effects of elimination of milk allergens and azo dyes. *Ann. Rheum. Dis.* 1992;51:298-302.

[194] Denman, AM; Mitchell, B; Ansell, BM. Joint complaints and food allergic disorders. *Ann. Allergy.* 1983;51:260-263.

[195] Karatay, S; Erdem, T; Yildirim, K; et al. The effect of individualized diet challenges consisting of allergenic foods on TNF-α and IL-1β levels in patients with rheumatoid arthritis. *Rheumatology.* 2004;43:1429-1433.

[196] Bock, SA; Buckley, J; Holst, A; et al. Proper use of skin tests with food extracts in diagnosis of hypersensitivity to food in children. *Clin. Allergy*. 1977;7:375 -383.

[197] Sampson, HA. Food allergy. Part 2: diagnosis and management. *J. Allergy Clin. Immunol.* 1999;103:981-99.

[198] Sampson HA. Utility of food-specific IgE concentrations in predicting symptomatic food allergy. *J. Allergy Clin. Immunol.* 2001;107: 891-896.

[199] Bock, SA. Prospective appraisal of complaints of adverse reactions to foods in children during the first 3 years of life. *Pediatrics.* 1987;79:683-688.

[200] Burks, AW; Ballmer-Weber, BK. Food allergies. *Mol. Nutr. Food Res.* 2006;50:595-603.

[201] Nieuwenhuizen, N; Lopata, A. Fighting food allergy: current approaches. *Ann. N. Y. Acad. Sci.* 2005;1056:30-45.

[202] Lee, LA; Burks, AW. Food allergies: prevalence, molecular characterization, and treatment/prevention strategies. *Annu. Rev. Nutr.* 2006;26;539-565.

[203] Bock, SA; Munoz-Furlong, A; Sampson, HA. Fatalities due to anaphylactic reactions to foods. *J. Allergy Clin. Immunol.* 2001;107:191-193.

[204] Fiocchi, A; Martelli, A. Dietary management of food allergy. *Pediatr. Ann.* 2006;35:755-763.

[205] James, JM; Crespo, JF. Allergic reactions to foods by inhalation. *Curr. Allergy Asthma Rep.* 2007;7:167-174.

[206] Nowak-Wegrzyn, A. Immunotherapy for food allergy. *Inflamm. Allergy Drug Targets.* 2006;5:23-34.

[207] Altman, DR; Chiaramonte, LT. Public perception of food allergy. *J. Allergy Clin. Immunol.* 1996;97:1247-1251.

[208] Opper, PH; Burakoff, R. Food allergy and intolerance. *Gastroenterologist.* 1993;1:211-220.

[209] Sicherer, SH; Leung, DY. Advances in allergic skin disease, anaphylaxis, and hypersensitivity reactions to foods, drugs, and insects. *J. Allergy Clin. Immunol.* 2007;119:1462-1469.

[210] Venter, C; Pereira, B; Grundy, J; et al. Incidence of parentally reported and clinically diagnosed food hypersensitivity in the first year of life. *J. Allergy Clin. Immunol.* 2006;117:1118-1124.

[211] Grimshaw, KE. Dietary management of food allergy in children. *Proc. Nutr. Soc.* 2006;65:412-417.

[212] Joint Task Force on Practice Parameters; American Academy of Allergy, Asthma and Immunology; American College of Allergy, Asthma and Immunology; Joint Council of Allergy, Asthma and Immunology. The diagnosis and management of anaphylaxis: an updated practice parameter. *J. Allergy Clin. Immunol.* 2005;115:S483-S523.

[213] Muňoz-Furlong, A. Daily coping strategies for patients and their families. *Pediatrics.* 2003;111:1654-1661.

[214] Joshi, P; Mofidi, S; Sicherer, SH. Interpretation of commercial food ingredient labels by parents of food-allergic children. *J. Allergy Clin. Immunol.* 2002;109:1019-1021.

[215] Taylor, SL; Hefle, SL. Food allergen labeling in the USA and Europe. *Curr. Opin. Allergy Clin. Immunol.* 2006;6:186-190.

[216] European Commission. Directive 2003/89/EC of the European Parliament and of the Council of 10 November 2003 amending Directive 2000/13/EC as regards indication of the ingredients present in foodstuffs. *Official J. Euro. Communities*. 2003;308:15-18.

[217] Lee, BW. Food and allergy. *Ann. Acad. Med. Singapore.* 1995;24:238-241.

[218] Steinman, HA. "Hidden" allergens in foods. *J. Allergy Clin. Immunol.* 1996;98:241-250.

[219] Dannaeus, A. Food allergy in infancy and children. *Ann. Allergy.* 1987;59:124-126.

[220] Leung, AK; Bowen, TJ. Seasonal allergic rhinitis and food allergy. In: Bergman, AB. (ed). *Twenty Common Problems in Pediatrics.* New York: McGraw-Hill. 2001, pp. 219-233.

[221] Oren, E; Banerji, A; Clark, S; et al. Food-induced anaphylaxis and repeated epinephrine treatments. *Ann. Allergy Asthma Immunol.* 2007;99:429-432.

[222] Kelso, JM. A second dose of epinephrine for anaphylaxis: how often needed and how to carry. *J. Allergy Clin. Immunol.* 2006;117:464-465.

[223] Clark, S; Camargo, CA, Jr. Emergency management of food allergy: systems perspective. *Curr. Opin. Allergy Clin. Immunol.* 2005;5:293-298.

[224] Baral, VR; Hourihane, JO. Food allergy in children. *Postgrad. Med. J.* 2005;81:693-701.

[225] Muraro, A; Roberts, G; Clark, A; et al. The management of anaphylaxis in childhood: position paper of the European Academy of Allergology and Clinical Immunology. *Allergy*. 2007;62:857-871.

[226] Wang, J; Sampson, HA. Food anaphylaxis. *Clin. Exp. Allergy*. 2007;37:651-660.

[227] Simons, FE; Roberts, JR; Gu, X; et al. Epinephrine absorption in children with a history of anaphylaxis. *J. Allergy Clin. Immunol.* 1998;101:33-37.

[228] Brown, SG. Cardiovascular aspects of anaphylaxis: implications for treatment and diagnosis. *Curr. Opin. Allergy Clin. Immunol.* 2005;5:359-364.

[229] Simons, FE. First-aid treatment of anaphylaxis to food: focus on epinephrine. *J. Allergy Clin. Immunol.* 2004;113:837-844.

[230] Du Toit, G; Fox, A; Morris, A. Managing food allergy in children. *Practitioner.* 2006;250:45-46, 49-52.

[231] Metcalfe, DD. Food hypersensitivity. *J. Allergy Clin. Immunol.* 1984;73:749-762.

[232] Leung, AK; Hon, KL; Robson, WL. Atopic dermatitis. *Adv. Pediatr.* 2007;54:241-273.

[233] Bailey, M; Haverson, K; Inman, C; et al. The development of the mucosal immune system pre- and post-weaning: balancing regulatory and effector function. *Proc. Nutr. Soc.* 2005;64:451-457.

[234] Kalliomäki, M; Kirjavainen, P; Eerola, E; et al. Distinct patterns of neonatal gut microflora in infants in whom atopy was and was not developing. *J. Allergy Clin. Immunol.* 2001;107:129-134.

[235] Watanabe, S; Narisawa, Y; Arase, S; et al. Differences in fecal microflora between patients with atopic dermatitis and healthy control subjects. *J. Allergy Clin. Immunol.* 2003;111:587-591.

[236] Björkstén, B; Sepp, E; Julge,K; et al. Allergy development and the intestinal microflora during the first year of life. *J. Allergy Clin. Immunol.* 2001;108:516-520.

[237] Laitenen, K; Isolauri, E. Management of food allergy: vitamins, fatty acids or probiotics? *Eur. J. Gastroenterol. Hepatol.* 2005;17:1305-1311.

[238] Boyle, RJ; Tang, ML. The role of probiotics in the management of allergic disease. *Clin. Exp. Allergy*. 2006;36:568-576.

[239] He, F; Morita, H; Hashimoto, H; et al. Intestinal *Bifidobacterium* species induce varying cytokine production. *J. Allergy Clin. Immunol.* 2002;109:1035-1036.

[240] Kirjavainen, PV; Apostolou, E; Salminen, SJ, et al. New aspects of probiotics – a novel approach in the management of food allergy. *Allergy.* 1999;54:909-915.

[241] O'Sullivan, GC; Kelly, P; O'Halloran, S; et al. Probiotics: an emerging therapy. *Curr. Pharm. Des.* 2005;11:3-10.

[242] Rosenfeld, V; Benfeldt, E; Valerius, NH; et al. Effect of probiotics on gastrointestinal symptoms and small intestinal permeability in children with atopic dermatitis. *J. Pediatr.* 2004;145:612-616

[243] Williams, HC. Two "positive" studies of probiotics for atopic dermatitis – or are they? *Arch. Dermatol.* 2006;142:1201-1203.

[244] Kalliomäki, M; Salminen, S; Arvilommi, H; et al. Probiotics in primary prevention of atopic disease: a randomized placebo-controlled trial. *Lancet.* 2001;357:1076-1079.

[245] Kalliomäki, M; Salminen, S; Poussa, T; et al. Probiotics and prevention of atopic disease: 4-year follow-up of a randomized placebo-controlled trial. *Lancet.* 2003;361:1869-1871.

[246] Lodinová-Zádníková, R; Cukrowska, B; Tlaskalova-Hogenova, H. Oral administration of probiotic *Escherichia coli* after birth reduces frequency of allergies and repeated infections later in life (after 10 and 20 years). *Int. Arch. Allergy Immunol.* 2003;131:209-211.

[247] Rosenfeld, V; Benfeldt, E; Nielsen, SD; et al. Effect of probiotic *lactobacilli* strains in children with atopic dermatitis. *J. Allergy Clin. Immunol.* 2003;111:389-395.

[248] Viljanen, M; Savilahti, E; Haahtela, T; et al. Probiotics in the treatment of atopic eczema/dermatitis syndrome in infants: a double-blind placebo-controlled trial. *Allergy.* 2005;60:494-500.

[249] Tamura, M; Shikina, T; Morihana, T; et al. Effects of probiotics on allergic rhinitis induced by Japanese cedar pollen: randomized double-blind, placebo-controlled clinical trial. *Int. Arch. Allergy Immunol.* 2007;143:75-82.

[250] Taylor, AL; Dunstan, JA; Prescott, SL, et al. Probiotic supplementation for the first 6 months of life fails to reduce the risk of atopic dermatitis and increases the risk of

allergen sensitization in high-risk children: a randomized controlled trial. *J. Allergy Clin. Immunol.* 2007;119:184-191.

[251] Kukkonen, K; Savilahti, E; Haahtela, T; et al. Probiotic and prebiotic galacto-oligosaccharides in the prevention of allergic diseases: a randomized, double-blind, placebo-controlled trial. *J. Allergy Clin. Immunol.* 2007;119:192-198.

[252] Weston, S; Halbert, A; Richmond, P; et al. Effects of probiotics on atopic dermatitis: a randomized controlled trial. *Arch. Dis. Child.* 2005;90:892-897.

[253] Passeron, T; Lacour, JP; Fontas, E; et al. Prebiotics and synbiotics: two promising approaches for the treatment of atopic dermatitis in children above 2 years. *Allergy.* 2006;61:431-437.

[254] Greer, FR; Sicherer, SH; Burks, AW; and the Committee on Nutrition and Section on Allergy and Immunology. Effects of early nutritional interventions on the development of atopic disease in infants and children: The role of maternal dietary restriction, breastfeeding, timing of introduction of complementary foods and hydrolyzed formulas. *Pediatrics.* 2008;121:183-191.

[255] Greer, FR; Sicherer, SH; Burks, AW. Effects of early nutritional interventions on the development of atopic disease in infants and children: the role of maternal dietary restriction, breastfeeding, timing of introduction of complementary foods, and hydrolyzed formulas. *Pediatrics.* 2008; 121:183-91.

[256] Zeiger, RS; Heller, S. The development and prediction of atopy in high-risk children: follow-up at age seven years in a prospective randomized study of combined maternal and infant food allergen avoidance. *J. Allergy Clin. Immunol.* 1995; 95:1179-90.

[257] Björkstén, B; Kjellman, NI. Does breast-feeding prevent food allergy? *Allergy Proc.* 1991;12:233-237.

[258] Bahna, SL. Management of food allergies. *Ann. Allergy.* 1984;53:678-682.

[259] Kramer, MS; Kakuma, R. Maternal dietary antigen avoidance during pregnancy and/or lactation for preventing or treating atopic disease in the child. *Cochrane Database Syst. Rev.* 2006;(3): CD000133

[260] Zutavern, A; Brockow, I; Schaaf, B; et al. Timing of solid food introduction in relation to eczema, asthma, allergic rhinitis, and food and inhalant sensitization at the age of 6 years: results from the prospective birth cohort study LISA. *Pediatrics.* 2008;121:e44-e52.

[261] Kull, I; Bergström, A, Lilja, G; et al. Fish consumption during the first year of life and development of allergic diseases during childhood. *Allergy.* 2006;61:1009-1015.

[262] Poole, JA; Barriga, K; Donald, Y; et al. Timing of initial exposure to cereal grains and the risk of wheat allergy. *Pediatrics.* 2006;117:2175-2182.

[263] Fiocchi, A; Assa'ad, A; Bahna, S; et al. Food allergy and the introduction of solid foods to infants: a consensus document. Adverse Reactions to Foods Committee, American College of Allergy, Asthma and Immunology. *Ann Allergy Asthma Immunol.* 2006;97(1):10-20

[264] Hodge, L; Salome, CM; Peat, JK; et al. Consumption of oily fish and childhood asthma risk. *Med. J. Aust.* 1998;164:137-140.

[265] Mayser, P; Mayer, K; Mahloudjian, M; et al. A double-blind, randomized, placebo-controlled trial of n-3 versus n-6 fatty acid-based lipid infusion in atopic dermatitis. *J. Parent. Enter. Nutr.* 2002;26:151-158.

[266] Nafstad, P; Nystad, W; Magnus, P; et al. Asthma and allergic rhinitis at 4 years of age in relation to fish consumption in infancy. *J. Asthma*. 2003;40:343-348.

[267] Thien, FCK; Woods, R; de Lucas S; et al. Dietary marine fatty acids (fish oil) for asthma in adults and children. *Cochrane Database Sys. Rev*. 2002;3:CD001283.

[268] Gool, CJ; Zeegers, MP; Thijs, C. Oral essential fatty acid supplementation in atopic dermatitis – a meta-analysis of placebo-controlled trials. *Br. J. Dermatol*. 2004;150:728-740.

[269] Host, A; Halken, S. Primary prevention of food allergy in infants who are at risk. *Curr. Opin. Allergy Clin. Immunol*. 2005;5:255-259.

[270] Hays, T; Wood, RA. A systematic review of the role of hydrolysed infant formulas in allergy prevention. *Arch. Pediatr. Adolesc. Med*. 2005;159:810-816.

[271] Osborn, DA; Sinn, J. Formulas containing hydrolysed protein for prevention of allergy and food intolerance in infants (review). *Cochrane Database Syst. Rev*. 2006 18;(4):CD003664.

[272] Zeiger, RS. Food allergen avoidance in the prevention of food allergy in infancy and children. *Pediatrics*. 2003;111:1662-1671.

[273] Osborn, DA; Sinn, J. Soy formula for prevention of allergy and food intolerance in infants (review). *Cochrane Database Syst. Rev*. 2006;4:CD003741.

[274] American Academy of Pediatrics, Committee on Nutrition. Hypoallergenic infant formulas. *Pediatrics*. 2000;106:346-349.

[275] Siltanen, M; Kajosaari, M; Poussa, T; et al. A dual long-term effect of breastfeeding on atopy in relation to heredity in children at 4 years of age. *Allergy*. 2003;58:524-530.

[276] Kajosaari, M; Saarinen, UM. Prophylaxis of atopic disease by six months' total solid foods elimination. *Acta Paediatr. Scand*. 1983;72:411-421.

[277] Morgan, J; Williams, P; Norris, F; et al. Eczema and early solid feeding in preterm infants. *Arch. Dis. Child*. 2004;89:309-314.

[278] Fiocchi, A; Assa'ad, A; Bahna, S; et al. Food allergy and the introduction of solid foods to infants: a consensus document. *Ann. Allergy Asthma Immunol*. 2006;97:10-21.

[279] Marini, A; Agosti, M; Motta, G; et al. Effects of a dietary and environmental prevention programme on the incidence of allergic symptoms in high atopic risk infants: three years follow-up. *Acta Paediatr*. 1996;414:S1-S22.

[280] Halken, S; Host, A; Hansen, LG; et al. Effect of an allergy prevention programme on incidence of atopic symptoms in infancy: a prospective study of 159 "high-risk" infants. *Allergy*. 1992;47:545-553.

[281] Leung, AK; Sauve, RS. Whole cow's milk in infancy. *Paediatr. Child. Health*. 2003;8:419-421.

[282] Duggan, C; Walker, WA. Protein intolerance. In: Oski, FA; DeAngelis, CD; Feigin, RD. (eds). *Principles and Practice of Pediatrics*. Philadelphia: JB Lippincott. 1994; pp.1887-1890.

[283] Rozenfeld, P; Docena GH; Anon, MC; et al. Detection and identification of a soy protein that cross-reacts with caseins from cow's milk. *Clin Exp Immunol*. 2002;130:49-58.

[284] Crittenden, RG; Bennett, LE. Cow's milk allergy: a complex disorder. *J. Am. Coll. Nutr*. 2005;24:S582-S591.

[285] Bellioni-Businco, B; Paganelli, R; Lucenti, P; et al. Allergenicity of goat's milk in children with cow's milk allergy. *J. Allergy Clin. Immunol*. 1999;103:1191-1194.

[286] Committee on Nutrition, American Academy of Pediatrics. Food sensitivity. In: Kleinman, RE. (ed). *Pediatric Nutrition Handbook*. Elk Grove Village, Ill: American Academy of Pediatrics. 2004; pp.593-607.

[287] Sampson, HA; Bernhisel-Broadbent, J; Yang, E; et al. Safety of casein hydrolysate formula in children with cow milk allergy. *J. Pediatr.* 1991;118:520-525

[288] Sampson, HA; James, JM; Bernhisel-Broadbent, J. Safety of an amino acid-derived infant formula in children allergic to cow's milk. *Pediatrics.* 1992;90:463-465.

[289] Chehade, M; Magid, MS; Mofidi, S; et al. Allergic eosinophilic gastroenteritis with protein-losing enteropathy: intestinal pathology, clinical course, and long-term follow-up. *J. Pediatr. Gastroenterol. Nutr.* 2006;42:516-521.

[290] Kagalwalla, AF; Sentongo, TA; Ritz, S; et al. Effect of six-food elimination diet on clinical and histologic outcomes in eosinophilic esophagitis. *Clin. Gastroenterol. Hepatol.* 2006;4:1097-1102.

[291] Liacouras, CA. Eosinophilic esophagitis: treatment in 2005. *Curr. Opin. Gastroenterol.* 2006;22:147-142.

[292] Nelson, HS; Lahr, J; Rule, R, et al. Treatment of anaphylactic sensitivity to peanuts by immunotherapy with injections of aqueous peanuts extract. *J. Allergy Clin. Immunol.* 1997;99:744-751.

[293] Pons, L; Burks, W. Novel treatments for food allergy. *Expert Opin. Investig. Drugs.* 2005;14:829-834.

[294] Allen, KJ; Hill, DJ, Heine, RG. 4. Food allergy in childhood. *MJA.* 2006;185:394-400.

[295] Enrique, E; Cisteró-Bahíma, A. Specific immunotherapy for food allergy: basic principles and clinical aspects. *Curr. Opin. Allergy Clin. Immunol.* 2006;6:466-469.

[296] Leung, DY; Sampson, HA; Yunginger, JW; et al. Effect of anti-IgE therapy in patients with peanut allergy. *N. Engl. J. Med.* 2003;348:986-993.

[297] Li, XM; Zhang, TF; Huang, CK; et al. Food Allergy Herbal Formula-1 (FAHF-1) blocks peanut-induced anaphylaxis in a murine model. *J. Allergy Clin. Immunol.* 2001;108:639-646.

[298] Li, XM; Srivastava, K; Grishin, A; et al. Persistent protective effect of heat-killed *Escherichia coli* producing "engineered," recombinant peanut proteins in a murine model of peanut allergy. *J. Allergy Clin. Immunol.* 2003;112:159-167.

[299] Mankad, VS; Burks, AW. Omalizumab: other indications and unanswered questions. *Clin. Rev. Allergy Immunol.* 2005;29:17-30.

[300] Okubo, K; Ogino, S; Nagakura, T; et al. Omalizumab is effective and safe in the treatment of Japanese cedar pollen-induced seasonal allergic rhinitis. *Allergol. Int.* 2006;55:379-386.

[301] Crespo, JF; James, JM; Rodriguez J. Diagnosis and therapy of food allergy. *Mol. Nutr. Food Res.* 2004;48:347-355.

[302] MacGlashan, DW; Bochner, BS; Adelman, DC; et al. Down-regulation of Fc (epsilon) RI expression on human basophils during vivo treatment of atopic patients with anti-IgE antibody. *J. Immunol.* 1997;158:1438-1445.

[303] Stein, ML; Collins, MH; Villanueva, JM; et al. Anti-IL-5 (mepolizumab) therapy for eosinophilic esophagitis. *J. Allergy Clin. Immunol.* 2006;118:1312-1319.

[304] Enrique, E; Pineda, F; Malek, T; et al. Sublingual immunotherapy for hazelnut food allergy: a randomized double-blind placebo-controlled study with a standardized hazelnut extract. *J. Allergy Clin. Immunol.* 2005;116:1073-1079.

[305] King, N; Helm, R; Stanley, JS; et al. Allergenic characteristics of a modified peanut allergen. *Mol. Nutr. Food Res*. 2005;49:963-971.

[306] Peng, HJ; Su, SN; Chang, ZN; et al. Induction of specific Th1 responses and suppression of IgE antibody formation by vaccination with plasmid DNA encoding Der f 11. *Vaccine*. 2002;20:1761-1768.

[307] Horn, AA; Raz, E. Immunostimulatory sequence oligodeoxynucleotide-based vaccination and immunomodulation: two unique but complementary strategies for the treatment of allergic diseases. *J. Allergy Clin. Immunol*. 2002;110:706-712.

[308] Marshall, JD; Abtahi, S; Eiden, JJ; et al. Immunostimulatory sequence DNA linked to the Amb a 1 allergen promotes T(H)1 cytokine expression while downregulating T(H)2 cytokine expression in PBMCs from human patients with ragweed allergy. *J. Allergy Clin. Immunol*. 2001;108:191-197.

[309] Hsieh, KY; Hus, CI; Lim JY; et al. Oral administration of an edible-mushroom-derived protein inhibits the development of food-allergic reactions in mice. *Clin. Exp. Allergy*. 2003;33:1595-1602.

[310] Li, XM; Srivastava, K; Huleatt, JW; et al. Engineered recombinant peanut proteins and heat-killed *Listeria monocytogenes* coadministration protects against peanut-induced anaphylaxis in a murine model. *J. Immunol*. 2003;170:3289-3295.

[311] Srivastava, KD; Kattan, JD; Zou, ZM; et al. The Chinese herbal medicine formula FAHF-2 completely blocks anaphylactic reactions in a murine model of peanut allergy. *J. Allergy Clin. Immunol*. 2005;115:171-178.

[312] James, JM; Burks, AW; Robertson, PK; et al. Safe administration of the measles vaccine to children allergic to eggs. *N. Engl. J. Med*. 1995;332:1262-1266.

[313] Lacksman, R; Finn, A. MMR vaccine and allergy. *Arch. Dis. Child*. 2000;82:93-95.

[314] American Academy of Pediatrics. Allergic reactions to egg-related antigens. In: Pickering, LK; Baker, CJ; Kimberlin, DW; et al. (eds). *Red Book: 2009 Report of the Committee on Infectious Diseases*. Elk Grove Village, IL: American Academy of Pediatrics, 2009, pp.48-49.

In: Food Allergies: Symptoms, Diagnosis, and Treatment ISBN: 978-1-61728-748-0
Editor: Patricia M. Rodgers

Chapter 2

FISH ALLERGY – A COMPREHENSIVE REVIEW OF RECENT DEVELOPMENTS IN FISH ALLERGY DIAGNOSIS AND FISH ALLERGEN DETECTION

Annette Kuehn[1], Hilger Christiane[1] and Hentges François[1, 2]
[1]CRP-Santé, Laboratory of Immunogenetics and Allergology, Luxembourg
[2]CHL, Unit of Immunology and Allergology, Luxembourg

ABSTRACT

Allergy to fish is one of the most common IgE-mediated food allergies, especially in geographical regions where fish is frequently consumed. Most fish-allergic patients are sensitized to β-parvalbumin, a highly stable protein of 11-12 kDa. Several isoforms of parvalbumins can be found in the same muscle tissue. These isoforms share conserved protein domains. Common IgE epitopes have been considered as an explanation for the extensive allergic cross-reactivity to different fish species. However, frequency and intensity of allergic reactions to fish are highly variable in sensitized patients.

The diagnosis of fish allergy has made progress over the last decade. New approaches have been investigated for component-resolved diagnosis. Parvalbumin molecules from different species are being produced as recombinant proteins and become available for use in allergen-specific serum IgE quantification. Component-resolved diagnosis provides also the opportunity to test IgE for fish allergens other than parvalbumin. The availability of well-characterized minor allergens in routine assays is important to improve the future clinical diagnosis of fish allergy. Diagnostic tools like the microarray system are being commercialized addressing the challenge of patient-specific allergy profiling.

To date, specific immunotherapy is not available for fish-allergic patients. A new EU project aims now to test a hypo-allergenic variant of recombinant parvalbumin in a clinical immunotherapy trial. For the time being, patients are advised to avoid any kind of fish and fish products, unless it was shown that some fish were tolerated by the individual. In the US and Europe, fish and fish-derived ingredients are included in the list of important food allergens. In order to protect fish-allergic consumers, regulatory food authorities require manufacturers to label fish and fishery products. Food monitoring and tracing became a legal issue. In the recent past, the need for reliable assays motivated research to develop analytical assays for fish allergen detection. Detection of fish allergens has been approached by a number of studies both on the protein level as well as on the DNA level, so that it can be expected that commercial assays will be available soon.

This chapter will provide a general overview of fish allergy and of the relevant molecular biology background. Recent developments in diagnosis of fish allergy and detection of fish allergens will be discussed.

INTRODUCTION

Allergy to fish is a frequent cause of IgE-mediated adverse reactions to food. Fish is considered one of the so-called "big eight" of major allergenic foods causing over 90 % of all IgE-mediated food allergies [1, 2]. In the United States, about 0.4 % of the adult population is affected by allergy to fish [3]. A similar percentage has been reported for European countries [4-6]. The prevalence of fish allergy in children was found to be slightly higher than in adults [5, 7]. In contrast to some other food allergies, fish allergy tends to persist into adult age in fish-sensitized children [8].

The diagnosis of fish allergy is based on the patient's clinical history, skin-prick tests, *in-vitro* determination of specific immunoglobulin E (IgE) antibodies and only to some extent oral food challenge tests. This diagnostic procedure allows predicting with some certainty a clinically relevant fish allergy, but it has also clear disadvantages. Skin testing for food allergy has often been described to be of variable significance. Food challenge tests bear a certain risk of systemic allergy reactions for the sensitized patient [9, 10]. *In-vitro* diagnosis has limitations due to the poor correlation of IgE reactivity and clinical symptoms [11]. This mismatch has been attributed to a significant heterogeneity of the extracts used as diagnostic reagents [12]. The current reagents in fish allergy diagnosis are protein extracts prepared from fish muscle. Food extracts can vary considerably in their content of allergenic protein and biological potency [13, 14].

A promising trend is the component-resolved diagnosis (CRD) using purified allergens as well characterized and standardized reagents [13, 15]. In CRD of fish allergy, the target molecule is the major fish allergen, represented currently by parvalbumins from carp and cod. For most patients, the availability of these molecules will improve considerably the current diagnosis in terms of sensitivity, specificity and correlation to clinical reality.

For some fish-allergic patients, the poor correlation between specific IgE testing to fish extracts and clinical sensitivity can be also explained by allergens which are missing in the diagnostic reagents. These allergens are usually different from parvalbumin. IgE reactivity to new fish allergens has been investigated and identified in several studies [16, 17]. Their clinical relevance is still not well understood. Recently, food allergy to fish gelatin has been shown by *in-vitro* and *in-vivo* assays [18]. Although these additional, usually minor allergens are critical for a precise diagnosis, they are missing in current reagents. Therefore, some patients might not have detectable IgE despite their clinical reactivity to fish and fish-derived food. The recent development of new instrumental tools will address the need for improved diagnosis. High through-put systems like the microarray allow simultaneous testing of allergen panels including major and minor fish allergens. This technique will be useful for the analysis of patients with multiple sensitizations.

Currently, the management of fish allergy relies on a strict elimination diet of all kind of fish as the main treatment approach [19]. This may contribute to an imbalanced nutrition in affected patients. Some fish-allergic patients tolerate several fish species, an aspect which is not taken into account in current fish allergy diagnosis. The improvement of diagnosis could help to ease the strict avoidance diet of fish-allergic patients which is not only of the individuals' but also of a socio-economic interest. Regulatory food authorities require manufacturers to label specifically fish and fish ingredients on product labels [1]. To date, this is the only possibility to assure safety of food products for fish-allergic consumers. Several studies have developed assays for fish allergen detection, but only a limited number of methods have been validated.

In summary, the development of tools for fish allergy diagnosis, therapy and fish allergen detection is still in progress. It will substantially change the management of fish allergy in the near future.

FISH ALLERGY

Fish as an Important Food Source

Fish is an important food component in human nutrition. It is a source of essential amino acids, unsaturated long-chain fatty acids and lipid-soluble vitamins. In the past decades, global fish consumption increased considerably, which tallies with general trends of healthy human nutrition [20]. The world fish production has even nearly doubled since the 1970s. As a consequence, most native fish stocks are today overexploited and more than 40 % of the current demand has to be covered by fish species farmed in aquaculture [21]. Today, over 700 fish species are commercially available on the international market. Nevertheless, the consumption of fish species varies substantially between different countries and even between geographical regions, which reflects the local fishery and traditional habits of eating in theses areas [22]. In European countries, major differences in the consumption of fish are apparent. Although cod, herring, salmon and tuna belong to the most common fish species eaten, Swedish consumers prefer cod, the Germans herring, the Dutch salmon and the Spanish tuna [22, 23]. Particularly, plaice is popular in Denmark, eel in the Netherlands and hake and sole in Spain. Regional eating habits of fish concerning frequency and fish species represent a cause for species-specific sensitization pattern of fish-allergic patients [24, 25].

Prevalence of Fish Allergy

Food allergies including fish allergy have increased steadily all over the world in the past decades. In general, hypersensitivity to fish is more often diagnosed in coastal regions, where the population has a frequent exposure to fish, for instance because of a daily fish consumption [26]. A high risk for allergic respiratory diseases is given in the work environment of fish processing factories, where the workers inhale aerosols containing fish allergens, especially during the production of fishmeal and bagging [27].

The prevalence of fish allergy was investigated in various studies around the world, but these studies differ by their design and therefore, are difficult to compare [11, 28]. Fish allergy was estimated to have a prevalence of 0.5 % in the United Kingdom, 0.3 % in Sweden and 0.1 % in Norway in the general population [4, 29]. In the United States, a random digit-dial telephone survey reported a prevalence of 0.4 % for fish allergy [30]. Fish allergy appears often at early stage and it tends to persist in most patients. A follow-up study with Greek children showed that over 50 % of the fish-allergic children maintained their sensitization as adult persons [8]. In a children population, a study from Finland estimated a prevalence of 3 %, a study from Spain a prevalence of 30.4 % and in an Italian study, the prevalence of 4.5 % was described for a population of atopic children [5, 7, 31]. For Swedish schoolchildren, a self-reported food allergy study estimated a prevalence of 8-16 % in wheezers and 2-3 % in non-wheezers [32].

Many studies have shown that the prevalence is often overestimated in studies with self-reported symptoms [11]. Therefore, these data have to be considered cautiously. Although the exact prevalence of fish allergy is not well established, fish is listed among the eight most common allergenic foods which are cow's milk, egg, peanut, tree nuts, shellfish, soy, and wheat [33].

Adverse Reactions to Fish

Food intolerance and food allergy are two different types of pathophysiological adverse reactions to food [11]. Food intolerance is caused by food-specific, pharmacologically active contaminants or components. Scombroid fish poisoning is a clinically important type of fish intolerance. Fish of the Scombroid family like tuna, mackerel and bonito contain naturally high levels of the amino acid histidine [34]. Caused by inadequate storage and bacterial contamination of fish, non-toxic histidine is decarboxylated to toxic histamine by bacterial biocatalysis. Ingestion of fish contaminated with heat-resistant histamine results in intoxication symptoms. This intoxication is often misinterpreted in the diagnostic procedure as fish allergy [35].

In contrast, fish allergy is triggered by a specific immune response to fish which is mediated by IgE antibodies. Most adverse reactions to fish are attributed to the IgE-mediated immunological mechanism.

The first step in the development of fish allergy is the sensitization to fish. This occurs mostly in childhood when fish is introduced into the diet. The second step of the allergic progress occurs when the sensitized patient is re-exposed to fish and the allergic reaction is elicited [36]. Clinical symptoms of fish allergy appear generally minutes to an hour later after exposure and vary from mild reactions to severe anaphylaxis. Allergic reactions to fish depend often on the type of exposure. Fish allergens as volatile molecules can be present in vapours or steam from fish processing [27]. Upon inhalation, sensitized patients may suffer from respiratory reactions like allergic rhinitis or allergic asthma. Upon ingestion, allergenic proteins may elicit directly allergic reactions by interacting with mucosal mast cells in the mouth which results in a frequent type of contact urticaria, the oral allergy syndrome (OAS). Gastrointestinal reactions are also often observed within minutes after fish ingestion. The uptake of the allergenic proteins from the digestive tract depends on different factors such as the food matrix, digestive stability of the allergens and the mucosal integrity. Fish allergens are highly resistant to digestion which is a key attribute of their allergenic potency [37]. Following the uptake of allergenic proteins from the digestive tract, allergens can directly interact with the mast cells of the intestinal mucosa causing gastrointestinal reactions. Allergens may be further transported to effector cells such as basophils in the blood or to any other effector tissue eliciting IgE-mediated, systemic reactions like urticaria, angioedema or anaphylaxis [36].

Threshold Dose of Allergenic Fish

In food allergy, only small quantities of the allergenic food can elicit an allergic IgE-mediated reaction in the sensitized individual. This has been also reported for patients with fish allergy, even by indirect contact [38, 39]. The so-called threshold dose reflects the lowest amount of food required to elicit allergic symptoms in most patients. It has been shown that threshold doses for food allergens vary considerably in a population of food-sensitized patients [36]. A few double-blind placebo-controlled food challenge (DBPCFC) studies report allergenic amounts of fish in a wide milligram range. The doses, which elicited allergic symptoms varied between 6 mg and 6 g fish in fish-sensitized subjects [40, 41]. Fish muscle compositions varies highly depending on the fish species and the fish preparation. In the recent past, no further data have been published on threshold doses from food challenge studies. Since food challenge studies have been performed with different fish, there is an obvious lack of clinical data preventing the definition of exact threshold doses [28].

Cross-Reactivity among Fish Species

Fish-allergic patients often react to multiple fish species and therefore, they are usually advised to avoid all kinds of fish. The cross-reactivity among fish species has been investigated in studies with different designs [42]. Some studies analyzed only the serological cross-reactivity and other studies correlated the serological and clinical cross-reactivity in common fish species. In a DBPCFC and open challenge study, all of the patients cross-reacted to 4 to 6 fish species, but all patients tolerated also at least one of the fish [43]. Most of the patients did tolerate tuna in this study. Hansen et al. showed cross-reactivity among cod, mackerel, herring and plaice, in a population of cod-allergic subjects [44]. Helbling et al. found clinically relevant cross-reactivity among taxonomically distinct fish species, but also tolerance to single fish species in some patients [45]. The existence of clinical mono-sensitivity to single fish species has been proven, such as for tropical sole, swordfish, pangasius/tilapia and tuna/marlin [46-49]. Today, advising fish-allergic patients which fish species to consume is an unsolved issue that seems to be only feasible by *in-vivo* provocation challenge.

PARVALBUMINS

Parvalbumin Lineages and Isoforms

In 1934, the occurrence of parvalbumin was for the first time described in the muscle of fish and amphibians [50]. Parvalbumin is a low-molecular weight protein (11-12 kDa) which was named according to its small size (parvus = small) and its albumin-like solubility, although it is not functionally related to serum albumin [51]. Two phylogenetic lineages of parvalbumins have been classified according to the comparison of the amino acid sequences, the so-called α- and the β-subtype parvalbumins [52]. Parvalbumins of the α-subtype contain less acidic residues then the β-subtype. The α-parvalbumins have been defined by an isoelectric point (pI) of 5.0 and higher and the β-parvalbumins by pI value of 4.5 and lower [53]. Mass spectrometric analysis has shown that α- and β-parvalbumins both have generally no post-translational modifications, except for an acetylation of the N-terminal methionine [54]. Protein identities among parvalbumins are often higher within the same lineage than between α- and β-subtypes of the same organism (**Chart 1**). Frog α- and β-parvalbumins are 51 % identical, but the identity of the frog α-parvalbumin ranges from 58 to 72 % when compared with α-homologs from distantly related species such as shark, rat, horse and chicken. The protein sequences of both α- and β-isotypes differ in characteristic amino acid positions. In fishes, at least four highly conserved amino acids as well as the lack of a C-terminal residue have been reported as a specific feature of β-parvalbumins [55, 56]. These conserved residues are highlighted and explained in the comparative sequence alignment of **Figure 1**. With the increasing number of characterized parvalbumins, it turned out that this rule is not applicable to each molecule.

Chart. 1. Protein identities of parvalbumins from distantly related species. α- and β-parvalbumins from pike (P02628, P02619), frog (CAC83046, CAC95152), human (P20472, P32930) were compared with α-parvalbumins from shark (P30563), rat (P02625), horse (CAX32964), chicken (CAX32963) and β-parvalbumins from carp (AJ292211), cod (AY035584), mouse (P51879), snake (P02615).

		pike		frog		human		shark	rat	horse	chicken	carp	cod	mouse	snake
		α	β	α	β	α	β	α				β			
pike	α		61	60	58	64	51	60	62	66	67	59	63	50	50
	β			54	62	58	47	50	58	58	59	77	73	47	64
frog	α				52	68	42	58	65	69	72	49	52	41	47
	β					57	46	52	60	56	56	66	62	46	58
human	α						51	58	91	88	79	56	58	50	49
	β							50	53	51	51	47	44	89	50
shark	α								59	60	68	52	54	46	40
rat										88	77	55	51	51	52
horse											83	55	57	48	49
chicken												55	54	47	47
carp	β												81	49	70
cod														45	66
mouse															51
snake															

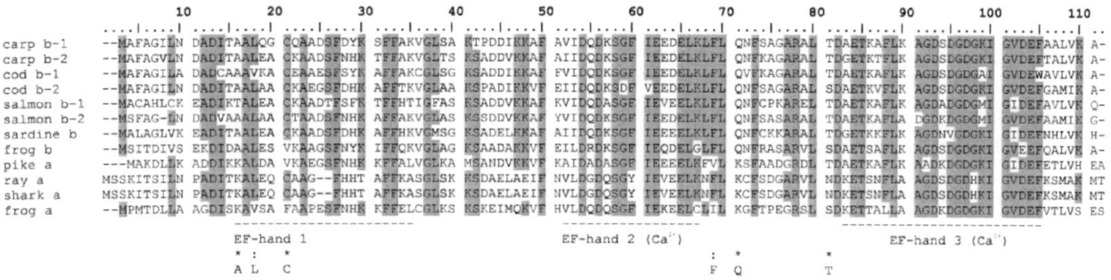

Figure 1. Comparison of fish parvalbumin from the α- and β-lineage. β-parvalbumins from carp (AJ292211, AJ292212) and cod (AY035584, AY035585), salmon (X97824, X97825) and sardine (FM177701) were compared with α-parvalbumins from pike (P02628), ray (P02630) and shark (P30563). The 3 EF-hand motives are underlined, identical amino acids are highlighted in grey, conserved residues for β-parvalbumins are marked with * and conserved residues for α-and β-parvalbumins are marked with :.

Parvalbumins occur in a wide range of species, such as fish and amphibians, but also in birds and higher vertebrates. In mammals, immunohistochemical studies have shown that parvalbumins are well distributed in the body such as in muscles, the central nervous system, bones and the skin [54]. Both α- and β-subtypes are found in the same mammalian tissues, but in tissue- and organ-specific ratios. In frogs, parvalbumins occur in the muscle tissue, but also in exocrine secretions of the cutaneous mucus proteome [57]. In fish, α- and β-parvalbumins are found in white and dark muscle tissue as well as in the swimbladder [58]. The β-subtype is the predominant parvalbumin found in bony fishes. In contrast to α-parvalbumin, several isoforms of β-parvalbumin can be present in a single muscle cell of fish. Recently, seven isoforms have been reported in the carp muscle. The expression level of these different isoforms varies along the longitudinal axis of the fish [59, 60]. For tuna, it has been reported that parvalbumin levels differ not only along the fish body, but also in the dorsal and ventral muscle tissue [60].

Remarkably, the wide-spread distribution of parvalbumin, the species-specific expression and the development of isoforms makes parvalbumins a useful marker in phylogenetic studies. This feature has been utilized in phylogenetic analysis of relationships between animals, such as fish and amphibians [56, 61].

Parvalbumin Distribution in Fish Muscle

Fish muscle proteins can be divided into three groups. 60-70 % of the total protein is composed of myofibrillar proteins, 2-5 % are connective tissue proteins and about 30 % are sarcoplasmic proteins. Sarcoplasmic proteins fulfill diverse biological functions in the cellular metabolism. Two calcium-binding proteins are found in the intracellular sarcoplasmic fraction of fish muscle, calmodulin and parvalbumin [62].

In bony fish, the muscle composition is characteristically composed of two types of tissues, white and dark muscle. The white muscle enables rapid movements and the dark muscle for continuous swimming [21]. Both muscle types differ in physiological metabolism. The dark muscle contains more myofibrillar and less sarcoplasmic protein, the white muscle has a higher proportion of sarcoplasmic protein. Most bony fishes have more light than dark muscle tissue. However, the latter is more developed in pelagic fish species like tuna, herring and mackerel. The protein composition of fish muscle differs among fish species. Fish proteins extracted from muscle tissue reveal characteristic, species-specific patterns which can be useful in identification of fish species [21]. An example for the variation of protein patterns in different fish species is visualized in Figure 2.

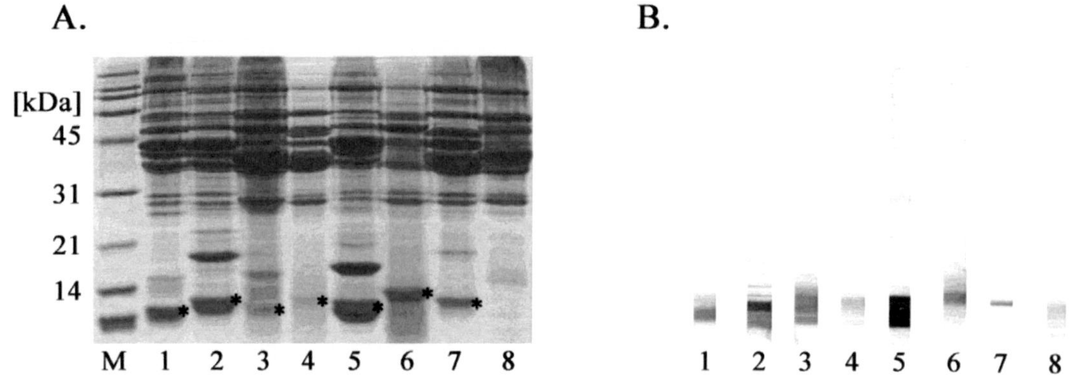

Figure 2. Protein pattern of muscle proteins in different fish species. A. Fish extracts were separated by SDS-PAGE (15 %) and proteins stained by Coomassie blue. Parvalbumin-like bands vary in number and intensity in the different extracts. Lanes: marker M, cod 1, carp 2, salmon 3, mackerel 4, herring 5, redfish 6, trout 7, tuna 8. Parvalbumin-like bands are marked with *. B. Following Western blotting, proteins were detected using an anti-fish parvalbumin antibody (Swant, Bellinzona, Swiss). The expression pattern of parvalbumins varies in the different fish species. Lanes: marker M, cod 1, carp 2, salmon 3, mackerel 4, herring 5, redfish 6, trout 7, tuna 8.

Both white and dark fish muscle tissues are commonly ingested and therefore, implicated in allergic reactions to fish. Dark muscles are less allergenic than the white muscles, because they contain less parvalbumin [63]. Parvalbumin levels were estimated to be about four times lower in dark muscle. In tuna, it has been reported that some muscle sections contain no detectable parvalbumin [60].

Parvalbumin as a Member of the EF-Hand Protein Family

Animal food allergens are mainly members of three protein superfamilies, the tropomyosins, the caseins and the EF-hand proteins [64]. Parvalbumins belong to the family of EF-hand proteins. This family comprises divalent metal ion-binding proteins which are characterized by helix-loop-helix binding domains, the so-called EF-hands. The helix-loop-helix domain consists of a 12 amino acid long binding loop, flanked on both sides by α-helices of 12 amino acids length [65]. Three EF-hand motifs are found in parvalbumin, one silent, stabilizing domain ("AB-site") and two calcium- or magnesium-binding domains, the so-called CD- and EF-site. It has been reported that β-parvalbumin has a higher binding affinity to calcium-ions than α-parvalbumin [54]. Moreover, the parvalbumin subtypes bind divalent metal-ions with different specificities. The CD-site of α-parvalbumin is specific for calcium ion-binding, while this domain binds either calcium or magnesium ions in β-parvalbumins. The difference in ion-binding has been explained by resolving the protein structures of both complexes. In α-parvalbumins, the CD- and EF-domains form highly rigid structures with very similar protein structures of the apo- and calcium-loaded form. In β-parvalbumins, calcium-binding and release results in major structural rearrangements and a general flexibility in the CD- and EF-domains. This remodeling of the ion-binding site enables magnesium-binding only in β-parvalbumins [65].

Important allergens belong to the family of calcium-binding protein such as Bet v 4 from birch pollen, Phl p 7 from grass pollen, Bra n 1 from mustard as well as parvalbumins from fish [64]. Within the group of calcium-binding allergens, protein comparison reveals a strict conservation of amino acids residues and protein domains involved in calcium-binding. The insight of these high conservations of protein sequence and structure contributed to the understanding of cross-reactivity among allergens. Parvalbumins can be found in two conformations, the calcium-free form with a closed protein structure and the calcium-bound form with an open protein structure [66]. It has been shown that calcium-depletion of parvalbumin results in a considerable reduction of IgE-binding [67]. This could be explained by changes in the protein conformation induced by calcium-binding. Thus, calcium-binding is an important factor influencing the allergenicity of parvalbumins. The reduction of IgE reactivity has been reported in parvalbumin mutants with mutations in the calcium-binding sites [68]. The calcium-binding regions of parvalbumins may partly be explained by the IgE cross-reactivity among these fish allergens by motif-specific epitopes. There is no evidence for a general cross-reactivity between calcium-binding allergens from different species. Indeed, the structural comparison of Bet v 4 and fish parvalbumin shows even matching EF-hand motives, but the considerable difference of the overall structure seem to be the reason for the lack of IgE cross-reactivity between the plant and the animal allergen [69]. In conclusion, EF-hand calcium binding sites cannot be considered epitopes causing general cross-reactivity.

Parvalbumins of the Beta-Subtype

In the past decades, β-parvalbumins have been described and characterized in a number of species, such as in fish, amphibians, birds and mammals.

One of the first in-depth studies on fish β-parvalbumins have been performed in Baltic cod (*Gadus callarias*) [70, 71]. The studies on cod parvalbumin have been complemented later on with research on recombinant molecules [72, 73].

Parvalbumins of the β-subtype have been purified and their molecular properties analyzed in a number of fish spcies. These muscle proteins were found in fish species such as hake (*Merluccius bilineanis*), eel (*Anguilla anguilla*), bigeye tuna (*Thunnus obesus*), red snapper (*Lutjanus compechanus*), pike (*Esox lucius*) and catfish (*Heterobranchus longifilis, Clarias gariepinus, Chrysichthys auratus*) [62, 74-78].

A panel of fish β-parvalbumins has been characterized and produced as recombinant molecules over the past decades. Parvalbumins have been identified and cloned from carp (*Cyprinus carpio*), salmon (*Salmo salar*), mackerel (*Scomber japonicus*) and Alaska Pollack (*Theragra chalcogramma*) [55, 79-81]. More recently, parvalbumins have been identified and cloned from tilapia (*Oreochromis mossambicus*), Pacific pilchard (*Sardinops sagax*), whiff (*Lepidorhombus whiffiagonis*) and swordfish (*Xiphias gladius*) [82-85].

Today, 3D-protein structures are available of β-parvalbumins from carp (4CPV), whiting (1A75), silver hake (1BU3) and pike (1PAL).

Parvalbumins of the Alpha-Subtype

Parvalbumins of the α-subtype have been identified and characterized from different species, mainly in mammals, birds and amphibians, but also in some fish.

The molecular properties of α-parvalbumins have been reported in a number of fish. These muscle proteins were found in some cartilaginous fish such as dogfish (*Scyliorhinus canicula*), shark and stingray (*Dasyatis sabina*) [86-88]. In bony fish, different isoforms of α-parvalbumin were analyzed from pike (*Esox lucius*) [89].

The X-ray protein structures are determined for α-parvalbumins from shark (5PAL) and pike (1PVA).

Physiological Function of Parvalbumins

Parvalbumins play an important role in biological systems in various functions. Different physiological functions have been discussed for parvalbumin of the α- and β-subtype. According to their ion-binding characteristic, α-parvalbumins may be pure Ca^{2+}-buffer proteins and β-parvalbumins may have the additional function as Ca^{2+}-sensors [65]. So far, no interaction between parvalbumin and other sarcoplasmic protein targets could be identified which would suggest the active role in down-stream processes of the muscle contraction and function.

In fish, parvalbumins are involved in muscle function by regulating the intracellular calcium concentration. Moreover, parvalbumin expression correlates with muscle relaxation. It has been shown that cod parvalbumin levels are higher in the faster relaxing anterior white muscle than in the slower relaxing posterior muscle [90]. Future studies are required to discover the exact role of parvalbumin in cell physiology of muscle function. Fish muscle may represent a useful model system for these future examinations.

Parvalbumins as Food Allergens

Food allergens are characterized by specific biochemical properties such as primary protein stability to proteolysis and thermal treatment. Class I food allergens are stable to digestion and food processing. Examples of class I food allergens are proteins of 10-70 kDa, such as the milk allergen Bos d 5 or the peanut allergen Ara h 1. In contrast, class II food allergens are labile to thermal and enzymatic treatment, for instance the birch pollen allergen Bet v 1 or the apple allergen Mal d 1, which are implicated in the so-called "birch pollen-fruit syndrome" [91]. As highly stable proteins of low molecular weight, parvalbumins from the β-subtype belong to the class I of food allergens.

Parvalbumin was defined as the main fish allergen in various fish species. More than 95 % of the fish-allergic patients have specific IgE to purified β-parvalbumin [69]. The first parvalbumin was characterized from Baltic cod (*Gadus callarias*) and designated as "fish allergen M" [92].

Meanwhile, β-parvalbumins have been studied as allergens in an extensive range of bony fishes, such as salmon, mackerel, carp and Alaska pollock (**Chart 2**). Parvalbumins have been also reported as the major allergen in four tropical fish species, threadfin (*Polynemus* *indicus*), Indian anchovy (*Stolephorus indicus*), pomfret (*Pampus chinensis*) and tengirri (*Scomberomorus guttatus*) [93].

Chart. 2. Entries of fish allergens in allergen databases. Official parvalbumin allergens and additional, non-parvalbumin allergens are shown.

www.allergen.org (January, 25, 2010):

order	species	fish	allergen	accession no.
Clupeiformes	*Clupea harengus*	herring	Clu h 1.0101	FM178220
			Clu h 1.0201	FM178221
			Clu h 1.0301	FM178222
	Sardinops sagax	sardine	Sar sa 1.0101	FM177701
Gadiformes	*Gadus callarias*	cod	Gad c 1.0101	P02622
Perciformes	*Thunnus albacares*	tuna	Thu a 1.0101	FM178217
	Xiphias gladius	swordfish	Xip g 1.0101	FM202668
Pleuronectiformes	*Lepidorhombus whiffiagonis*	whiff	Lep w 1.0101	AM904681
Salmoniformes	*Salmo salar*	salmon	Sal s 1.0101	X97824
Scorpaeniformes	*Sebastus marinus*	redfish	Seb m 1.0101	FM178218
			Seb m 1.0201	FM178219

www.allergome.org (January, 25, 2010):

order	species	fish	allergen	allergome code
Anguilliformes	*Anguilla anguilla*	eel	Ang a 1	783
Cypriniformes	*Cyprinus carpio*	carp	Cyp c 1	263
	Engraulis encrasicolus	anchovy	Eng e 1	7685
Siluriformes	*Ictalurus punctatus*	catfish	Ict p 1	2947
Gadiformes	*Gadus morhua*	cod	Gad m gelatin	7711
	Merluccius bilinearis	hake	Mer bi 1	6265
	Theragra chalcogramma	pollock	The c 1	1084
Pleuronectiformes	*Hippoglossus hippoglossus*	halibut	Hip h 1	2826
Perciformes	*Lates calcarifer*	barramundi	Lat c 1	7686
	Thunnus albacares	tuna	Thu a collagen	1253
Salmoniformes	*Salmo salar*	salmon	Sal s gelatin	7709
	Oncorhynchus mykiss	trout	Onc m vitellogenin	7654

Until today, the official list of allergens maintained by the International Union of Immunological Societies Allergen nomenclature subcommittee contains 11 β-parvalbumins as fish allergens (www.allergen.org). Currently, the Allergome database contains over 80 fish allergens including parvalbumins and other fish allergens (www.allergome.org) (**Chart 2**).

Molecular properties have been determined for parvalbumins as reasons for their allergenicity. Parvalbumins have a high allergenic potency as food allergens, because they are resistant to heat, chemical denaturation and enzymatic proteolysis. Food processing can also affect and reduce the allergenicity of parvalbumin, as described for different fish preparations [43, 94]. Fish parvalbumin may form oligomers under specific conditions, which might influence the allergenicity of the proteins [72]. Furthermore, the specific IgE-binding is sensitive to calcium-binding so that the apo-parvalbumin (calcium-free) is generally less allergenic than the calcium-bound form [69].

Fish α-parvalbumins have not yet been assessed in the context of fish allergy. Generally, α-parvalbumins are assumed to be non-allergenic proteins. This has been explained by their evolutionary proximity to the human homolog. Proteins with a sequence identity of 62 % and higher to the human homolog were presumed of low allergenicity [95]. A few exceptions from this rule have been reported. Frog α-parvalbumin was identified as food allergen causing anaphylaxis in a case of food allergy to fried frog legs [96]. Later on, IgE cross-reactivity to fish β-parvalbumin and frog α-parvalbumin has been shown in some fish-allergic patients [97]. Chicken α-parvalbumin was reported as meat allergen in a case of food allergy to chicken leg [98]. Particularly, this chicken meat-allergic patient did not show IgE cross-reactivity to fish β-parvalbumin (**Figure 3**). The protein identity of frog and chicken α-parvalbumin to the human homolog is 68 % and 79 % respectively, against the "similarity rule" in these particular cases.

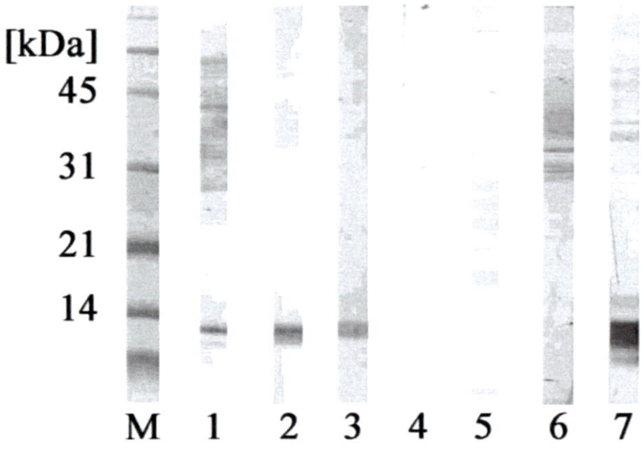

Figure 3. Chicken α-parvalbumin as a new meat allergen. Allergens were detected at 14 kDa and >30 kDa by the patients IgE antibodies in chicken leg extract (1). Specific IgE recognize purified native (2) and recombinant (3) chicken α-parvalbumin, but not native cod (4) or salmon β-parvalbumin (5). IgE binding to the 14 kDa protein in chicken leg extract is inhibited by preincubation of the serum with recombinant chicken parvalbumin (6). (7) chicken parvalbumin detection by a commercial antibody, (M) marker.

Other Fish Allergens

IgE-Reactive Fish Muscle Proteins

In the past, various studies have shown that β-parvalbumins are not the only fish allergens. Additional allergens have been described, but they have not been identified, characterized nor tested in *in-vivo* experiments. One of the first studies on new fish allergens reported a new 63 kDa allergen in cod [99]. An extensive range of IgE-reactive protein bands was detected in cod extract [100]. Some bands were considered new allergens, while others were identified as parvalbumin oligomers [72]. A 25 kDa protein has been published as a putative allergen in a case of monosensitivity to swordfish [47]. In cod, a 41 kDa aldehyde phosphate dehydrogenase has been described as a putative new allergen [16]. A 40 kDa protein was reported in eel and eelpout as cross-reactive allergen [101]. In two species of snapper, different allergens of 35-90 kDa have been identified in a patient population where parvalbumin seemed to play a minor role as responsible allergen [102]. Cross-reactivity between tuna and marlin was explained by a new 94-105 kDa allergen [49]. In addition to parvalbumin, allergens of 46 kDa and 51 kDa were described in Indian scad [103]. IgE-reactive proteins of 29-54 kDa have been reported in tropical fish species [93]. In salmon, a 26 kDa triose-phosphate isomerase, a 41 kDa fructose-bis-phosphate aldolase and a 70 kDa serum albumin were published as new fish allergens [104]. Putative cross-reactive allergens of 18 kDa and 45 kDa were reported in pangasius and tilapia [48]. In conclusion, identification of new fish allergens was the issue of a number of studies in the past decade, but a definite proof and conclusive outcome is still missing.

Fish-Related Allergens

A parasitic nematode, *Anisakis spp*, can infect fish and cephalopods living in sea water. This infection is transmitted to humans upon consumption of the infected fish or seafood [105]. Allergic symptoms appear when the larvae are deposited in the digestive tract. Allergy to Anisakis can contribute to severe symptoms such as urticaria, angioedema and anaphylaxis. Nine different proteins (Ani s 1-9) have been identified as triggers for the fish-induced Anisakis allergy [106]. Important cross-reactivity has been reported between Anisakis and house dust mite allergens [107, 108]. Today, Anisakis allergens are available for routine specific IgE testing.

Fish allergies have been reported in the literature for decades, but food allergy to fish roe has been only recently published. IgE-mediated fish allergy does not appear concomitant with adverse reactions to fish roe [109]. Vitellogenin, a 118 kDa fish roe yolk protein, has been identified as allergen causing allergy to fish roe [110]. Cross-reactivity among different fish roes and the chicken egg homologs has been shown [111, 112]. Currently, there is no routine diagnostic available for patients with food allergy to fish roe.

Fish Gelatin

Fish gelatin and collagen are important ingredients in different applications of the cosmetic, pharmaceutical, medical or food industry. Fish gelatin is a good alternative to mammalian gelatins, particularly because of its physicochemical properties, increased safety (e.g. outbreak of bovine spongiform encephalopathy in Europe) and compatibility with religious restrictions from both Islam and Judaism [28]. The production of fish gelatin is still only about 1% of the annual world gelatin production, but the demand is increasing. Fish gelatin is processed in food products such as for the encapsulation of vitamins or as a low-calorie stabilizer in food [113]. Fish collagen is extracted from skins, bones and fins from warm- and cold-water fish. Fish gelatin is produced from fish collagen by acidic or alkaline hydrolysis resulting in a heterogenic peptide mix. Among fish species, fish gelatins differ by their characteristic amino acid compositions.

There are only a few reports on food allergic reactions to gelatin, mainly with mammalian gelatins. Two studies reported adverse food reactions to gelatin in a population of children with gelatin-specific IgE [114]. Another report showed the clinical case of food allergy to fruit gum candy cause by gelatin [115]. Adverse food reactions to fish gelatin had not been reported in the past. Specific IgE to fish gelatin were reported without further evidence of its clinical relevance [17, 116]. Two studies with *in-vivo* experiments did not prove the allergenicity of fish gelatin in fish-allergic patients, except for in one patient with a mild reaction to a cumulative dose of 7.6 g fish gelatin [117, 118]. Recently, a first case report showed that fish gelatin can be a trigger for life-threatening anaphylaxis [18]. Evidence for an anaphylactic reaction to fish gelatin resulted from the obvious clinical history, strong and specific IgE binding to fish gelatin and positive skin tests (**Figure 4**). Today, there is no routine test available for fish gelatin, neither for specific IgE testing nor for skin prick tests.

As fish gelatin is a product derived from an allergenic source, this food ingredient must be declared in the United States [119]. In the European Union, fish gelatin is still exempted from labelling regulations. This temporary exemption is based on the rationale that there is no evidence for the presence of parvalbumin in fish gelatin so far. Indeed, the contamination of fish gelatin with parvalbumin is an important issue in food safety. In a recent study, different commercial fish gelatins and products were tested for the presence of parvalbumin in fish gelatin [120]. No parvalbumin could be detected in any of the analyzed fish gelatins. In contrast, isinglass, a product produced from the swim bladder of some fishes, contained considerable levels of parvalbumin.

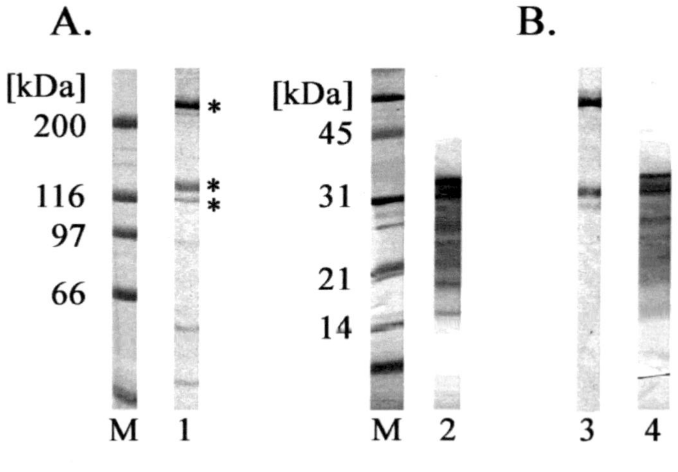

Figure 4. Fish collagen and fish gelatin as new fish allergens. Fish collagen isolated from tuna skin and food grade fish gelatin was separated by SDS-PAGE (7.5 % gel in lane 1, 3; 15 % gel in lane 2, 4). A. Coomassie staining visualizes collagen bands at 110/210 kDa (1, marked with *) and a protein pattern of fish collagen bands at <30 kDa (2). B. The patients IgE strongly detect the tuna collagen bands (3) and the protein pattern of fish gelatin bands (4) in immunoblot. (M) marker.

DIAGNOSIS OF FISH ALLERGY

Scombroid Fish Poisoning and Anisakis Allergy

The differentiation between IgE-mediated fish allergy and intoxication by bacterially contaminated fish, the Scombroid fish poisoning, can be an issue in diagnosis. Inappropriate storage of fish can lead to formation of high histamine levels in the muscle of Scombroid fish by enterobacteria [34]. The term 'Scombroid poisoning' is misleading, since also fish from other families have been reported to cause this intoxication [121]. The symptoms are similar to those of an IgE-mediated food allergy so that fish poisoning can be misdiagnosed as food allergy. Today, the correct diagnosis of scombroid poisoning is still a challenge. Several hours after the incidence, plasma histamine concentrations can be determined by commercial assays [122]. Recording the clinical history and the fish species consumed provides important indications, in combination with negative results for fish-specific IgE. Symptoms upon ingestion of particular fish such as canned tuna may point to an intoxication, because these processed fish have been reported with a low allergenicity [43]. Histamine is heat stabile and survives fish processing such as canning. Toxin analysis of the fish muscle is still one of the most important steps in approaching a confirmed diagnosis.

In recent years, Anisakis simplex has been recognized as an important cause of allergic disease in sensitized patients. Even when fish is cooked or fried, Anisakis is still a health risk as a fish-borne allergen source. Anisakis extracts contain multiple allergens that may cross-react with antibodies to unrelated allergens (microorganisms, parasites, insects) resulting in serological IgE diagnosis with false-positive results [123]. However, positive skin tests to Anisakis often indicate positive results to other allergens [105]. An antigen-capture ELISA using a monoclonal antibody has been proposed as an alternative to common laboratory test [123]. The identification and characterization of Anisakis allergens improved the understanding of the cross-reactivity with other allergens, but laboratory diagnosis requires still an improvement of sensitivity and specificity of the serological test.

Allergen Databases and IgE Epitopes

In the past decades, the number of identified and characterized fish allergens increased tremendously. Bioinformatics contributed to the development of allergen-specific databases. Meanwhile, several allergen databases are available which differ by their bioinformatics' approaches of allergen classification [124]. These databases provide important sets of molecular, biochemical and clinical data of allergens [64]. New allergens, such as gelatin from fish, are included into the databases being available to the research community. Furthermore, data comparison allows identification of evolutionary, structural and sequence-based relationships among allergens [125]. The prediction of potential IgE cross-reactivity is an important issue which has been successfully applied to a number of parvalbumin molecules [126]. Finally, this systematic analysis of allergen fosters improvements of allergy diagnosis and therapy.

The cross-reactivity among fish species is of clinical relevance for sensitized patients. Different studies investigated the IgE-reactive epitopes of parvalbumins [127, 128].

Conformational epitopes are most probably relevant for IgE binding to parvalbumin [129]. Today, the availability of parvalbumin sequences and the elucidation of parvalbumin structures, followed by 3D molecular modelling of common epitopes help to explain this cross-reactivity in a pool of parvalbumin molecules. However, the application of IgE epitope mapping is limited because of the clinical relevance of in-vitro IgE-binding. More research is needed to explain, why fish-allergic patients tolerate single fish species. In the future, cell-based assays such as basophil activation tests may address the clinical relevance of IgE-binding [130].

Component-Resolved Diagnosis

Currently, the diagnosis of fish allergy is almost exclusively performed using crude extracts which allow identifying and quantifying allergen-specific IgE antibodies in the serum [14]. Fish extracts consist of a variable mixture of allergenic and non-allergenic components, therefore only some of the proteins bind to IgE. In different studies it has been shown that the protein composition of fish muscle varies considerably depending on different factors such as the fish species and the type of fish muscle [21, 60, 63].

Meanwhile, fish allergens can be produced by advanced molecular technologies such as recombinant molecules in appropriate host organisms such as *E. coli* [131]. A panel of parvalbumin molecules is now available as recombinant allergens, such as Cyp c 1 from carp, Gad m 1 from cod, Sars sa 1 from sardine or The c 1 from Pollock (**Chart 2**). These molecules have to be subjected to strict a quality control analysis confirming amongst others the identity, purity, structure in comparison to the native counterparts. Finally, recombinant fish allergens will be useful tools in diagnostic assays as recombinants are generally highly standardized molecules of significant availability.

Nowadays, high-throughput techniques like microarray systems enable large-scale testing for specific IgE. Individual sensitization patterns can be determined using purified, recombinant allergens [132]. Only a small amount of serum is required for simultaneous testing of multiple allergens. In fish allergy diagnosis, this tool is appropriate to test IgE-binding to parvalbumins, which become more and more available as recombinant molecules. Recent publications have shown that, besides the known β parvalbumins, there are additional important allergens present in fish. These new allergens are lacking completely as characterized reagents for component-resolved diagnosis (CRD) purposes. Microarray systems will enable testing of a complete set of major and minor fish allergens from the allergenic source. Recently, a new basophil-mediated microarray immunoassay was developed for diagnostic purposes [133]. Allergens were not detected with patient's serum, but with human basophils passively sensitized with patient's serum. This system may improve the clinical relevance of chip technologies in food diagnosis.

Therapy of Fish Allergy

Immunotherapy of Fish Allergy

As fish allergy is an increasing burden, the interest in immunotherapy and the induction of tolerance grows steadily in the affected population. In allergen-specific immunotherapy, the antigen is delivered to the immune system via the oral or sublingual route [134]. In principle, the antigen dose can be the food itself or heat-denaturated food, purified allergen or engineered recombinant protein. A successful treatment of a fish-allergic patient by intradermal immunotherapy using codfish extract has been reported in the past [135]. Another study reported the oral desensitization of fish-allergic patients with cooked cod. The desensitization was successfully completed in 9 from 11 patients. It has been concluded that oral tolerance may be mediated by the same mechanisms as those involved in therapeutic desensitisations for respiratory allergies [136].

IgE-mediated allergy to fish is mainly caused by parvalbumin, the major fish allergen. It has been reported, that IgE-binding epitopes are located in highly conserved regions of parvalbumins. A hypoallergenic variant of carp parvalbumin has been produced as a recombinant molecule and proposed for application in immunotherapy of fish allergy [137]. In this study, the hypoallergenicity of parvalbumin mutants was confirmed in IgE-binding experiments, histamine release assays, skin prick tests and animal experiments with vaccinated mice. An EU-funded project (FAST, Food Allergy Specific ImmunoTherapy) was recently initiated targeting the immunotherapy of food allergy to fish and fruit. In this study, a subcutaneously administered hypoallergenic variant of fish parvalbumin will be tested. This project is a promising approach to improve the medical care of food-allergic patients.

Food Allergen Labelling of Fish

Today, the management of fish allergy still relies mainly on avoidance. Fish has been recognized as an important food allergen by labelling authorities in the US and in Europe. In order to protect allergic consumers and increase market transparency, labelling of packaged foods containing ingredients derived from fish is now mandatory for producers. In the US, this new labelling law, the Food Allergen Labelling & Consumer Protection Act (FALCPA), came into effect in 2006. In the European Union, the so-called '25 % rule' was in effect until 2005 [119]. The labelling of any food ingredient was only required for contents of more than 25 % of the product. The new food labelling legislation changed the '25 % rule' to the '5 % rule', which is applicable for any food component. The labelling is mandatory for ingredients derived from commonly allergenic food, regardless of the percentage in the food [138]. Allergic consumers clearly benefit from this development. In contrast to the US, several ingredients such as fish gelatin are still temporarily exempted from the labelling law in the European Union. Decisions on permanent inclusion or exemption will depend on evaluation of the allergenicity of these fish-derived ingredients. However, the labelling requirements only apply to food allergens which are intentionally introduced into the packaged food. Accidental cross-contaminations during the production process are a frequent reason for the introduction of hidden and unlabelled food allergens [119].

The complex food allergen labelling regulations created a need for fast and reliable analytical methods for fish allergen detection.

Fish Allergen Detection

The development of fish allergen detection assays lags behind commercial tests for other food allergens [139]. Generally, the detection of parvalbumin is a difficult challenge as these proteins show biochemical and immunological variability among the fish species [140]. Protein- as well as DNA-based assays have been described for the detection of parvalbumins.

Fish proteins have been detected in a colorimetric ELISA using immunostick tubes for rapid fish detection [141]. In this study, the used polyclonal antibody was raised against total fish muscle proteins. Fish parvalbumins have significant advantages as tracer molecules in allergen detection assays because of their high resistance to food processing. Several anti-parvalbumin antibodies have been produced in the past, while some are already commercially available. The use of commercial anti-parvalbumin antibodies for allergen detection has been evaluated in several studies. It has been reported that a frog anti-parvalbumin antibody can be used as a reagent for fish parvalbumin detection [142]. Fish parvalbumins have been quantified using an anti-cod parvalbumin antibody in ELISA [143]. A competitive indirect ELISA has been developed for the detection of parvalbumin in fish gelatin products using a commercial anti-parvalbumin antibody [120]. A monoclonal anti-catfish parvalbumin antibody has been reported as a useful reagent for allergen detection assays [144]. Parvalbumin has been even quantified in environmental samples by an antibody-based assay [145]. A rapid method for parvalbumin detection, which does not rely on immunodetection, has been reported using a biosensor technique. The detection level was a limiting factor for routine usage [146]. As fish-derived products such as isinglass have been shown to be allergenic, this food matrix has been targeted in a first detection assay [147].

DNA-based methods offer advantages over protein-based systems, because they can be applied to processed food samples. DNA fragments which are degraded down to 100-200 bp are still detectable in DNA-based assays. A parvalbumin gene-specific PCR has been developed for Japanese mackerel (*Scomber japonicus*) in food [148]. A common real-time polymerase chain reaction (PCR) was reported for the detection of fish parvalbumins [149]. A specific PCR for salmon parvalbumin gene has been developed which has been recently modified to a real time PCR [150]. PCR methods are highly sensitive and specific for detection of low levels of DNA in food. However these assays do not detect the allergen, but indicate the presence of the allergenic food component even in processed food.

Summary

A rapid development in molecular and clinical research has considerably advanced the diagnosis and management of fish allergy. The recent research on known and new fish allergens, allergen expression levels and allergen processing in food, together with novel high through-put methods and fish allergen detection assays, are milestones in this field. Taking all together, it will be of great benefit for the fish-allergic consumer.

REFERENCES

[1] FDA. Questions and answers regarding food allergen, including the food allergen labeling and consumer protection act of 2004., *Food and drug administration*, Editor. 2005.

[2] Sicherer, S.H. & Sampson, H.A. (2006). 9. Food allergy. *J Allergy Clin Immunol*, 117 (2 Suppl): S470-5.

[3] Sicherer, S.H., Munoz-Furlong, A., & Sampson, H.A. (2004). Prevalence of seafood allergy in the United States determined by a random telephone survey. *J Allergy Clin Immunol*, 114 (1): 159-65.

[4] Aas, K. ed. Fish allergy and the cod fish allergen model. Food allergy and intolerance. *Food allergy and intolerance*, ed. C.S. Brostoff J. 1987: London. 356-66.

[5] de Martino, M., Peruzzi, M., de Luca, M., Amato, A.G., Galli, L., Lega, L., Azzari, C., & Vierucci, A. (1993). Fish allergy in children. *Ann Allergy*, 71 (2): 159-65.

[6] Rance, F., Grandmottet, X., & Grandjean, H. (2005). Prevalence and main characteristics of schoolchildren diagnosed with food allergies in France. *Clin Exp Allergy*, 35 (2): 167-72.

[7] Saarinen, U.M. & Kajosaari, M. (1980). Does dietary elimination in infancy prevent or only postpone a food allergy? A study of fish and citrus allergy in 375 children. *Lancet*, 1 (8161): 166-7.

[8] Priftis, K.N., Mermiri, D., Papadopoulou, A., Papadopoulos, M., Fretzayas, A., & Lagona, E. (2008). Asthma symptoms and bronchial reactivity in school children sensitized to food allergens in infancy. *J Asthma*, 45 (7): 590-5.

[9] de Martino, M., Novembre, E., Galli, L., de Marco, A., Botarelli, P., Marano, E., & Vierucci, A. (1990). Allergy to different fish species in cod-allergic children: in vivo and in vitro studies. *J Allergy Clin Immunol*, 86 (6 Pt 1): 909-14.

[10] Eckman, J., Saini, S.S., & Hamilton, R.G. (2009). Diagnostic evaluation of food-related allergic diseases. *Allergy Asthma Clin Immunol*, 5 (1): 2.

[11] Cianferoni, A. & Spergel, J.M. (2009). Food allergy: review, classification and diagnosis. *Allergol Int*, 58 (4): 457-66.

[12] Fernandez-Rivas, M., Aalbers, M., Fotisch, K., de Heer, P., Notten, S., Vieths, S., & van Ree, R. (2006). *Immune reactivity of candidate reference materials*. Arb Paul Ehrlich Inst Bundesamt Sera Impfstoffe Frankf A M, (95): 84-8

[13] Scheurer, S. (2006). Improvement of the diagnosis of allergy by using purified allergens. *Clin Exp Allergy*, 36 (12): 1483-6.

[14] Ballmer-Weber, B.K., Lidholm, J., & Vieths, S. (2007). Recombinant allergens in the diagnosis of food allergy: Which are the advantages? *Rev Fr Allergol*, 49.

[15] Valenta, R., Lidholm, J., Niederberger, V., Hayek, B., Kraft, D., & Gronlund, H. (1999). The recombinant allergen-based concept of component-resolved diagnostics and immunotherapy (CRD and CRIT). *Clin Exp Allergy*, 29 (7): 896-904.

[16] Das Dores, S., Chopin, C., Romano, A., Galland-Irmouli, A.V., Quaratino, D., Pascual, C., Fleurence, J., & Gueant, J.L. (2002). IgE-binding and cross-reactivity of a new 41 kDa allergen of codfish. *Allergy*, 57 Suppl 72: 84-7.

[17] Hamada, Y., Nagashima, Y., & Shiomi, K. (2001). Identification of collagen as a new fish allergen. *Biosci Biotechnol Biochem*, 65 (2): 285-91.

[18] Kuehn, A., Hilger, C., & Hentges, F. (2009). Anaphylaxis provoked by ingestion of marshmallows containing fish gelatin. *J Allergy Clin Immunol*, 123 (3): 708-9.

[19] Kagan, R.S. (2003). Food allergy: an overview. *Environ Health Perspect*, 111 (2): 223-5.

[20] FAO, Food and Agriculture Organization (2008). *The State of World Fisheries and Aquaculture - Sofia* 2008.

[21] Rehbein, H. & Oehlenschlaeger, J. eds. Fishery products. *Quality, safety and authenticity.* 2009, Wiley-Blackwell.

[22] Welch, A.A., Lund, E., Amiano, P., Dorronsoro, M., Brustad, M., Kumle, M., Rodriguez, M., Lasheras, C., Janzon, L., Jansson, J., Luben, R., Spencer, E.A., Overvad, K., Tjonneland, A., Clavel-Chapelon, F., Linseisen, J., Klipstein-Grobusch, K., Benetou, V., Zavitsanos, X., Tumino, R., Galasso, R., Bueno-De-Mesquita, H.B., Ocke, M.C., Charrondiere, U.R., & Slimani, N. (2002). Variability of fish consumption within the 10 European countries participating in the European Investigation into Cancer and Nutrition (EPIC) study. *Public Health Nutr*, 5 (6B): 1273-85.

[23] FAO, Food and Agriculture Organization (2009). *International seafood trade: challenges and opportunities* - Rome 2009.

[24] Pascual, C., Martin Esteban, M., & Crespo, J.F. (1992). Fish allergy: evaluation of the importance of cross-reactivity. *J Pediatr*, 121 (5 Pt 2): S29-34.

[25] Zinn, C., Lopata, A., Visser, M., & Potter, P.C. (1997). The spectrum of allergy to South African bony fish (Teleosti). Evaluation by double-blind, placebo-controlled challenge. *S Afr Med J,* 87 (2): 146-52.

[26] Hourihane, J.O. (1998). Prevalence and severity of food allergy--need for control. *Allergy*, 53 (46 Suppl): 84-8.

[27] Jeebhay, M.F., Robins, T.G., Seixas, N., Baatjies, R., George, D.A., Rusford, E., Lehrer, S.B., & Lopata, A.L. (2005). Environmental exposure characterization of fish processing workers. *Ann Occup Hyg*, 49 (5): 423-37.

[28] Taylor, S.L. (2004). Fish allergy: fish and products thereof. J Food Sci, 69 (8).

[29] Bjornsson, E., Janson, C., Plaschke, P., Norrman, E., & Sjoberg, O. (1996). Prevalence of sensitization to food allergens in adult Swedes. *Ann Allergy Asthma Immunol*, 77 (4): 327-32.

[30] Munoz-Furlong, A. & Sampson, H.A. (2004) Prevalence of self-reported seafood allergy in the US. *J Allergy Clin Immunol*, 113.

[31] Crespo, J.F., Pascual, C., Burks, A.W., Helm, R.M., & Esteban, M.M. (1995). Frequency of food allergy in a pediatric population from Spain. *Pediatr Allergy Immunol,* 6 (1): 39-43.

[32] Sandin, A., Annus, T., Bjorksten, B., Nilsson, L., Riikjarv, M.A., van Hage-Hamsten, M., & Braback, L. (2005). Prevalence of self-reported food allergy and IgE antibodies to food allergens in Swedish and Estonian schoolchildren. *Eur J Clin Nutr*, 59 (3): 399-403.

[33] Bousquet, J., Bjorksten, B., Bruijnzeel-Koomen, C.A., Huggett, A., Ortolani, C., Warner, J.O., & Smith, M. (1998). Scientific criteria and the selection of allergenic foods for product labelling. *Allergy*, 53 (47 Suppl): 3-21.

[34] McLauchlin, J., Little, C.L., Grant, K.A., & Mithani, V. (2006). Scombrotoxic fish poisoning. *J Public Health* (Oxf), 28 (1): 61-2.

[35] Attaran, R.R. & Probst, F. (2002). Histamine fish poisoning: a common but frequently misdiagnosed condition. *Emerg Med J*, 19 (5): 474-5.

[36] Taylor, S.L., Gendel, S.M., Houben, G.F., & Julien, E. (2009). The Key Events Dose-Response Framework: a foundation for examining variability in elicitation thresholds for food allergens. *Crit Rev Food Sci Nutr*, 49 (8): 729-39.

[37] Untersmayr, E., Poulsen, L.K., Platzer, M.H., Pedersen, M.H., Boltz-Nitulescu, G., Skov, P.S., & Jensen-Jarolim, E. (2005). The effects of gastric digestion on codfish allergenicity. *J Allergy Clin Immunol*, 115 (2): 377-82.

[38] Monti, G., Bonfante, G., Muratore, M.C., Peltran, A., Oggero, R., Silvestro, L., & Mussa, G.C. (2003). Kiss-induced facial urticaria and angioedema in a child allergic to fish. *Allergy*, 58 (7): 684-5.

[39] Caiaffa, M.F., De Serio, A., Lotti, A., Kourtis, G., & Macchia, L. (2008). Indirect food contact in severe fish allergy. *Rev Fr Allergol*, 48: 111-112.

[40] Hansen, T.K. & Bindslev-Jensen, C. (1992). Codfish allergy in adults. Identification and diagnosis. *Allergy*, 47 (6): 610-7.

[41] Sicherer, S.H., Morrow, E.H., & Sampson, H.A. (2000). Dose-response in double-blind, placebo-controlled oral food challenges in children with atopic dermatitis. *J Allergy Clin Immunol*, 105 (3): 582-6.

[42] Hentges, F. (2009). Fish and shellfish allergens. *Rev Fr Allergol*, 49: 156-9.

[43] Bernhisel-Broadbent, J., Strause, D., & Sampson, H.A. (1992). Fish hypersensitivity. II: Clinical relevance of altered fish allergenicity caused by various preparation methods. *J Allergy Clin Immunol*, 90 (4 Pt 1): 622-9.

[44] Hansen, T.K., Bindslev-Jensen, C., Skov, P.S., & Poulsen, L.K. (1997). Codfish allergy in adults: IgE cross-reactivity among fish species. *Ann Allergy Asthma Immunol*, 78 (2): 187-94.

[45] Helbling, A., Haydel, R., Jr., McCants, M.L., Musmand, J.J., El-Dahr, J., & Lehrer, S.B. (1999). Fish allergy: is cross-reactivity among fish species relevant? Double-blind placebo-controlled food challenge studies of fish allergic adults. *Ann Allergy Asthma Immunol*, 83 (6 Pt 1): 517-23.

[46] Asero, R., Mistrello, G., Roncarolo, D., Casarini, M., & Falagiani, P. (1999). True monosensitivity to a tropical sole. *Allergy*, 54 (11): 1228-9.

[47] Kelso, J.M., Jones, R.T., & Yunginger, J.W. (1996). Monospecific allergy to swordfish. *Ann Allergy Asthma Immunol*, 77 (3): 227-8.

[48] Ebo, D., Kuehn, A., Bridts, C.H., Hilger, C., Hentges, F., & Stevens, W.J. (2010). Monosensitivity to pangasius and tilapia caused by allergens other than parvalbumin. *J Investig Allergol Clin Immunol*, 20(1): 84-88

[49] Kondo, Y., Komatsubara, R., Nakajima, Y., Yasuda, T., Kakami, M., Tsuge, I., & Urisu, A. (2006). Parvalbumin is not responsible for cross-reactivity between tuna and marlin: A case report. *J Allergy Clin Immunol,* 118 (6): 1382-3.

[50] Deuticke, H.J. (1934). Über die Sedimentationskonstante von Muskelproteinen. *Physiol Chem,* 224: 216-28.

[51] Pechere, J.F. (1968). Muscular parvalbumins as homologous proteins. *Comp Biochem Physiol,* 24 (1): 289-95.

[52] Moncrief, N.D., Kretsinger, R.H., & Goodman, M. (1990). Evolution of EF-hand calcium-modulated proteins. I. Relationships based on amino acid sequences. *J Mol Evol*, 30 (6): 522-62.

[53] Goodman, M., Pechere, J.F., Haiech, J., & Demaille, J.G. (1979). Evolutionary diversification of structure and function in the family of intracellular calcium-binding proteins. *J Mol Evol*, 13 (4): 331-52.

[54] Arif, S.H. (2009). A Ca(2+)-binding protein with numerous roles and uses: parvalbumin in molecular biology and physiology. *Bioessays*, 31 (4): 410-21.

[55] Lindstrom, C.D., van Do, T., Hordvik, I., Endresen, C., & Elsayed, S. (1996). Cloning of two distinct cDNAs encoding parvalbumin, the major allergen of Atlantic salmon (Salmo salar). *Scand J Immunol*, 44 (4): 335-44.

[56] Kretsinger, R.H. (1980). Structure and evolution of calcium-modulated proteins. CRC *Crit Rev Biochem*, 8 (2): 119-74.

[57] Leroy, B., Toubeau, G., Falmagne, P., & Wattiez, R. (2006). Identification and characterization of new protein chemoattractants in the frog skin secretome. *Mol Cell Proteomics,* 5 (11): 2114-23.

[58] Schoenman, E.R., Chiaro, J.A., Jones, A., Bastin, L.D., & Coughlin, D.J. (2010). A comparative analysis of parvalbumin expression in pinfish (Lagodon rhomboides) and toadfish (Opsanus sp.). *Comp Biochem Physiol A Mol Integr Physiol*, 155 (1): 91-9.

[59] Brownridge, P., de Mello, L.V., Peters, M., McLean, L., Claydon, A., Cossins, A.R., Whitfield, P.D., & Young, I.S. (2009). Regional variation in parvalbumin isoform expression correlates with muscle performance in common carp (Cyprinus carpio*). J Exp Biol,* 212 (Pt 2): 184-93.

[60] Lim, D.L., Neo, K.H., Goh, D.L., Shek, L.P., & Lee, B.W. (2005). Missing parvalbumin: implications in diagnostic testing for tuna allergy. *J Allergy Clin Immunol*, 115 (4): 874-5.

[61] Bobak, P. & Slechta, V. (1988). Comparison of parvalbumins of some species of family Cyprinidae. *Comp Biochem Physiol B*, 91 (4): 697-9.

[62] Gazzaz, S.S. & Rasco, B.A. (1993). Parvalbumins in fish and their role as food allergens: a review. *Rev Fisheries Sci*, 1 (1): 1-26.

[63] Kobayashi, A., Tanaka, H., Hamada, Y., Ishizaki, S., Nagashima, Y., & Shiomi, K. (2006). Comparison of allergenicity and allergens between fish white and dark muscles. *Allergy*, 61 (3): 357-63.

[64] Radauer, C., Bublin, M., Wagner, S., Mari, A., & Breiteneder, H. (2008). Allergens are distributed into few protein families and possess a restricted number of biochemical functions. *J Allergy Clin Immunol*, 121 (4): 847-52 e7.

[65] Schwaller, B. (2009). The continuing disappearance of "pure" Ca2+ buffers. *Cell Mol Life Sci*, 66 (2): 275-300.

[66] Valenta, R., Hayek, B., Seiberler, S., Bugajska-Schretter, A., Niederberger, V., Twardosz, A., Natter, S., Vangelista, L., Pastore, A., Spitzauer, S., & Kraft, D. (1998). Calcium-binding allergens: from plants to man. *Int Arch Allergy Immunol*, 117 (3): 160-6.

[67] Bugajska-Schretter, A., Grote, M., Vangelista, L., Valent, P., Sperr, W.R., Rumpold, H., Pastore, A., Reichelt, R., Valenta, R., & Spitzauer, S. (2000). Purification, biochemical, and immunological characterisation of a major food allergen: different immunoglobulin E recognition of the apo- and calcium-bound forms of carp parvalbumin. *Gut*, 46 (5): 661-9.

[68] Tomura, S., Ishizaki, S., Nagashima, Y., & Shiomi, K. (2008). Reduction in the IgE reactivity of Pacific mackerel parvalbumin by mutations at Ca^{2+}-binding sites. *Fisheries Sci*, 74 (2): 411-7.

[69] Wopfner, N., Dissertori, O., Ferreira, F., & Lackner, P. (2007). Calcium-binding proteins and their role in allergic diseases. *Immunol Allergy Clin North Am,* 27 (1): 29-44.

[70] Rao, K.S., Focant, B., Gerday, C., & Hamoir, G. (1969). Low molecular weight albumins of cod white muscle (Gadus callarias L.). *Comp Biochem Physiol*, 30 (1): 33-48.

[71] Apold, J. & Elsayed, S. (1979). The effect of amino acid modification and polymerization on the immunochemical reactivity of cod allergen M. *Mol Immunol*, 16 (8): 559-64.

[72] Das Dores, S., Chopin, C., Villaume, C., Fleurence, J., & Gueant, J.L. (2002). A new oligomeric parvalbumin allergen of Atlantic cod (Gad mI) encoded by a gene distinct from that of Gad cI. *Allergy*, 57 Suppl 72: 79-83.

[73] Ma, Y., Griesmeier, U., Susani, M., Radauer, C., Briza, P., Erler, A., Bublin, M., Alessandri, S., Himly, M., Vazquez-Cortes, S., de Arellano, I.R., Vassilopoulou, E., Saxoni-Papageorgiou, P., Knulst, A.C., Fernandez-Rivas, M., Hoffmann-Sommergruber, K., & Breiteneder, H. (2008). Comparison of natural and recombinant forms of the major fish allergen parvalbumin from cod and carp. *Mol Nutr Food Res,* 52 Suppl 2: S196-207.

[74] Pechere, J.F., Capony, J.P., & Ryden, L. (1971). The primary structure of the major parvalbumin from hake muscle. Isolation and general properties of the protein. *Eur J Biochem,* 23 (3): 421-8.

[75] Dubois, I. & Gerday, C. (1990). Soluble calcium-binding proteins: parvalbumins and calmodulin from eel skeletal muscle. *Comp Biochem Physiol B,* 95 (2): 381-5.

[76] Shiomi, K., Hamada, Y., Sekiguchi, K., Shimakura, K., & Nagashima, Y. (1999). Two classes of allergens, parvalbumins and higher molecular weight substances, in Japanese eel and bigeye tuna. *Fisheries Sci*, 65: 943-8.

[77] Permyakov, E.A., Medvedkin, V.N., Kalinichenko, L.P., & Burstein, E.A. (1983). Comparative study of physiochemical properties of two pike parvalbumins by means of their intrinsic tyrosyl and phenylalanyl fluorescence. *Arch Biochem Biophys*, 227 (1): 9-20.

[78] Huriaux, F., Vandewalle, P., & Focant, B. (2002). Immunological study of muscle parvalbumin isotypes in three African catfish during development. *Comp Biochem Physiol B Biochem Mol Biol*, 132 (3): 579-84.

[79] Bugajska-Schretter, A., Pastore, A., Vangelista, L., Rumpold, H., Valenta, R., & Spitzauer, S. (1999). Molecular and immunological characterization of carp parvalbumin, a major fish allergen. *Int Arch Allergy Immunol*, 118 (2-4): 306-8.

[80] Hamada, Y., Tanaka, H., Ishizaki, S., Ishida, M., Nagashima, Y., & Shiomi, K. (2003). Purification, reactivity with IgE and cDNA cloning of parvalbumin as the major allergen of mackerels. *Food Chem Toxicol*, 41 (8): 1149-56.

[81] Van Do, T., Hordvik, I., Endresen, C., & Elsayed, S. (2005). Characterization of parvalbumin, the major allergen in Alaska pollack, and comparison with codfish *Allergen M. Mol Immunol*, 42 (3): 345-53.

[82] Lee, S.J., Ju, C.C., Chu, S.L., Chien, M.S., Chan, T.H., & Liao, W.L. (2007). Molecular cloning, expression and phylogenetic analyses of parvalbumin in tilapia, Oreochromis mossambicus. *J Exp Zool A Ecol Genet Physiol*, 307 (1): 51-61.

[83] Beale, J.E., Jeebhay, M.F., & Lopata, A.L. (2009). Characterisation of purified parvalbumin from five fish species and nucleotide sequencing of this major allergen from Pacific pilchard, Sardinops sagax. *Mol Immunol*, 46 (15): 2985-93.

[84] Griesmeier, U., Bublin, M., Radauer, C., Vazquez-Cortes, S., Ma, Y., Fernandez-Rivas, M., & Breiteneder, H. (2009). Physicochemical properties and thermal stability of Lep w 1, the major allergen of whiff. *Mol Nutr Food Res.*, DOI10.1002/mnfr.200900043

[85] Griesmeier, U., Vazquez-Cortes, S., Bublin, M., Radauer, C., Ma, Y., Briza, P., Fernandez-Rivas, M., & Breiteneder, H. (2010). Expression levels of parvalbumins determine allergenicity of fish species. *Allergy*, 65 (2): 191-8.

[86] Conlon, J.M., O'Harte, F., Smith, D.D., Balment, R.J., & Hazon, N. (1992). Purification and characterization of urotensin II and parvalbumin from an elasmobranch fish, Scyliorhinus canicula (common dogfish). *Neuroendocrinology*, 55 (2): 230-5.

[87] Rabbani-Chadegani, A., Abdossamadi, S., Bargahi, A., & Yousef-Masboogh, M. (2008). Identification of low-molecular-weight protein (SCP1) from shark cartilage with anti-angiogenesis activity and sequence similarity to parvalbumin. *J Pharm Biomed Anal*, 46 (3): 563-7.

[88] Heffron, J.K. & Moerland, T.S. (2008). Parvalbumin characterization from the euryhaline stingray Dasyatis sabina. *Comp Biochem Physiol A Mol Integr Physiol,* 150 (3): 339-46.

[89] Permyakov, S.E., Karnoup, A.S., Bakunts, A.G., & Permyakov, E.A. (2009). Sequence microheterogeneity of parvalbumin pI 5.0 of pike: a mass spectrometric study. *Biochim Biophys Acta*, 1794 (1): 129-36.

[90] Thys, T.M., Blank, J.M., & Schachat, F.H. (1998). Rostral-caudal variation in troponin T and parvalbumin correlates with differences in relaxation rates of cod axial muscle. *J Exp Biol*, 201 (Pt 21): 2993-3001.

[91] Breiteneder, H. & Ebner, C. (2000). Molecular and biochemical classification of plant-derived food allergens. *J Allergy Clin Immunol,* 106 (1 Pt 1): 27-36.

[92] Aas, K. & Elsayed, S.M. (1969). Characterization of a major allergen (cod). Effect of enzymic hydrolysis on the allergenic activity. *J Allergy,* 44 (6); 333-43

[93] Lim, D.L., Neo, K.H., Yi, F.C., Chua, K.Y., Goh, D.L., Shek, L.P., Giam, Y.C., Van Bever, H.P., & Lee, B.W. (2008). Parvalbumin--the major tropical fish allergen. *Pediatr Allergy Immunol,* 19 (5): 399-407.

[94] Sletten, G., Van Do, T., Lindvik, H., Egaas, E., & Florvaag, E. (2009). Effects of industrial processing on the immunogenicity of commonly ingested fish species. *Int Arch Allergy Immunol*, 151 (3): 223-236.

[95] Jenkins, J.A., Breiteneder, H., & Mills, E.N. (2007). Evolutionary distance from human homologs reflects allergenicity of animal food proteins. *J Allergy Clin Immunol*, 120 (6): 1399-405.

[96] Hilger, C., Grigioni, F., Thill, L., Mertens, L., & Hentges, F. (2002). Severe IgE-mediated anaphylaxis following consumption of fried frog legs: definition of alpha-parvalbumin as the allergen in cause. *Allergy*, 57 (11): 1053-8.

[97] Hilger, C., Thill, L., Grigioni, F., Lehners, C., Falagiani, P., Ferrara, A., Romano, C., Stevens, W., & Hentges, F. (2004). IgE antibodies of fish allergic patients cross-react with frog parvalbumin. *Allergy*, 59 (6): 653-60.

[98] Kuehn, A., Lehners, C., Hilger, C., & Hentges, F. (2009). Food allergy to chicken meat with IgE reactivity to muscle alpha-parvalbumin. *Allergy*, 64 (10): 1557-8.

[99] Mata, E., Favier, C., Moneret-Vautrin, D.A., Nicolas, J.P., Han Ching, L., & Gueant, J.L. (1994). Surimi and native codfish contain a common allergen identified as a 63-kDa protein. *Allergy*, 49 (6): 442-7.

[100] Dory, D., Chopin, C., Aimone-Gastin, I., Gueant, J.L., Guerin, L., Sainte-Laudy, J., Moneret-Vautrin, D.A., & Fleurence, J. (1998). Recognition of an extensive range of IgE-reactive proteins in cod extract. *Allergy*, 53 (1): 42-50.

[101] Sten, E., Hansen, T.K., Stahl Skov, P., Andersen, S.B., Torp, A., Bindslev-Jensen, U., Bindslev-Jensen, C., & Poulsen, L.K. (2004). Cross-reactivity to eel, eelpout and ocean pout in codfish-allergic patients. *Allergy*, 59 (11): 1173-80.

[102] Rosmilah, M., Shahnaz, M., Masita, A., Noormalin, A., & Jamaludin, M. (2005). Identification of major allergens of two species of local snappers: Lutjanus argentimaculatus (merah/ red snapper) and Lutjanus johnii (jenahak/ golden snapper). *Trop Biomed*, 22 (2): 171-7.

[103] Misnan, R., Murad, S., Jones, M., Taylor, G., Rahman, D., Arip, M., Abdullah, N., & Mohamed, J. (2008). Identification of the major allergens of Indian scad (Decapterus russelli). *Asian Pac J Allergy Immunol*, 26 (4): 191-8.

[104] Nakamura, R., Satoh, R., Nakajima, Y., Kawasaki, N., Yamaguchi, T., Sawada, J., Nagoya, H., & Teshima, R. (2009). Comparative study of GH-transgenic and non-transgenic amago salmon (Oncorhynchus masou ishikawae) allergenicity and proteomic analysis of amago salmon allergens. *Regul Toxicol Pharmacol*, 55 (3): 300-8.

[105] Valls, A., Pascual, C.Y., & Martín Esteban, M. (2005). Anisakis allergy: an update. *Rev Fr Allergol*, 45: 108-113.

[106] Lopata, A.L. & Lehrer, S.B. (2009). New insights into seafood allergy. *Curr Opin Allergy Clin Immunol,* 9 (3): 270-7.

[107] Johansson, E., Aponno, M., Lundberg, M., & van Hage-Hamsten, M. (2001). Allergenic cross-reactivity between the nematode Anisakis simplex and the dust mites Acarus siro, Lepidoglyphus destructor, Tyrophagus putrescentiae, and Dermatophagoides pteronyssinus. *Allergy*, 56 (7): 660-6.

[108] Guarneri, F., Guarneri, C., & Benvenga, S. (2007). Cross-reactivity of Anisakis simplex: possible role of Ani s 2 and Ani s 3. *Int J Dermatol*, 46 (2): 146-50.

[109] Makinen-Kiljunen, S., Kiistala, R., & Varjonen, E. (2003). Severe reactions from roe without concomitant fish allergy. *Ann Allergy Asthma Immunol*, 91 (4): 413-6.

[110] Perez-Gordo, M., Sanchez-Garcia, S., Cases, B., Pastor, C., Vivanco, F., & Cuesta-Herranz, J. (2008). Identification of vitellogenin as an allergen in Beluga caviar allergy. *Allergy*, 63 (4): 479-80.

[111] Kondo, Y., Kakami, M., Koyama, H., Yasuda, T., Nakajima, Y., Kawamura, M., Tokuda, R., Tsuge, I., & Urisu, A. (2005). IgE Cross-reactivity between Fish Roe(Salmon, Herring and Pollock) and Chicken Egg in Patients Anaphylactic to Salmon Roe. *Allergol Int*, 54: 317-23.

[112] Shimizu, Y., Nakamura, A., Kishimura, H., Hara, A., Watanabe, K., & Saeki, H. (2009). Major allergen and its IgE cross-reactivity among salmonid fish roe allergy. *J Agric Food Chem,* 57 (6): 2314-9.

[113] Karim, A.A. & Bhat, R. (2009). Fish gelatin: properties, challenges, and prospects as an alternative to mammalian gelatins. *Food Hydrocolloids*, 23 (3): 563-76.

[114] Sakaguchi, M., Nakayama, T., & Inouye, S. (1996). Food allergy to gelatin in children with systemic immediate-type reactions, including anaphylaxis, to vaccines. *J Allergy Clin Immunol,* 98 (6 Pt 1): 1058-61.

[115] Wahl, R. & Kleinhans, D. (1989). IgE-mediated allergic reactions to fruit gums and investigation of cross-reactivity between gelatine and modified gelatine-containing products. *Clin Exp Allergy*, 19 (1): 77-80.

[116] Sakaguchi, M., Toda, M., Ebihara, T., Irie, S., Hori, H., Imai, A., Yanagida, M., Miyazawa, H., Ohsuna, H., Ikezawa, Z., & Inouye, S. (2000). IgE antibody to fish gelatin (type I collagen) in patients with fish allergy. *J Allergy Clin Immunol*, 106 (3): 579-84.

[117] Andre, F., Cavagna, S., & Andre, C. (2003). Gelatin prepared from tuna skin: a risk factor for fish allergy or sensitization? *Int Arch Allergy Immunol*, 130 (1): 17-24.

[118] Hansen, T.K., Poulsen, L.K., Stahl Skov, P., Hefle, S.L., Hlywka, J.J., Taylor, S.L., Bindslev-Jensen, U., & Bindslev-Jensen, C. (2004). A randomized, double-blinded, placebo-controlled oral challenge study to evaluate the allergenicity of commercial, food-grade fish gelatin. *Food Chem Toxicol*, 42 (12): 2037-44.

[119] Taylor, S.L. & Hefle, S.L. (2006). Food allergen labeling in the USA and Europe. *Curr Opin Allergy Clin Immunol,* 6 (3): 186-90.

[120] Weber, P., Steinhart, H., & Paschke, A. (2009). Competitive indirect ELISA for the determination of parvalbumins from various fish species in food grade fish gelatins and isinglass with PARV-19 anti-parvalbumin antibodies. *J Agric Food Chem*, 57 (23): 11328-34.

[121] Auerswald, L., Morren, C., & Lopata, A. (2006). Histamine levels in seventeen species of fresh and processed South African seafood. *Food Chem*, 98.

[122] Bedry, R., Gabinski, C., & Paty, M.C. (2000). Diagnosis of scombroid poisoning by measurement of plasma histamine. *N Engl J Med*, 342 (7): 520-1.

[123] Lorenzo, S., Iglesias, R., Leiro, J., Ubeira, F.M., Ansotegui, I., Garcia, M., & Fernandez de Corres, L. (2000). Usefulness of currently available methods for the diagnosis of Anisakis simplex allergy. *Allergy*, 55 (7): 627-33.

[124] Mari, A., Scala, E., Palazzo, P., Ridolfi, S., Zennaro, D., & Carabella, G. (2006). Bioinformatics applied to allergy: allergen databases, from collecting sequence information to data integration. The Allergome platform as a model. *Cell Immunol*, 244 (2): 97-100.

[125] Marti, P., Truffer, R., Stadler, M.B., Keller-Gautschi, E., Crameri, R., Mari, A., Schmid-Grendelmeier, P., Miescher, S.M., Stadler, B.M., & Vogel, M. (2007). Allergen motifs and the prediction of allergenicity. *Immunol Lett*, 109 (1): 47-55.

[126] Saha, S. & Raghava, G.P. (2006). AlgPred: prediction of allergenic proteins and mapping of IgE epitopes. *Nucleic Acids Res*, 34: W202-9.

[127] Elsayed, S., Apold, J., Holen, E., Vik, H., Florvaag, E., & Dybendal, T. (1991). The structural requirements of epitopes with IgE binding capacity demonstrated by three

major allergens from fish, egg and tree pollen. *Scand J Clin Lab Invest Suppl*, 204: 17-31.

[128] Yoshida, S., Ichimura, A., & Shiomi, K. (2008). Elucidation of a major IgE epitope of Pacific mackerel parvalbumin. *Food Chem*, 111 (4): 857-61.

[129] Untersmayr, E., Szalai, K., Riemer, A.B., Hemmer, W., Swoboda, I., Hantusch, B., Scholl, I., Spitzauer, S., Scheiner, O., Jarisch, R., Boltz-Nitulescu, G., & Jensen-Jarolim, E. (2006). Mimotopes identify conformational epitopes on parvalbumin, the major fish allergen. *Mol Immunol*, 43 (9): 1454-61.

[130] Lin, J. & Sampson, H.A. (2009). The role of immunoglobulin E-binding epitopes in the characterization of food allergy. *Curr Opin Allergy Clin Immunol*, 9 (4): 357-63.

[131] Egger, M., Hauser, M., Himly, M., Wopfner, N., Wallner, M., & Ferreira, F. (2009). Development of recombinant allergens for diagnosis and therapy. *Front Biosci* (Elite Ed), 1: 77-90.

[132] Wohrl, S. (2008). The potential of allergen biochips. *Recent Pat Inflamm Allergy Drug Discov*, 2 (3): 186-90.

[133] Lin, J., Renault, N., Haas, H., Schramm, G., Vieths, S., Vogel, L., Falcone, F.H., & Alcocer, M.J. (2007). A novel tool for the detection of allergic sensitization combining protein microarrays with human basophils. *Clin Exp Allergy*, 37 (12): 1854-62.

[134] Skripak, J.M. & Sampson, H.A. (2008). Towards a cure for food allergy. *Curr Opin Immunol*, 20 (6): 690-6.

[135] Casimir, G., Cuvelier, P., Allard, S., & Duchateau, J. (1997). Life-threatening fish allergy successfully treated with immunotherapy. *Pediatr Allergy Immunol*, 8 (2): 103-5.

[136] Patriarca, G., Nucera, E., Pollastrini, E., Roncallo, C., De Pasquale, T., Lombardo, C., Pedone, C., Gasbarrini, G., Buonomo, A., & Schiavino, D. (2007). Oral specific desensitization in food-allergic children. *Dig Dis Sci,* 52 (7): 1662-72.

[137] Swoboda, I., Bugajska-Schretter, A., Linhart, B., Verdino, P., Keller, W., Schulmeister, U., Sperr, W.R., Valent, P., Peltre, G., Quirce, S., Douladiris, N., Papadopoulos, N.G., Valenta, R., & Spitzauer, S. (2007). A recombinant hypoallergenic parvalbumin mutant for immunotherapy of IgE-mediated fish allergy. *J Immunol*, 178 (10): 6290-6.

[138] Cheftel, J. (2005). Food allergen labelling in the European Union. *Food Chem* 93: 531-50.

[139] Poms, R.E., Klein, C.L., & Anklam, E. (2004). Methods for allergen analysis in food: a review. *Food Addit Contam*, 21 (1): 1-31.

[140] Koppelman, S.J. & Hefle, S.L. eds. *Detecting allergens in food.* 2006, Woodhead publishing.

[141] Carrera, E., García, T., Céspedes, A., González, I., Sanz, B., Hernández, P.E., & Martín, R. (1997). Immunostick Colorimetric ELISA Assay for the Identification of Smoked Salmon, Trout and Bream. *J Sci Food Agric*, 74: 547-50.

[142] Chen, L., Hefle, S.L., Taylor, S.L., Swoboda, I., & Goodman, R.E. (2006). Detecting fish parvalbumin with commercial mouse monoclonal anti-frog parvalbumin IgG. *J Agric Food Chem*, 54 (15): 5577-82.

[143] Faeste, C.K. & Plassen, C. (2008). Quantitative sandwich ELISA for the determination of fish in foods. *J Immunol Methods*, 329 (1-2): 45-55.

[144] Gajewski, K.G. & Hsieh, Y.H. (2009). Monoclonal antibody specific to a major fish allergen: parvalbumin. *J Food Prot*, 72 (4): 818-25.

[145] Lopata, A.L., Jeebhay, M.F., Reese, G., Fernandes, J., Swoboda, I., Robins, T.G., & Lehrer, S.B. (2005). Detection of fish antigens aerosolized during fish processing using newly developed immunoassays. *Int Arch Allergy Immunol*, 138 (1): 21-8.

[146] Lu, H.Y., Ohshima, T., & Ushio, H. (2004). Rapid detection of the major allergen parvalbumin by surface Plasmon resonance biosensor. *J Food Sci*, 69: 652-58.

[147] Lifrani, A., Dos Santos, J., Dubarry, M., Rautureau, M., Blachier, F., & Tome, D. (2009). Development of animal models and sandwich-ELISA tests to detect the allergenicity and antigenicity of fining agent residues in wines. *J Agric Food Chem*, 57 (2): 525-34.

[148] Choi, K.Y. & Hong, K.W. (2007). Genomic DNA sequence of mackerel parvalbumin and a PCR test for rapid detection of allergenic mackerel ingredients in food. *Food Sci Biotechnol*, 16: 67-70.

[149] Sun, M., Liang, C., Gao, H., Lin, C., & Deng, M. (2009). Detection of parvalbumin, a common fish allergen gene in food, by real-time polymerase chain reaction. *J AOAC Int*, 92 (1): 234-40.

[150] Hildebrandt, S. & Garber, E. (2009). Effects of processing on detection and quantification of the parvalbumin gene in Atlantic salmon (Salmo salar). *Food Chem*, 119: 75-80.

In: Food Allergies: Symptoms, Diagnosis, and Treatment
Editor: Patricia M. Rodgers
ISBN: 978-1-61728-748-0

Chapter 3

IMMUNOMODULATION BY FOOD: ALLERGY MITIGATION BY DIETARY COMPONENTS

Harry J. Wichers*[*] *and Jurriaan J. Mes
Wageningen University and Research Centre, Wageningen, The Netherlands

ABSTRACT

Proper and well-balanced immune functioning is of pivotal importance to health and well-being. In the past decades, there has been an apparent decrease in the prevalence of classical infectious diseases, with a concomitant increase in immune-related disorders, including allergies. Causally, a relationship with changes in life-style-related factors, amongst which hygienic practice, is often laid.

Diet and nutrition can affect functioning of various immune parameters. This concept can be explored to prevent or mitigate allergic reactions via the development of targeted food products or ingredients. This review describes recent findings with respect to food products and ingredients that show potential in this respect, with special emphasis on pro- and prebiotics, ß-glucans, fungal immunomodulatory proteins and ω-3 polyunsaturated fatty acids. The micro-organism-related products appear to strengthen Th1-mediated immunity, thus possibly restoring defective immune maturation due to overly hygienic living conditions.

Also ω-3-PUFAs may hold promise to attenuate allergic symptoms, although this concept appears to function via mechanisms that are clearly distinct from the micro-organism derived compounds.

Keywords: Immunity, immunomodulation, allergy, probiotics, prebiotics, ß-glucans, fungal immunomodulatory proteins, ω-3 polyunsaturated fatty acids, diet, nutrition

* Wageningen University and Research Centre, PO Box 17, 6700, A Wageningen, The Netherlands, e-mail harry.wichers@wur.nl, phone +31 317 480175, fax +31 317 483011

BACKGROUND

A properly functioning and balanced immune system is pivotal to maintain health and well-being. Roughly since world war II, the prevalence of 'traditional' infectious diseases, such as tuberculosis, hepatitis, or measles, has decreased, with a concomitant increase in immune-related disorders, such as multiple sclerosis, Crohn's disease, type 1 diabetes and various allergic diseases. Also, disease incidence decreased in North-South direction in the Northern hemisphere, and vice versa in the Southern hemisphere [1]. This suggests non-genetic factors playing a role, such as health care and medical practice (e.g. vaccination programmes), living environment and life style, welfare, dietary patterns, and the like. In particular for the strongly increased prevalence of asthma and allergic disease, a connection to hygienic practice and subsequent reduced exposure to microbes, which is supposed to result in a 'not fully ripened' immune system, was hypothesised [2]. This may include hygienic practice in food preparation, of which the virtue for public health is not to be disputed, but that may have contributed to impaired or delayed immune maturation. In addition, the development of food products that are composed of highly refined ingredients has probably led to decreased consumption of micronutrients that may be relevant for immune maturation [3]. It is interesting to note, that the incidence of tuberculosis appeared inversely related to the incidence of asthma and rhinoconjunctivitis. This could confirm the importance of a vigilant Th1-compartment in disease aetiology, as mycobacteria are known to elicit particularly strong Th1-responses [4], adding to the Th1/2-paradigm as being at the immunological basis of allergic disease [5]. In many other chronic diseases, for instance cardiovascular diseases, neoplastic malignancies, and metabolic syndrome, chronic inflammatory processes contribute to the development of associated health problems. Also in such clinical situations, an important role for immune interventions may be found [6-10]. The prophylactic and therapeutic relevance of immune modulation is illustrated by the possibility to develop antitumor strategies via vaccination e.g. as has been described for *Mycobacterium*-based vaccines and lung tumours, an effect supposedly based on selective enhancement of Th1-mediated immunity [11]. Another example is the claimed prophylactic effect of the Th1-stimulating mushroom-derived ß-glucan lentinan on malaria [12]. Altogether, immune modulation, e.g. via dietary strategies, is not only relevant for such specific clinical conditions, but holds promise for maintaining immune homeostasis in the healthy population as well, despite the heterogeneity of the concept of 'health'. Immune functioning strongly varies in distinguishable life stages. For instance, with increasing age, there is a decline in the functional capacity to elicit generalised and specific immune responses, accompanied by a decrease in production and functional response of regulatory cells. Overall, these developments result in impaired innate and adaptive immune responses, elicited self-antigen reactivity, a higher susceptibility towards infection and the development of malignant tissue. Overall implications of such senescence phenomena of immunity are that specific health parameters may vary with age, immune impairment eventually leading to increased risk of mortality [13-17].

IMMUNE FUNCTIONING AND DIETARY COMPONENTS

For quite a few dietary components, clear effects on immune functioning have been described. Protein energy malnutrition (PEM), for instance, has a profound effect on immune functioning, in particular in the elderly. The properties of T-cell and B-cell subsets and functions and of innate immunity are clearly linked to protein nutritional status. Immune responses can be restored by intervening in this protein shortage, where patients that suffer from inflammatory processes respond slower. The imbalance between normal macrophage functions and decreased T-cell functions is partly responsible for chronic inflammatory processes in vulnerable patients, because of which acute phase responses are more detrimental to nutritional status and nutrient reserves in elderly patients than in adults [18, 19]. Not only protein status, but also dietary protein-carbohydrate ratio is likely important in maintaining immune responsiveness: a low protein-high carbohydrate ratio for prolonged intervals seemed beneficial for immune status in a rat model [20].

Specific nutritional preparations have been developed, for clinical use in critically ill patients with a jeopardised immune functioning. Usually, such preparations contain at the least specific amino acids such as arginine and glutamine, nucleotides, and specific poly-unsaturated fatty acids, notably ω-3 PUFAs such as docosahexaenoic acid (22:6n-3; DHA) and eicosapentaenoic acid (20:5n-3; EPA) [21, 22]. Next to ω-3-PUFAs there is a clear interest in vitamins, such as A, C, D en E, and minerals as Zn and Se, which have been associated with modulating immune functions. A number of recent reviews and research papers addresses these concepts in detail [21-26]. For a number of other nutrients and products, research is still in a less advanced stage, e.g. at best in the stage of *in vitro* experimentation, animal models, and (limited) human trials. Some issues of research will be dealt with below.

Despite all knowledge and promising results on food and nutrition that can support and maintain immune homeostasis, research into the possible role of functional foods to mitigate (human) immune functioning is still in its infancy. Controversies around food health claims will remain as long as no improvement in e.g. identification of suitable biomarkers, and a more detailed comprehension of individual phenotypic responses in relation to underlying physiological and biochemical mechanisms to nutrients have emerged. In this context, immune modulating functional foods should be addressed as food products with health benefits for specific groups of consumers, for instance those with an unbalanced or skewed immune system or for those in which the immune system needs to be challenged similar to vaccination. As the balance and skewing can be in different directions, the immunomodulatory properties of products should match the specific needs of (groups of) individuals. This implies that products that are of benefit to e.g. allergic consumers do not necessarily have a beneficial effect on other consumers; requirements for neonates likely differ from those of the elderly, and so on. In research and intervention studies and positioning the eventual product, immunomodulatory properties of food products should therefore be approached and tuned with immunological specifications of target groups.

Targets and Prerequisites

The objectives of the research area are to develop dietary or food products to support vital and balanced immune functioning in various life stages, for specific groups of consumers. In order to develop these products immunological read-outs are essential because:

1. Many chronic health threats, with enormous impact on quality of life as well as economic impact, is related to immune functioning, such as auto-immune diseases, allergies and asthma, or immune deficiencies [1].
2. The immune system plays a, in some cases (perhaps partial) causal, role in pathology of at the least quite a few chronic and age-related anomalies.
3. Food components can modulate immune responses, both positively as well as negatively (e.g. food allergy), as becomes increasingly evident from randomised double blind intervention studies as well as from clinical trials (see below).

Immune functioning as a paradigm offers advantages that may facilitate the translation from an experimental setting to possible application and implementation, as immune functioning may well serve as a theoretical framework for assessment of health impact. Already for a long time the pivotal role of immunity in health and well-being has been acknowledged resulting in:

- Many available immune parameters, diagnostically validated *in vitro* or *in vivo* test systems
- Many available animal models and cell lines for *in vitro* analysis
- Standard clinical practice and pathology of many chronic conditions in which the role of the immune system is relatively well documented
- An increased interest to link individual immune functionality to life style-and age-related parameters, where particularly food and nutrition show the best documented effects.

Further mechanistic underpinning of health effects of food intake appears a prerequisite to achieve further progress in the development of dietary tools for enhancing health homeostasis. Lack of sufficient scientific basis for such will result in contradictory claims and statements, confusion and loss of trust and confidence amongst consumers. Addressing this lacuna will contribute to a solid basis for food that can enhance maintenance of health and quality of life, including food that can successfully pass food health claims.

Research into Immunomodulation by Food, with a Focus on Allergy

Probiotics

According to the currently adopted definition by FAO/WHO, probiotics are: 'Live microorganisms which, when administered in adequate amounts, confer a health benefit on the host'. Some years ago, relationships between the composition of intestinal microbiota and the occurrence and incidence of allergic diseases were noted [27-29]. For Estonian and Swedish school children it was demonstrated that allergic children were less often colonised with *Lactobacilli* and more often with aerobic coliforms and *Staphylococcus aureus* [27, 28], or lower *Bifidobacterium*-counts and higher *Clostridium* colonisation numbers were found [29]. This was supposed to be relevant for proper maturation of intestinal immunity, and in particular to have impact on the balance between Th1 and Th2-cells [28, 29]. Such observations led to the hypothesis that nutritional and dietary intervention, via probiotics, were possible for this type of condition.

In a Finnish study, *Lactobacilli* (LGG), were given to 159 atopic pregnant women for 2 weeks and to their babies for 6 months. This resulted in 50% decreased incidence in atopic eczema, at 2 years of age, in infants in the LGG group compared to the placebo group [30]. Similarly, LGG and *Bifidobacterium lactis* Bb12 were shown to decrease severity of atopic eczema [31]. Suggesting a possible mechanism, another study illustrated that the tolerance-related cytokine IL-10 was elevated significantly in serum from patients in the LGG group [32]. Sometimes a combination of probiotics was beneficial in the management of atopic dermatitis [33] but sometimes this was not reproducible elsewhere [34].

In a group of teenagers and young adults, *Lactobacillus rhamnosis* did not lead to reduced birch-pollen allergy symptoms [35]. In addition, dietary LGG-supplementation a few weeks before delivery did not appear to have an effect on proliferation of PBMCs from atopic or control neonates. This suggested that there was no impact on sensitisation potential [36]. It however has to be kept in mind that specific probiotic strains can have different effects [37], that matrix and formulation can have effect on bioactivity of the product, that exposure and intervention may have been to short to reveal an effect and that there is a variation in the width of unbalances in natural skewing and therefore the composition of the test population is relevant. A good standardisation of strains, process and formulation, combined with (*in vitro*) product bioactivity quality control should be addressed before interventions are conducted. A more detailed genotyping and phenotyping practise of biological parameters in the study population is extremely relevant to analyse effects on the sub-group or individual level. This supports the idea that both product and population should be studied in depth before and during intervention studies.

Summarising, results of probiotics in allergy prevention are variable and heavily debated. *In vitro* observations suggest that a possible mechanism for positive effects on allergy-related immunity is the consequence of or leading to the restoration of imbalances between various T-cell subsets, possibly indirectly via TLR signalling in innate immune cells. *In vitro* effects are for certain, and *in vivo* results therefore likely are as well, strongly strain-dependent; *in vitro* screening of probiotics strains resulted in strain-dependent immune-effects, e.g. IL-10 inducing (tolerance enhancing?) or Th1-skewing [37]. Apart from this, effects on gut permeability or intestinal allergen processing cannot be ruled out as yet. In addition, responses may be dependent of individual patient characteristics as well, e.g. whether allergies have already fully developed or not and immune aberrancies are still prone to modulation. Recently, interactions between (inducible) *Lactobacillus*-S-layer protein and gut-DCs were described, which may contribute to the mechanism of action [38], in particular primarily on innate immunity.

The conclusion is that stringent requirements for experimental design are imperative to avoid contradictory data, and to further elaborate this promising area of research.

ß-Glucans

ß-(1→3)-(1→6)-Glucans are cell wall components that occur in a wide variety of organisms, such as bacteria, yeasts, algae, cereals (mainly containing (1→4)-cross-links [39]), fungi and lichens. It concerns polymers of glucose with a ß-(1→3)-backbone and ß-(1→6)-cross-links. Molecular weights are typically in the range of several hundreds of kDa, which indicates a polymerisation degree of several thousands of glucose units. ß-glucans gain particular research interest for their anticipated effects on immunity. A supposed mechanism for this is for instance via binding to cells from the innate immune compartment such as macrophages and to NK-cells, for which also receptors have been described (see below) [40, 41].

A number of studies into the effect of ß-glucans on allergic reactions has been published. The mitigating effect of a ß-glucan from *Aureobasidium pullulans* strain A1 on allergic reactions in ovalbumin-allergic Balb/C mice has been described by Kimura *et al.* [42]. It was found that feeding 0.5-1.0% of a ß-glucan from *Aureobasidium pullulans* strain A1 in the diet of ovalbumin-allergic Balb/C mice considerably reduced ova-specific IgE, and stimulated IL-4, IFN- and IL-12 production in ConA-stimulated splenocytes from the mice.

The ß-glucan (lentinan) from shiitake was evaluated in a human trial with cedar-pollen allergic patients. The ß-glucans, orally applied as superfine dispersed β-1, 3-glucans before symptom onset, exhibited significant alleviation of symptoms of Japanese cedar pollen–induced rhinitis, such as sneezing, nasal congestion, and conjunctivitis [43]. Allergic symptoms were not only relieved for seasonal allergy to cedar pollen but also for perennial allergy. Oral ingestion of ß-(1→3)-glucan in allergic individuals reduced the spontaneous increase in both allergen-specific and total IgE titres. Clinical responses to treatment correlated well with the capacity of monocytes to bind to ß-(1→3)-glucan [43]. Both the route of application (nasal application of ß-glucans resulting in the glucans acting as an allergen, [42]), and the degree of dispersion appeared important, as non-dispersed lentinan did not give the desired effects [43].

Similar allergy-mitigating effects have been observed for crude fungal extracts, such as from *Ganoderma lucidum* (Japanese lacquer mushroom), in a murine (C3H/HeJ) model for peanut allergy [44], and a model for house dust mite allergy [45].

ß-Glucans are able to activate innate pathways, e.g. in macrophages [40, 41] and were found to stimulate the production of TNF-α, IFN-γ and IL-12 when injected into ICR-mice [46]. Similar observations were made for models of human peripheral blood mononuclear cells in which various fungal extracts were screened [47]. A slightly different observation was made for the ß-glucan from *Aureobasidium pullulans*, that was found to particularly induce IL-8 production in PBMCs and in a monocyte cell line [48]. Activated innate immune cells may subsequently activate T-cells, also in PBMC-cultures, thus stimulating Th1-like responses, which is corroborated by the above cited studies. Characteristics of such stimulation may depend on typical characteristics of ß-glucans such as the molecular weight (the *Aureobasidium*-glucan being relatively small, ca. 100 kDa) and degree of branching (50-80%) [42], which may account for different observations. Various receptors for ß-glucans (dectin-1, complement receptor 3, TLR2 and TLR6, scavenger receptors and lactosylceramide) have been identified. Dectin-1 is particularly expressed on immune cells, such as dendritic cells, macrophages, monocytes, neutrophils, eosinophils, some T-cells and in humans also on B-cells. Possible expression of dectin-1 in intestinal cells is under debate

[40]. Interaction of dectin-1 and TLR2 after binding to ß-glucan-type ligands leads to synergistic effects on the production of cytokines such as TNF-α and IL12, a process in which NF-kB [49] and spleen tyrosine kinase are thought to be involved [50]. Dectin-1 preferentially binds to the ß-(1→3)-part of the glucan. Receptor binding studies, in which the Ig-labelled polysaccharide-binding domains of dectin-1 were used to detect glucan-binding, indicated that the minimally required length to allow binding to dectin-1 is 10-11 glucose residues [51]. It is important to realise that these observations were based on a rather abstracted experimental model, and that the possible physiological significance of the ß-(1→6)-branches is as yet not clarified. Binding of ß-glucans to dectin-1 and TLR-2 shows synergistic effects, which perhaps indicates a role for the ß-(1→6)-branched structure [49]. Single-chain ß-glucans appear to induce stronger responses (NF-kB, iNOS-production, TNF-α) in (murine) macrophages compared to oligomeric chains [41]. Increased solubility of ß-glucans enhances their effectiveness, as demonstrated for instance by the impact of sulphated, carboxymethylated, methylated, hydroxyethylated or hydroxypropylated derivatives on Sarcoma-180 tumour cells [52]. The relevance of increased solubility on allergy mitigation is as yet not clear, but the effect of degree of dispersion points in a similar direction [43].

The synthesis, modifications and breakdown of ß-glucans in food crops is a dynamic process. Genotypic variation, growing conditions, developmental stage at harvest, post harvest treatment and processing all can have effects on ß-glucan concentrations, bioavailability and bioactivity [53, 54 and own studies, in preparation]. This illustrates that product quality control, preferably based on bioactivity, should be included when conducting feeding or intervention trials.

In conclusion, there appear to be clear indications, from animal models as well as from a human study, that orally applied ß-glucans or glucan-containing preparations can be of help in relieving food and respiratory allergy-related symptoms. Taking this concept further, it might be promising to analyse possible effects also in other settings in which Th1-stimulation might be relevant, such as stimulation of cell-mediated immunity, vaccine adjuvant development, support of chemotherapy, and improved infection resistance. It appears as if ß-glucans activate, indirectly via innate activation, Th1-mediated immunity, in which TLR/CLR (dectin-)-signalling is involved.

A number of research issues is still open, such as e.g. how and where interactions between ß-glucans and immune cells take place (intestinally via microfold-(M-) cells? Via, into the intestinal lumen perturbing, dendritic cells? Through transport via tight junctions? And/or via para-cellular transport?). Also structure-function studies and research on application and delivery methods, for instance incorporation into food products or supplements, are required to develop this promising research direction.

Fungal Immunomodulatory Proteins (FIPs)

FIPs may be relevant for allergy mitigation, as these proteins were found to be able to inhibit food allergic, as well as respiratory allergic, reactions in mouse models, either applied orally or nasally.

When the FIP from *Flammulina velutipes* (golden needle mushroom; FIP-fve) was fed (at 200 μg/mouse, i.e. ca. 10 $mg.kg^{-1}$, every other day, for details see [55]) to ovalbumin-allergic Balb/c-mice, allergy symptoms, including symptom score, histamine release and intestinal damage, were strongly suppressed. The Th2-dominant phenotype shifted towards a strongly elevated Th1-response (measured in splenocytes) [55]. This indicates potential application in allergy prophylaxis. Liu *et al.* reported that FIP-fve could be applied in local nasal immune therapy, suppressing allergic responses to house dust mite allergy in Balb/c mice [56]. Also in this study the cytokine profile shifted towards a stronger Th1-response.

FIPs are relatively small, ca. 15 kDa, proteins of fungal origin. FIP-fve, and FIPs from *Volvariella volvacea* ((paddy) straw mushroom; FIP-vvo), *Ganoderma lucidum* and *G. tsugae* (Japanese lacquer mushroom; LZ-8 and FIP-gts, resp.) have been described in some detail. These proteins are composed of resp. 114 (FIP-fve), 110 (LZ-8 and FIP-Gts) and 112 (FIP-vvo) amino acids, and share high sequence homology [57]. FIPs showed lectin-like properties, as they are able to agglutinate erythrocytes, and were proposed to be classified as such [59].

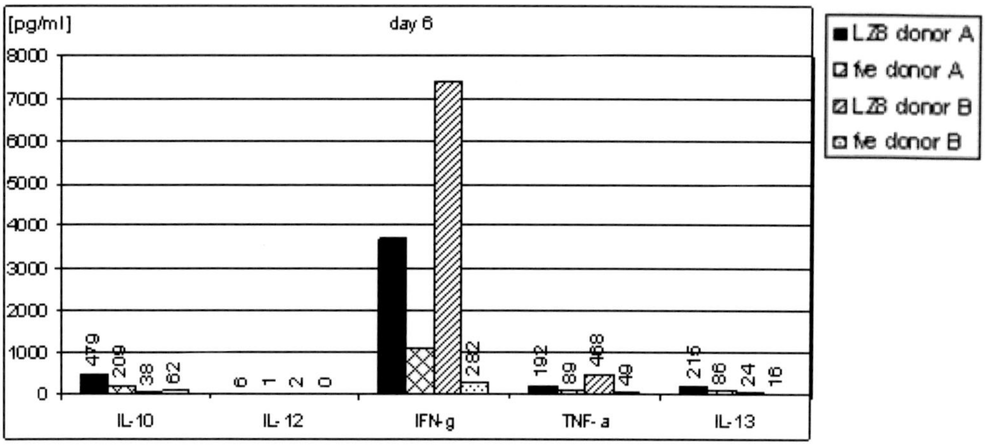

Figure 1. N-terminally His-tagged FIP-LZ8 and FIP-fve were cloned into the pET101/D-TOPO vector, with which E. coli was transfected. PBMC-cultures, prepared as in [62], were cultured in the presence of 25 μg/ml of rec-FIPs, and after 6 days, cytokine production was measured flow cytometrically.

The X-ray structure of FIP-fve indicated this protein to be a homodimer of which each subunit comprises a pair of N-terminal secondary structural elements, an α-helix followed by a β-strand, linked to a domain consisting almost exclusively of β-sheets adopting an Ig-like fold. Percentages of α-helix, ß-strand and loop were resp. 11.3, 42.6 and 46.1 [58, 59]. The α-helices H_A and H_B are amphipathic and the side chains of the amino acids on the hydrophobic face of one helix pack well against those of the other α-helix. This enables binding to each other via hydrophobic interactions, which may be important for immunomodulatory activity (see below). Lin *et al.* [60] predicted that the N-terminal residues 1-13 of FIP-Gts formed an α-helix. Recombinant mutants of FIP-Gts in which residues 1-13 (the N-terminal a-helix) were deleted, were incapable of dimerisation. Triple mutants in which Leu5, Phe7 and Leu9 were deleted no longer possessed the amphipathic character, the ability to form dimers with itself or with the wild type FIP-Gts protein and also lost the ability to induce INF-γ and IL-2 in hPBLs. This suggests that the dimerisation property is important for immunomodulatory activity [59, 60]. With respect to the putative mode of action of FIPs, stimulation of IFN-γ production in human PBMCs via p38-MAPK-activation has been suggested [61]. Own observations [62, and unpublished results] indicated that natural FIPs or heterologously expressed FIPs (in *E. coli*) from *Flammulina* or *Ganoderma* have a moderate, questionably significant, effect on NO-production in RAW 264.7 cells (a murine monocyte cell line). A Th1-skewing effect in human PBMC-cultures from healthy volunteers could be observed (Figure 1).

In the heterologous expression system, the rec-LZ8 was produced as its monomer of approx. 15 kDa, whereas the FIP from *Flammulina* (rec-FIP-fve) occurred as a dimer of ca. 35 kDa in SDS-PAGE gels under denaturing conditions (Figure 2).

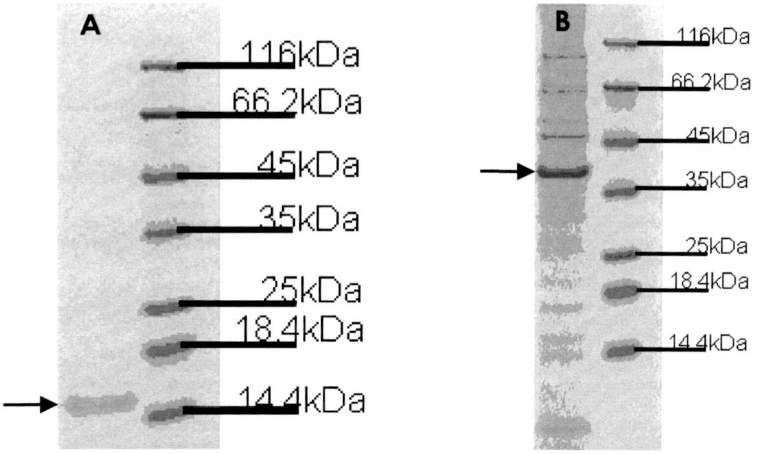

Figure 2. Isolation of FIP-LZ8 (panel A) and FIP-fve (panel B) (arrows) from inclusion bodies that were obtained from transfected E. coli. MW-markers are indicated.

Considering the apparent lower PBMC-stimulatory activity of rec-FIP-fve compared to that of rec-LZ8, it seems as if not only dimerisation is important for activity [60], but also the relative orientation towards each other of the units constituting the homodimer, as the α-helices appear to require a close contact to exert biological activity. The low activity towards NO-production in RAW 264.7 cells suggests that the primary site of action of FIPs may be towards cells from the adaptive immune compartment, particularly Th1-cells as IFN-γ production is most strongly upregulated (Figure 1).

Observations on an immunomodulatory protein from *Auricularia* (Jew's ear) mushroom, a protein that perhaps, but not (yet) confirmed, should also be considered as a FIP, partly corroborated the above findings for the Th1-skewing effect, but not for NO-production in RAW 264.7 cells [63].

FIPs, at the least their biological activities, were found to be relatively resistant towards common food processing conditions, such as freezing, thawing, dehydration, and acid/alkali-conditions [64, 65], which is interesting for their potential application as food or feed additive.

Questions as to their stability and bioactivity when incorporated in products or whether fresh mushroom can have the same effects as purified or recombinantly expressed proteins remain to be answered. Moreover the working mechanism should be further clarified. Recently, Ca^{2+}-transport and PKC-α-activation were proposed to be involved in subcellular activation mechanisms in PBMCs [66]. More animal model and human intervention studies will be required to study its effect *in vivo* and its benefit for specific groups or individuals.

Ω-3 Polyunsaturated Fatty Acids

A number of studies has used animal models to study the effect of ω-3-PUFAs on allergic reactions. Yin *et al.* [67] studied the effects of fish oil supplementation on airway inflammation, in a murine model of allergic inflammation produced by sensitization to ovalbumin. ω-3 Fatty acids were dose dependently built-in into mouse lung tissue after dietary supplementation. Oxidative stress was measured using isoprostane (IsoPs) levels (isomers of cyclooxygenase (COX)-derived prostaglandins). OVA challenge caused a significant increase of F2-IsoPs (from AA) in mouse lung, which suggests an increased level of oxidative stress. The fish oil supplementation group showed a significant decrease of F2-IsoPs and an increase of F3-IsoPs (from EPA) and of F4-IsoPs (from DHA). However, fish oil supplementation led to an increase in the production of proinflammatory cytokine IL-5 and IL-13. Furthermore, fish oil supplementation suppressed the production of PGE2 in the bronchoalveolar lavage [66].

Korotkova *et al.* [68] examined whether maternal intake of dietary fatty acids influences the induction of oral tolerance to OVA in neonatal rats. The results indicate that the dietary ratio of ω-6/ω-3 PUFA is important for the induction of neonatal oral tolerance. It was concluded that non-optimal feeding can have effects on the development of immunological tolerance to dietary antigen ingested by the mother, and that the ratio of ω-6/ω-3 FA in the diet may be relevant in the context of increased prevalence of allergy.

In human clinical trials, supplementing n-3 fatty FA to adults, with recognized allergies and bronchial asthma have so far been disappointing. This might indicate that once allergic immune responses are established, intervention is no longer able to mitigate these [69].

Woods *et al.* conducted a study to assess the influence of food and nutrient intake on asthma risk in young adults. Dietary intake was assessed by means of a validated semi quantitative food-frequency questionnaire. However, no association between fish intake and asthma was found [70].

Schnappinger *et al.* [71] conducted a study to assess the influence of fish consumption on allergic sensitisation and allergic diseases in adults. Allergic sensitisation was described as the presence of elevated serum levels of allergen-specific IgE antibodies, and is proposed to be fundamental to allergic diseases and is therefore considered a potential risk factor for the development of allergic diseases. The results of the study showed that fish and DHA intake are inversely related to allergic sensitisation in adult females, but not in males. No significant association was found between fish and DHA intake and allergic diseases. The gender-related differences in metabolism of PUFAs might be a possible explanation for the fact that a lower rate of allergic sensitisation was only found in women [72].

The immature immune system is still very susceptible to immunomodulatory environmental conditions, particularly in the pre- and postnatal period [73]. Therefore supplementation with anti-inflammatory ω-3 PUFAs during the pre-natal period might provide a non-invasive intervention window to modify immune development before any disease is established [69]. Dunstan et al. [69] performed a randomized double-blind controlled trial to determine whether maternal dietary supplementation with ω-3 PUFAs during pregnancy could alter the immune response in infants. Allergen-specific T-cell responses in cord-blood between fish-oil supplemented and control groups were compared. The fish oil supplementation group showed a significantly higher proportion of total ω-3

PUFAs in neonatal erythrocyte membranes as compared with the control group. At birth babies in the fish oil supplementation group generally had weaker cytokine (IL-5, IL-13, Il-10 and IFN-γ) responses to allergens (house dust mite, ovalbumin, and cat) and mitogens (phytohaemagglutinin) although this was not statistically significant [69].

Kull *et al.* [74] investigated the association between fish consumption during the first year of life and development of allergic diseases by four years of age. Data were obtained from a prospective birth cohort controlling for disease-related modification of exposure. Data on allergic heredity and various exposures were obtained when the infants were newborn by parental questionnaires. Subsequently information on diet, including consumption and time for introduction of fish was collected at 1 year of age. It was concluded that regular fish consumption before the age of 1 appears to be associated with a decreased risk of allergic disease and sensitization to food and inhalant allergens during the first four years of life.

In conclusion, there are some indications that ω-3-PUFA consumption has impacts on the development of allergy symptoms. Although important, it is not so easy to evaluate e.g. levels of ω-3-PUFA consumption in order to show some effect in the mitigation of rheumatic symptoms (3.5-4 g/day) [75], as exposure levels are not always reported unequivocally. A variety of mechanisms for the possible action of ω-3-PUFA on immune functioning has been proposed; for a review, see Kim *et al* [76].

PERSPECTIVES

The option of dietary immunomodulation appears to be feasible and realistic , at the least for the relatively well-defined immune responses such as in allergies. Considering the pivotal role of immune homeostasis in general health, and the very relevant and significant societal and economic perspectives, further pursuing this research avenue seems worthwhile. Some food components appear to exhibit effects on specific immune compartments This offers potential use in a variety of applications, depending on the specifications of underlying chronic processes and characteristics of consumers. Foods can thus play a significant role in fortifying and balancing immune responses.

As it becomes more and more clear that the aetiology and course of a given 'disease' various from person to person, the conclusion appears obvious that also treatments, or supporting dietary measures, should be matched with individual needs. This means that, for immunomodulatory foods, uniform approaches will not be maximally effective. This emphasises the need for more knowledge of individual consumers' responses, and the metabolic parameters that are connected to first signs of derailed homeostasis in order to re-establish this via food based intervention. Together with in-depth knowledge on underlying mechanisms it will pave the way for product development in the near future.

REFERENCES

[1] Bach JF (2002) The effect of infections on susceptibility to autoimmune and allergic diseases. *New Engl. J. Med* 347 911-20.

[2] Strachan DP (1989) Hay fever, hygiene, and household size. *Br. Med. J.* 299(6710) 1259-60.

[3] Rowbotham J, Clayton P (2008) An unsuitable and degraded diet? Part three: Victorian consumption patterns and their health benefits. *J R Soc Med* 101: 454–62.

[4] Von Mutius E, Pearce N, Beasley R, Cheng S, Von Ehrenstein O, Björkstén B, Weiland S (2000) International patterns of tuberculosis and the prevalence of symptoms of asthma, rhinitis, and eczema. *Thorax* 55:449–53.

[5] Coffman RL, Varkila K, Scott P, Chatelain R. (1991) Role of cytokines in the differentiation of CD4+ T-cell subsets in vivo. *Immunol Rev.* 123:189-207.

[6] Kabingu E, Vaughan L, Owczarczak B, Ramsey KD, Gollnick SO (2007) CD8+ T cell-mediated control of distant tumours following local photodynamic therapy is independent of CD4+ T cells and dependent on natural killer cells. *Br. J. Cancer* 96, 1839 – 48.

[7] Valdés-Ramos R, Benítez-Arciniega AD (2007) Nutrition and immunity in cancer. *Br J. Nutr.* 98, Suppl. 1, S127–32.

[8] Oda E. (2008) The metabolic syndrome as a concept of adipose tissue disease. *Hypertens Res.* 31(7):1283-91.

[9] Després JP, Lemieux I (2006) Abdominal obesity and metabolic syndrome. *Nature* 444(7121):881-7.

[10] Wisse BE (2004) The inflammatory syndrome: the role of adipose tissue cytokines in metabolic disorders linked to obesity. *J Am Soc Nephrol.* 15(11):2792-800.

[11] Grange JM, Bottasso O, Stanford CA, Stanford JL (2008) The use of mycobacterial adjuvant-based agents for immunotherapy of cancer. *Vaccine* 26 (2008) 4984–90.

[12] Zhou L-D, Zhang Q-H, Zhang Y, Liu J, Cao Y-M (2009) The shiitake mushroom-derived immuno-stimulant lentinan protects against murine malaria blood-stage infection by evoking adaptive immune-responses. *Int Immunopharmacol* 9(4) 455-62.

[13] Burns EA, Goodwin JS (2004) Effects of aging on immune function. *J. Nutr. Health Ageing* 8(1) 9-18.

[14] Derhovanessian E, Solana R, Larbi A, Pawelec G (2008) Immunity, Ageing and Cancer. *Immunity & Ageing 2008*, 5:11 doi:10.1186/1742-4933-5-11.

[15] Gardner EM, Murasko DM (2002) Age-related changes in Type 1 and Type 2 cytokine production in humans. *Biogerontology* 3: 271–89.

[16] Gorczynski RM, Terzioglu E (2008) Aging and the immune system. *Int Urol Nephrol* 40(4) 1117-25.

[17] Srivastava S, Lundqvist A, Childs R. (2008) Natural killer cell immunotherapy for cancer: a new hope. *Cytotherapy.*10(8):775-83.

[18] Lesourd B. (2004) Nutrition: a major factor influencing immunity in the elderly. *J Nutr Health Aging.* 8(1):28-37.

[19] Keusch GT. (2003) The history of nutrition: malnutrition, infection and immunity. *J Nutr* 133(1):336S-340S.

[20] Pal S, Poddar K (2008) Dietary protein-carbohydrate ratio: exogenous modulator of immune response with age. *Immunobiol* 213: 557-66.

[21] Calder PC (2007) Immunonutrition in surgical and critically ill patients. *Br J Nutr* 98(S1): S133-9.

[22] Fernandes G (2008) Progress in nutritional immunology. *Immunol Res* 40: 244–61.

[23] Harbige LS (1996) Nutrition and imunity with emphasis on infection and autoimmune disease. *Nutr Health* 10: 285-312.

[24] Calder PC, Kew S (2002) The immune system: a target for functional Foods? *Br J Nutr* 88: S165-76.

[25] López-Varela S, González-Gross M, Marcos A (2002) Functional foods and the immune system: a review. *Eur J Clin Nutr* 56(S3): S29-33.

[26] Hoyles L, Vulevic J (2008) Diet, immunity and functional foods. *Adv Exp Med Biol* 635: 79-92.

[27] Bjorksten B, Naaber P, Sepp E, Mikelsaar M (2000) The intestinal microflora in allergic Estonian and Swedish 2-year-old children. *Clin Exp Allergy* 29(3): 342-6.

[28] Bottcher MF, Nordin EF, Sandin A, Midtvedt T, Bjorksten B (2000) Microflora-associated characteristics in faeces from allergic and nonallergic infants. *Clin Exp Allergy* 30(11): 1590-6.

[29] Kalliomäki M, Kirjavainen P, Eerola E, Kero P, Salminen S, Isolauri E. (2001) Distinct patterns of neonatal gut microflora in infants in whom atopy was and was not developing. *J Allergy Clin Immunol.* 107(1):129-34.

[30] Kalliomäki M, Salminen S, Poussa T, Arvilommi H, Isolauri E. (2003) Probiotics and prevention of atopic disease: 4-year follow-up of a randomised placebo-controlled trial. *Lancet* 361(9372):1869-71.

[31] Isolauri E, Arvola T, Sütas Y, Moilanen E, Salminen S. (2000) Probiotics in the management of atopic eczema. *Clin Exp Allergy*. 30(11): 1604-10.

[32] Pessi T, Sütas Y, Hurme M, Isolauri E. (2000) Interleukin-10 generation in atopic children following oral Lactobacillus rhamnosus GG. *Clin Exp Allergy*. 30(12): 1804-8.

[33] Rosenfeldt V, Benfeldt E, Nielsen SD, Michaelsen KF, Jeppesen DL, Valerius NH, Paerregaard A (2003) Effect of probiotic Lactobacillus strains in children with atopic dermatitis. *J Allergy Clin Immunol.* 2003 Feb;111(2): 389-95.

[34] Brouwer ML, Wolt-Plompen SA, Dubois AE, van der Heide S, Jansen DF, Hoijer MA, Kauffman HF, Duiverman EJ (2006) No effects of probiotics on atopic dermatitis in infancy: a randomized placebo-controlled trial. *Clin Exp Allergy*. 36(7): 899-906.

[35] Helin T, Haahtela S, Haahtela T. (2002) No effect of oral treatment with an intestinal bacterial strain, *Lactobacillus rhamnosus* (ATCC 53103), on birch-pollen allergy: a placebo-controlled double-blind study. *Allergy*. 57(3): 243-6.

[36] Kopp MV, Goldstein M, Dietschek A, Sofke J, Heinzmann A, Urbanek R (2008) Lactobacillus GG has in vitro effects on enhanced interleukin-10 and interferon-gamma release of mononuclear cells but no in vivo effects in supplemented mothers and their neonates. *Clin Exp Allergy* 38(4): 602-10.

[37] Vissers YM, Snel J,. Zuurendonk PF, Smit BA, Wichers HJ, Savelkoul HFJ Differential effects of *Lactobacillus acidophilus* and *Lactobacillus plantarum* strains on cytokine induction in human peripheral blood mononuclear cells. *FEMS Immunol Med Microbiol, accepted article, doi: 10.1111/j.1574-695X.2010.00662.x.*

[38] Konstantinov SR, Smidt H, de Vos WM, Bruijns SC, Singh SK, Valence F, Molle D, Lortal S, Altermann E, Klaenhammer TR, van Kooyk Y. (2008) *S layer protein A of Lactobacillus acidophilus NCFM regulates immature dendritic cell and T cell functions.* Proc Natl Acad Sci U S A. 2008 Dec 9;105(49): 19474-9.

[39] Muralikrishna G, Subba Rao MVSST (2007) Cereal Non-Cellulosic Polysaccharides: Structure and Function Relationship—An Overview. *Crit Rev Food Sci Nutr* 47(6): 599-610.

[40] Volman JJ, Ramakers JD, Plat J. (2008) Dietary modulation of immune function by beta-glucans. *Physiol Behav*. 94(2): 276-84.

[41] Kataoka K, Muta T, Yamazaki S, Takeshige K (2002) Activation of macrophages by linear (1→3)-ß-D-glucans. *J Biol Chem* 277(39): 36825-31.

[42] Kimura Y, Sumiyoshi M, Suzuki T, Suzuki T, Sakanaka M (2007) Inhibitory effects of water-soluble low-molecular-weight ß-(1,3–1,6) D-glucan purified from *Aureobasidium pullulans* GM-NH-1A1 strain on food allergic reactions in mice. *Int. Immunopharmacol.* 7: 963–72.

[43] Yamada J, Hamuro J, Hatanaka H, Hamabata K, Kinoshita S (2007) Alleviation of seasonal allergic symptoms with superfine ß-1,3-glucan: A randomized study. *J Allergy Clin Immunol* 119: 1119-26.

[44] Li XM, Zhang TF, Huang CK, Srivastava K, Teper AA, Zhang L, Schofield BH, Sampson HA (2001). Food Allergy Herbal Formula-1 (FAHF-1) blocks peanut-induced anaphylaxis in a murine model. *J Allergy Clin Immunol.* 108: 639-46.

[45] Liu Y-H, Tsai C-F, Kao M-C, Lai Y-L, Tsai JJ (2003) Effectiveness of Dp2 nasal therapy for Dp-2 induced airway inflammation in mice: using oral *Ganoderma lucidum* as an immunomodulator. *J Microbiol Immunol Infect* 36: 236-42.

[46] Tada R, Tanioka A, Iwasawa H, Hatashima K, Shoji Y, Ishibashi K-I, Adachi Y, Yamazaki M, Tsubaki K, Ohno N (2008) Structural characterisation and biological activities of a unique type ß-D-glucan obtained from *Aureobasidium pullulans*. *Glycoconj J* 25(9): 851-61.

[47] Lull-Noguera C, Wichers HJ, Savelkoul HFJ (2005) Anti-inflammatory and immuno-modulating properties of fungal metabolites. *Mediat. Inflamm*. 2005(2): 63-80.

[48] Ikewaki N, Fujii N, Onaka T, Ikewaki S, Inoko H (2007) Immunological actions of Sophy ß-glucan (ß-1,3-1,6 glucan), currently available commercially as a health food supplement. *Microbiol Immunol* 51(9): 861-73.

[49] Meyer-Wentrup F, Cambi A, Adema GJ, Figdor CG (2005) "Sweet Talk": Closing in on C Type Lectin Signaling. *Immunity* 22: 399-400.

[50] Brown GD (2006) Dectin-1: a signalling non-TLR pattern-recognition receptor. *Nature Rev Immunol* 6: 33-43.

[51] Palma AS, Feizi T, Zhang Y, Stoll MS, Lawson AM, Diaz-Rodriguez E, Campanero-Rhodes MA, Costa J, Gordon S, Brown GD, Chai W (2006) Ligands for the ß-Glucan Receptor, Dectin-1, assigned using "designer" microarrays of oligosaccharide probes (neoglycolipids) generated from glucan polysaccharides. *J Biol Chem* 281: 5771–9.

[52] Wang Y, Zhang L, Li Y, Hou X, Zeng F (2004) Correlation of structure to antitumor activities of five derivatives of a ß-glucan from *Poria cocos* sclerotium. *Carb Res* 339: 2567–74.

[53] Brauer D, Kimmons T, Phillips M (2002) Effects of management on the yield and high-molecular-weight polysaccharides content of Shiitake (*Lentinula endodes*) mushrooms. *J. Agric. Food Chem*. 50: 5333-7.

[54] Minato K, Kawakami S, Nomura K, Tsuchida H, Mizuno M (2004) An exo ß-1,3-glucanase synthesized de novo degrades lentinan during storage of *Lentinula edodes*

and diminishes immunomodulating activity of the mushroom. *Carbohydrate Polymers* 56: 279-86.

[55] Hsieh KY, Hsu CI, Lin JY, Tsai CC, Lin RH (2003) Oral administration of an edible-mushroom-derived protein inhibits the development of food-allergic reactions in mice. *Clin Exp Allergy* 33: 1595-602.

[56] Liu Y-H, Kao M-C, Lai Y-L, Tsai J-J (2003) Efficacy of local nasal immunotherapy for Dp2-induced airway inflammation in mice: using Dp2-peptide and fungal immunomodulatory peptide. *J Allergy Clin Immunol* 112(2): 301-10.

[57] Hsu H-C, Hsu C-I, Lin R-H, Kao C-L, Lin J-Y (1997) Fip-vvo, a new fungal immunomodulatory protein isolated from *Volvariella volvacea*. *Biochem J* 323: 557-65.

[58] Seow SV, Kuo I-C, Paaventham P, Kolatkar PR, Chua KY (2003) Crystallisation and preliminary X-ray crystallographic studies on the fungal immunomodulatory protein Fve from the golden needle mushroom (*Flammulina velutipes*). *Acta Crystallog* 59: 1487-9.

[59] Paaventhan P, Jospeh JS, Seow SV, Vaday S, Robinson H, Chua KY, Kolatkar PR (2003) A 1.7Å structure of fve, a member of the new fungal immunomodulatory protein family. *J Mol Biol* 322: 461-70.

[60] Lin WH, Hung CH, Hsu CI, Lin JY (1997) Dimerization of the N-terminal amphiphatic α-helix domain of the fungal immunomodulatory protein from *Ganoderma tsugae* (Fip-gts) defined by a yeast two-hybrid system and site-directed mutagenesis. *J Biol Chem* 272: 20044-8.

[61] Wang PH, Hsu CI, Tang SC, Huang YL, Lin JY, Ko JL (2004) Fungal immunomodulatory protein from *Flammulina velutipes* induces interferon-γ production through p38 mitogen-activated protein kinase signaling pathway. *J Agric Food Chem* 52: 2721-5.

[62] Jeurink PV, Lull-Noguera C, Savelkoul HFJ, Wichers HJ (2008) Immunomodulatory capacity of fungal proteins on the cytokine production of human peripheral blood mononuclear cells. *Int. Immunopharmacol*. 8(8): 1124-33.

[63] Sheu F, Chien P-J, Chien A-L, Chen Y-F, Chin K-L (2004) Isolation and characterization of an immunomodulatory protein (APP) from the Jew's Ear mushroom *Auricularia polytricha*. *Food Chem* 87(4): 593-600.

[64] Chang H-H, Chien P-J, Tong M-H, Sheu F (2007) Mushroom immunomodulatory proteins possess potential thermal/freezing resistance, acid/alkali tolerance and dehydration stability. *Food Chem* 105: 597–605.

[65] Tong M-H, Chien P-J, Chang H-H, Tsai M-J, Sheu F (2008) High processing tolerances of immunomodulatory proteins in Enoki and Reishi mushrooms. *J Agric Food Chem* 56: 3160–6.

[66] Ou C-C , Hsiao Y-M, Wu W-J,. Tasy G-J, Ko J-L, Lin M-Y (2009) FIP-fve stimulates interferon-gamma production via modulation of calcium release and PKC-α activation. *J Agric Food Chem* 57: 11008–13.

[67] Yin H, Liu W, Goleniewska K, Porter NA, Morrow JD, Peebles RS Jr (2009) Dietary supplementation of [omega]-3 fatty acid-containing fish oil suppresses F2-isoprostanes but enhances inflammatory cytokine response in a mouse model of ovalbumin-induced allergic lung inflammation. *Free Radical Biol Med* 47: 622-8.

[68] Korotkova M, Telemo E, Yamashiro Y, Hanson LA, Strandvik B (2004) The ratio of n-6 to n-3 fatty acids in maternal diet influences the induction of neonatal immunological tolerance to ovalbumin. *Clin Exp Immunol* 137: 237-44.

[69] Dunstan JA, Mori TA, Barden A, Beilin LJ, Taylor AL, Holt PG, Prescott SL (2003) Fish oil supplementation in pregnancy modifies neonatal allergen-specific immune responses and clinical outcomes in infants at high risk of atopy: A randomized, controlled trial. *J Allergy Clin Immunol* 112: 1178-84.

[70] Woods RK, Walters EH, Raven JM, Wolfe R, Ireland PD, Thien FC, Abramson MJ (2003) Food and nutrient intakes and asthma risk in young adults. *Am J Clin Nutr* 78: 414.

[71] Laan MP, Baert MR, Bijl AM, Vredendaal AE, De Waard-van der Spek FB, Oranje AP, Savelkoul HF, Neijens HJ (2000) Markers for early sensitization and inflammation in relation to clinical manifestations of atopic disease up to 2 years of age in 133 high-risk children. *Clin Exp Allergy* 30: 944-53.

[72] Schnappinger M, Sausenthaler S, Linseisen J, Hauner H, Heinrich J (2009) Fish Consumption, Allergic Sensitisation and Allergic Diseases in Adults. *Ann Nutr Metab* 54: 67-74.

[73] Blümer N, Renz H (2007) Consumption of 3-fatty acids during perinatal life: role in immuno-modulation and allergy prevention. *J Perinatal Med* 35: 12-8.

[74] Kull I, Bergström A, Lilja G, Pershagen G, Wickman M (2006) Fish consumption during the first year of life and development of allergic diseases during childhood. *Allergy* 61:1009-15.

[75] Galli C, Calder PC (2009) Effects of fat and fatty acid intake on inflammatory and immune responses: a critical review. *Ann Nutr Metab* 55: 123-39.

[76] Kim W, Khan NA, McMurray DN, Prior IA, Wang N, Chapkin RS (2010) Regulatory activity of polyunsaturated fatty acids in T-cell signaling. *Prog Lipid Res doi:* 10.1016/j.plipress.2010.01.002.

In: Food Allergies: Symptoms, Diagnosis, and Treatment ISBN: 978-1-61728-748-0
Editors: Patricia M. Rodgers

Chapter 4

PATHOPHYSIOLOGY AND MECHANISMS OF FOOD ALLERGY

Patricia Olaya Paschoal
Centro Universitário Plínio Leite/ Universidade de São Paulo
Gerlinde Teixeira – Universidade Federal Fluminense

ABSTRACT

Food allergy, whose symptoms may vary widely from one patient to the other, has a wide prevalence, affecting 6% of children and 3 to 4% of adults (Benhamou, 2009; Simpson, 2008). It has a potential impact on family life and the accidental contact to food allergens is a latent risk for sudden and life-threatening reactions (Burks, 2008). To our knowledge, the best form of treatment is still food avoidance, which can further reduce quality of life for patients and their families. It is important for all health professionals working with these patients to gain understanding of the mechanisms of this disease, and thus diminish the difficulty in establishing the diagnosis.

In normal conditions, the physiological access of dietary macromolecules into the organism through the gut mucosa generally induces a phenomenon called oral tolerance (OT) in which the immunological reactions are mediated by regulatory lymphocytes in a non inflammatory milieu (Burks, 2008). On the other hand, the ingestion of food proteins may also result in abnormal responses, leading to immunological consequences such as food allergy and inflammatory gut reactions (Benhamou, 2009). Food allergies, characterized both by humoral and cellular mechanisms, are reactions initiated by immunological mechanisms and should be called food hypersensitivity. In many cases the immunological reaction is mediated by IgE - typified as a Th2 response - which accounts for most of the acute reactions that are not restricted to the gut. The cases in which the main mechanisms involve IgG and cellular reactions - typified as Th1 responses - the symptoms tend to be chronic and are frequently restricted to the gut (Eigenmann, 2009).

Accidental exposure remains a serious problem for individuals who are allergic to specific food allergens. Patients with severe forms of food allergy must not only be alert to situations in which exposure is possible but must also be prepared to treat reactions when they occur. This is particularly important when the individual has little control over their surroundings or cannot request medical attention (Comstock, 2008).

Food allergies have increased over the past decade and are an important problem in daily clinical practice. Adverse reactions to food may result in a large number of clinical signs involving skin, circulatory system, and the gastrointestinal tract. Food allergies can also lead to fatal final consequences such as hypotension an anaphylaxis. The diagnosis relies on a detailed history, an elimination diet, skin tests, laboratory tests, and food challenges. The basis of the food allergy treatment is the elimination diet.

INTRODUCTION

Regulation of the Immune Response by Mucosal Presentation of Antigen

The lumen of the gastrointestinal tract is daily exposed to a vast assortment of dietary proteins, of which an important part is absorbed in an immunologically significant manner. The fact that the majority of the population has lifelong clinical and immunological tolerance both to food antigens and to their gut flora demonstrates the effectiveness of the default or physiological immune response to food antigens. On the other hand, the entry of pathogenic bacteria or viruses in the gut leads to moderate to severe inflammatory reactions. Thus, the Gut Associated Lymphoid Tissue (GALT) has to balance between either tolerance to commensal bacteria and food antigens or protective (inflammatory) immune responses that are induced upon encounter of intestinal pathogens and toxins (Worbs, 2006).

Oral tolerance has long been used as a strategy for preventing allergic reactions. In 1829, Dakin reported that certain Native American populations ate poison ivy leaves to avoid contact hypersensitivity reaction in subsequent encounters to the plant. In classic experiments Besredka (1909) and Wells (1911) found that animals which were repeatedly fed milk or hen egg protein (Ovalbumin) were protected from anaphylaxis when injected with the protein. More recently, the molecular and cellular basis of oral tolerance has been extensively studied. The unique propensity of the intestinal immune system to evoke tolerance to orally administrated antigens offers attractive strategies to either prevent or treat autoimmune diseases (Worbs, 2006).

Although oral tolerance has been known for more than a century, the mechanisms of its induction have not been fully elucidated yet. Plausible mechanisms responsible for tolerance to orally administered antigens are either anergy or deletion of antigen-specific effector T cells, or the local generation of regulatory T cells (Treg) by GALT antigen-presenting cells (APC) (Park, 2008). These mechanisms are not mutually exclusive and more than one mechanism may be operative with the same protein. It is generally accepted that specialized professional APC located at strategic places in the gut are responsible for oral tolerance induction, especially those comprising mesenteric lymph nodes, lamina propria, Peyer's patches and mucosal epithelium. Among APCs, dendritic cells (DC's) are the ones that play a critical role. The microenvironment at the time of antigen uptake, the state of maturation or activation, and the cytokine profiles play a decisive role in determining immunity or tolerance (Kelsall, 2005). A subset of DC's that increase in number in Peyer's patches during the induction of tolerance is composed of CD11c+CD11b+ cells, and these suppress T-cell proliferation and induce CD4+CD25+ regulatory T cells. On the other hand, CD11c+CD8α+ DCs, which are predominant in inflammatory environments, promote T-cell proliferation (Min, 2006).

Treg's are crucial regulators of peripheral self-tolerance. They suppress the effector functions not only through the secretion of soluble mediators, such as transforming growth factor-β (TGF-β) and interleukin-10 (IL-10), but also through a cell-contact dependent manner involving monocytes / macrophages, T and B cells (Roncarolo, 2007). Treg's are generated by both central – in the thymus - and peripheral – in the secondary lymphoid tissues – mechanisms. Central tolerance occurs during lymphocyte maturation upon confrontation with self-antigens, and peripheral tolerance occurs under specific conditions involving antigen presentation in the absence of co-stimulation (Lee, 2007).

Several factors including antigen properties, route of exposure, genetics, and the age of the host contribute to the development of oral tolerance. In general, soluble antigens are more tolerogenic than particulate antigen. Yet paradoxically, most food allergens are soluble proteins (Burks, 2008). An increase in the incidence of adverse reactions to ingested foods, which may reflect a failure of oral tolerance induction or a breakdown of its maintenance, has been shown by epidemiological studies (Strachan, 2000).

It has been proposed that one of the determining factors in the induction of oral tolerance is due to the dose of ingested antigen (Ag). Lower doses of antigen favor active suppression, whereas higher doses favor anergy and T-cell depletion. In low-dose oral tolerance, Ag reactive CD4+ T-cells secrete regulatory cytokines such as TGF-β, IL-10 and IL-4, characteristic of Treg's, which not only suppress Ag-specific responses, but also mediate bystander suppression (Hyun, 2006).

A break in the mechanisms of induction or in the maintenance of oral tolerance taking place in the gut may result in an allergy type sensitization. In these patients, a small amount of the large load of potential food allergens may not only result in food allergies mediated by immunoglobulin E (IgE), but also through mechanisms which include eosinophil-driven disease and T-cell-mediated inflammation (Eigenmann, 2009). Furthermore, the understanding of oral immune tolerance and the results of some epidemiological studies are seriously demanding us thorough reconsideration concerning both the pathogenesis and our current policy to prevent or manage food allergy (Kurihara, 2010).

A question that rises is: What is the relative importance of antigenicity of food proteins and of the timing of the introduction of novel proteins in the gut? To address this question, we proposed an experimental protocol based on Teixeira's food allergy model (2009), in which animals received a systemic immunization with peanut protein extract (PPE) prior to a challenge diet containing exclusively raw peanuts (Paschoal 2009). Teixeira demonstrated that when animals are immunized to PPE and then eat the raw seeds they develop an inflammatory reaction of the gut that is time dependent (Teixeira 2009). To determine if the status of the gut influences the induction of oral tolerance or systemic sensitization, animals received sweetened egg white to drink ad libitum prior to or during exposure to the challenge diet. Our results demonstrate that OT was developed when ovalbumin was administrated to mice sensitized to peanuts before the induction of gut inflammation due to the exposure to a challenge diet containing the specific antigen. In contrast, a shift to systemic immunization was observed when the introduction of the novel protein occurred concomitantly to the introduction of the challenge diet in sensitized animals, which induces acute or chronic inflammation (Paschoal, 2009). Thus, although we believe that food antigenicity is important, the status of the gut upon receiving a novel protein is also determining in the outcome of the immune response.

FOOD PROTEINS

Most food proteins reaching the gut mucosa are already partially digested by proteases as well as by gastric acidity. It has been suspected that reduced gastric acidity plays an important role in the pathogenesis of food allergy as is seen in young infants, and in the use of proton pump inhibitors in the adult population (Moreno, 2007). Resistance of proteins to pepsin digestion has been proposed as a marker for potential allergenicity as it does not appear to be a characteristic shared by many food allergens. Thus, resistance to pepsin digestion using a simulated gastric fluid (SGF) has been included as criteria for the allergenicity assessment of novel proteins (Moreno, 2007).

During lifetime, great quantities of nutrients including potentially allergenic food proteins are processed through the gut. The mucus on the surface of the gut epithelial cells is an important barrier among the mechanisms regulating the absorption of food antigens into the sub-mucosa. It also plays a major role as a barrier to potential foreign antigens. This protection is reduced in the first weeks of life, as mucin is only present in low amounts in the newborn (Eigenmann, 2009). Although any food can cause an allergic reaction, only few of them such as peanuts, milk, eggs, tree nuts, fish, shellfish and wheat are responsible for the great majority of the symptoms (Cianferoni, 2009).

Regional dietary habits and methods of food preparation clearly play a role in the prevalence of specific food allergies in various countries around the world. Ingested dietary proteins when degraded by gastric acidity and luminal digestive enzymes lose conformational epitopes, which are often destroyed resulting in the diminishing of immunogenicity (Burks, 2008). Proteins that are not digested and processed in the lumen of the gut can contact both the epithelium and the cells of the mucosal immune system beneath it in various manners by cells such as, dendritic cells and M cells. The former sample antigens by extending processes through the epithelium and into the lumen; the latter, which overlie the Peyer's patches, take up particulate antigens and deliver them to subepithelial dendritic cells (Burks, 2008).

Food allergens are put into two categories, class 1 and class 2. Antigens identified as class 1 allergens are water-soluble glycoproteins, 10 to 60 kilo-Dalton in size and presumably comprised of sequential epitopes which are stable to heat, acid, and proteases. Although class 1 proteins are heat stable, cooking can either reduce or increase the allergenicity of certain food proteins of this class. Heating can increase the allergenicity through the induction of covalent modifications that lead to new antigens or improve stability of the proteins. Examples of class 1 antigens are peanuts, egg white, and cow's milk. On the other hand, as class 2 food allergens are comprised of conformational epitopes, they are highly heat labile, susceptible to enzymatic degradation and difficult to isolate. An example of a class 2 allergen is the birch pollen Bet v1. This allergen can induce sensitization through the respiratory tract and may result in the induction oral pruritus to homologous class 2 allergens present in raw apples (Mal d 1) or in carrots (Dau c 1) (Mansueto, 2006).

Microbiota

The increasing prevalence in the susceptibility to allergy has been linked to a concomitant reduction in childhood infectious diseases (the hygiene hypothesis). The relationship between microbes and allergy is of particular interest in the digestive tract, which is colonized by commensal bacteria that might also influence the mucosal immune response (Bashir, 2004). Gut microbiota is largely established in the first 24 hours after birth and is dependent on maternal microbiota and the local environment.

As mentioned before, the intestine is subjected to a constant flow of stimuli from microbiota, food and pathogens. Despite this constant antigenic challenge, the mucosal tissue lining the intestinal tract remains largely under control. Thus, another question that can be proposed is: Why does the microbiota mainly induce a tolerogenic response in the gut if it is composed of bacteria which present a similar profile of proteins that are able to stimulate a Th1 response? Mechanisms regulating the homeostatic balance in the gut have been investigated for many years by several groups, but the precise nature of the regulatory control still remains unclear (Arnett, 2010). This ambiguity has been put forward by different authors such as Mansueto (2006) who proposed that gut microbiota might enhance a Th1 cytokine response with secretion of interferon-γ (IFN-γ). On the other hand, Bashir (2004) argues that the Th2/Treg cell-dominant tone of the gut-associated lymphoid tissue (GALT) is shaped, in part, by antigenic stimulation by the luminal bacteria, and it protects against the development of intestinal inflammation.

The innate immune system's initial response to microorganisms involves the detection of broad microbial "signatures" by pattern recognition molecules such as Toll-like receptors (TLRs), and influences the nature of the subsequent adaptive response (Bashir, 2004). Probiotic therapy appears to alleviate allergic inflammation demonstrated by the control of clinical symptoms and reduction of local and systemic inflammatory markers. Based on experimental data, the mechanisms behind these outcomes may involve enhanced antigen elimination and down regulated inflammatory responses via direct effects on the immune system, as well as effects seen as modified degradation, permeation, and presentation of food antigens. The mechanisms of the probiotic action may be mediated via effects on the microbial composition and metabolic activity of the microbiota (Kirjavainen, 2002).

Dendritic cells in peripheral lymphoid organs were initially considered to be terminally differentiated, nondividing cells with a short half-life (Liu, 2007). It is now known that these cells are more dynamic, being able to expand in the periphery, and are involved in pushing T cells towards, either a tolerogenic state or an inflammatory immune response. Moreover, mucosal dendritic cells, residing either in the Peyer's patches or in the lamina propria of the intestine, appear to preferentially produce IL-10 rather than IL-12, and in particular have long been thought to promote tolerance in the gut. Expanding dendritic cells, including those present in the intestinal tissues, promote the ability to induce oral tolerance (Arnett, 2010).

Interleukin-10 (IL-10) is a cytokine originally identified by its ability to suppress the differentiation of Th1 cells through binding to its heterodimeric receptor, composed of the IL-10R1 and the IL-10R2 chains. IL-10 can be produced by a variety of hematopoietic cells including regulatory T cells, and is capable of profoundly inhibiting the effector function of a variety of activated cells. Mainly Th1 cells, macrophages, monocytes, and dendritic cells are affected by IL-10, whose effects are typically considered "anti-inflammatory", given that IL-10 has the ability to counter regulate interferon γ and other cytokines (Arnett, 2010).

Lymphocytes expressing IL-10 are found in the intestine of both immature and mature mice, suggesting that IL-10 may play a role in preventing activation of T cells in response to self and foreign antigens in the normal intestine (Arnett, 2010). One of the tolerogenic factors that mucosal dendritic cells appear to produce is indoleamine 2,3-dioxygenase (IDO), which is also produced by various tumor cells, and some alternatively activated macrophages, thus potently induced by IFNγ as well as TNFα, IL-12, IL-18, and CTLA-4:B7 signaling. IDO is an enzyme with an immunomodulatory function (Fig 1) and its immunosuppressive capability stems from its function as the initial and rate-limiting enzyme responsible for the breakdown of tryptophan with a concomitant build-up of several metabolites, referred to as kynurenines (Arnett, 2010).

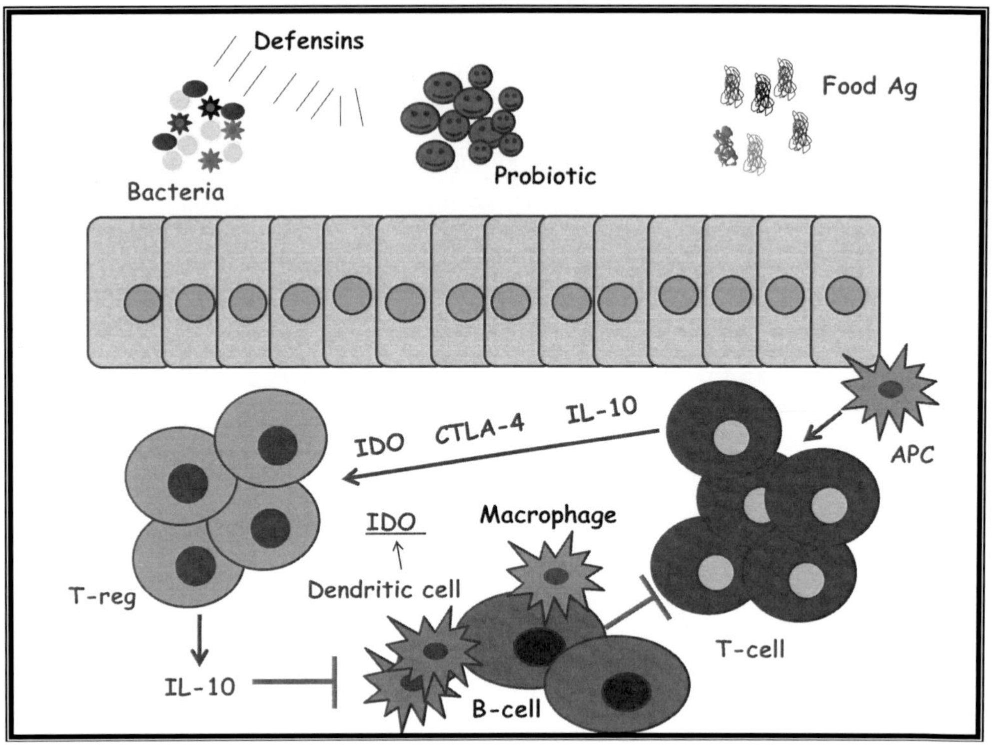

Figure 1. Mechanisms of negative regulation of intestinal inflammation.

The recent development in novel approaches in treating food allergies, which attempt to elicit a decreased Th2-like response and induce tolerance by the immune system in response to a specific food allergens, include peptide immunotherapy, traditional Chinese medicine, mutated or homologous protein immunotherapy, DNA immunization and immunization with immunostimulatory sequences (Li, 2009). Other approaches, such as the anti-IgE therapy, aim at preventing the release of mediators by mast cells. It is the combination of these different approaches that would probably offer the best treatment option for food-allergic patients in a not too distant future. Various options for the treatment of food allergy have been explored using allergens. These methods are being primarily developed for the treatment of respiratory allergies, and some may be potentially applied to the treatment of food allergies (Rancé, 2009).

PATHOPHYSIOLOGY AND MECHANISMS

If the tolerogenic balance in the intestine is lost, intestinal diseases may manifest. Adverse reactions to food, a broad term representing any abnormal clinical response associated with food ingestion can be further classified as food intolerance or food allergy based on the pathophysiological mechanism of the reaction. Allergic reactions can be caused by either IgE- or non-IgE-mediated mechanisms (Fig 2). Other consequences can be inflammatory bowel diseases (IBD), such as Crohn's disease (CD) or ulcerative colitis (UC) (Berin, 2009; Cianferoni, 2009)

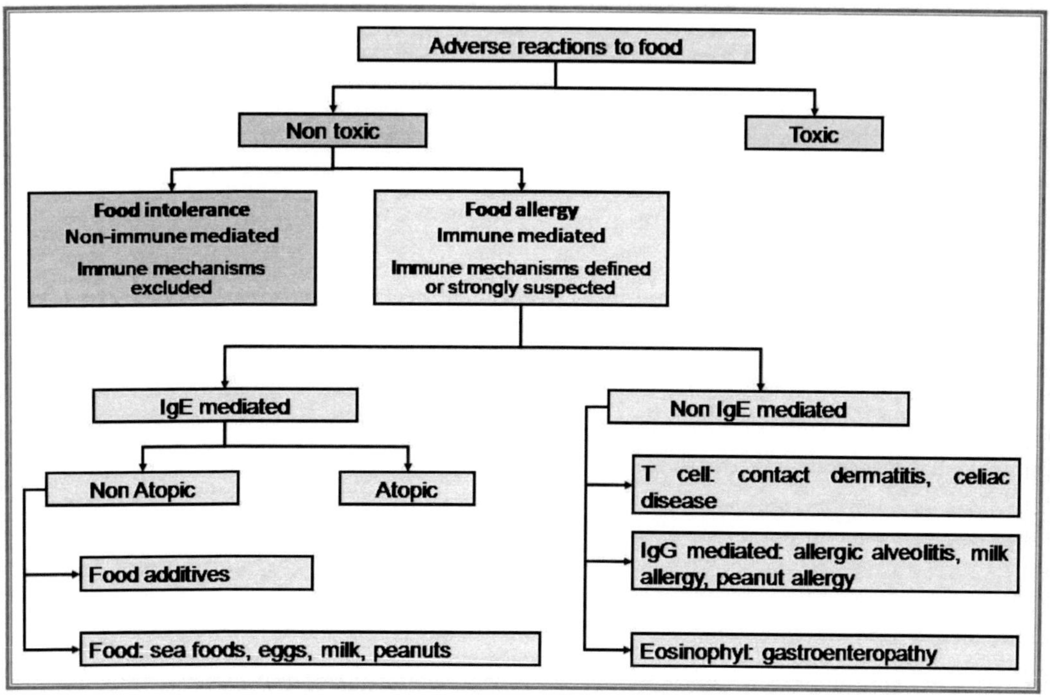

Figure 2. A possible classification tree of adverse reaction to food.

Food intolerance is defined as an adverse reaction to food for which no immunological mechanism has been demonstrated or suspected. Food intolerance can affect any system of the body. The most common symptoms include: irritable bowel, headaches, migraines, fatigue, behavioral problems, or urticaria. Asthma symptoms can also be triggered in some patients, and occasionally anaphylactoid reactions occur. Reactions are dose dependent and tend to be delayed (hours to days), making it difficult to identify the cause (Hodge, 2009). Food chemicals implicated include artificial food colors, preservatives, flavor enhancers, glutamates, vasoactive amines and salicylates (Hodge, 2009).

Typically an IgE-mediated allergy occurs when antigens activate a Th2 response with the secretion of cytokines that, acting upon B lymphocytes, induce a switch in immunoglobulin secretion to IgE. These antibodies bind to mast cells that, upon antigen cross-linking of at least 2 IgE molecules, degranulate releasing potent inflammatory mediators such as histamine and other vasoactive peptides, resulting in an immediate allergic reaction (Cianferoni, 2009).

Non-IgE-mediated allergic reactions are less well characterized and represent an increasing set of immunologic reactions to food. This group of allergies is likely to be multifactorial, which occurs in the absence of demonstrable food-specific IgE antibody in the skin or the serum. The pathophysiological mechanisms include the direct stimulation of T cells by the specific proteins and IgA and/or IgG immune complexes (antibodies bound to the food antigens) (Comstock, 2008). Typically, this type of allergy evolves in the presence of acute or chronic inflammation in the gastrointestinal tract, where eosinophils and T cells seem to play a major role. TNF-α appears to play an important part in the pathogenesis of food protein-induced enterocolitis, as has been shown by it's in vitro obtainment from the peripheral blood monocytes in infants with this syndrome (Cianferoni, 2009).

The presence of a single allergic disorder significantly increases the risk of developing other allergic disorders which can affect different organ systems (Simpson, 2008). An initial exposure to the food antigen by APC in this context may prime naive T cells into Th2 type response with secretion of interleukin (IL)-4 and IL-13. These two cytokines initiate class-switching towards an 'allergy phenotype' and will facilitate food-specific IgE production by plasmocytes. Circulating IgE will then bind to the Fcε RI receptor on mast cells present in potential target organs (Eigenmann, 2009).

Regulatory T cells suppress immune responses through soluble and / or cell surface–associated downregulatory cytokines such as IL-4, IL-10, and TGF-β. Suppression can also be carried out by either CD8+ cells or CD4+ cells. Antigen-specific regulatory cells migrate to both lymphoid and target organs. In the former, they inhibit the generation of effector cells, while in the latter they release cytokines that are not antigen-specific. Defects in regulatory T-cell activity likely contribute to the development of food allergy. CD41CD25 regulatory T cells mediate suppression through cell surface–bound TGF-β, although the suppressor function can possibly occur independently of TGF-β. CD41CD25 cells express the transcription factor forkhead box P3 (FOXP3), which is thought to help block Th1 and Th2 responses (Burks, 2008).

Prevalence of food allergy varies with age, and clinical onset is usually in the first year of life. It is often due to the first introduction of a food substituting maternal milk and is strongly associated with atopic eczema. Multiple food allergies are frequently involved in children but at the age of 5, the norm is being allergic to only one or two foods (Hodge, 2009). Most children outgrow milk, egg, soy and wheat allergies before they get to school age. In contrast, allergy to peanut, tree nuts, and fish typically persist to adulthood. However, if acquired early and with lower levels of specific IgE and less severe symptoms, it may remit in a minority (Zeiger, 2003; Hodge, 2009).

The basic feature of immediate type symptoms in general is the production of food-specific IgE. This type of food allergy may be confirmed by positive skin prick tests specific to peanuts, hen's egg white and cow's milk, in combination with a suggestive history. Proof of sensitization by in vitro techniques itself, without provocation is not diagnostic of food allergy, which should be based on a convincing history of allergic reactions or on the result of an oral food challenge test (Ito, 2009; Bidat, 2009).

Oral Allergy Syndrome

Oral allergy syndrome (OAS) is a condition characterized by IgE-mediated immediate allergic symptoms restricted to the oral mucosa, which may involve itching, stinging pain, and vascular edema of the lips, tongue, palate, and pharynx with a sudden onset, occasionally accompanied by itching of the ear and feeling of tightness of the throat. Usually, these symptoms gradually resolve. A typical example of OAS is oral mucosal symptoms that appear when a patient with birch pollen allergy eats a food of the Rosaceae family (apple, cherry, peach, etc.) (Kondo, 2009).

Conclusion

During lifetime, great quantities of nutrients including potentially allergenic food proteins are in contact with the immune system through the gut. However, the majority of the population has lifelong clinical and immunological tolerance both to food antigens and to their gut flora. When the effectiveness of the default or physiological immune response to food antigens is broken the clinical consequence is food allergy. The understanding of food allergy mechanisms is very important for a better quality of life for both patients and their families. Oral immunotherapy or induction of tolerance by oral route in food allergies seems a hopeful approach and patients could be free from persistent anxiety of sudden and serious symptoms. More studies are necessary to elucidate the underlying mechanisms and to begin safer and securer clinical methods urgently. Up to our knowledge the best approach to circumvent clinical symptoms of food allergy is still food avoidance.

References

Arnett, HA; Viney, JL. Gatekeepers of intestinal inflammation *Inflamm Res,* 2010;59(1):1-14

Bashir, MEH; Louie, S; Shi, HN; Anderson, CN. Toll-Like Receptor 4 Signaling by Intestinal Microbes Influences Susceptibility to Food Allergy. *The Journal of Immunology*, 2004,172: 6978–6987.

Benhamou, AH; Tempia, MGS; Belli, DC; Eigenmann, PA. An overview of cow's milk allergy in children *Swiss Med Wkly*, 2 0 0 9;13 9(2 1-2 2) :3 0 0-3 0 7.

Berin, MC; Mayer, L. Immunophysiology of experimental food allergy. *Mucosal Immunol,* 2009;Jan;2(1):24-32.

Besredka, A. "De. Sexiéme memoire de l'anaphylaxie latique." *Ann. Inst. Pasteur Lille*, 1909; 23: 166.

Bidat, E. Bilan allergologique d'allergie alimentaire. Archives de pédiatrie, 2009;16:65-72.

Burks, AW; Laubach, S; Jones, SM. Oral tolerance, food allergy, and immunotherapy: Implications for future treatment. *J Allergy Clin Immunol*, 2008;121:1344-50.

Cianferoni, A; Spergel, JM. Food Allergy: Review, Classification and Diagnosis. *Allergology International,* 2009;58:457-466.

Comstock, SS; DeMera, R; Vega, LC; Boren, EJ; Deane, S; Haapanen, LA D; Teuber, SS. Allergic reactions to peanuts, tree nuts, and seeds aboard commercial airliners. *Ann Allergy Asthma Immunol*, 2008;101:51–56.

Eigenmann PA. Mechanisms of food allergy. *Pediatr Allergy Immunol*, 2009. 20: 5-11.

Hodge, L; Swain, A; Faulkner-Hogg, K. *Food allergy and intolerance*. Australian Family Physician, 2009;Vol. 38, No. 9.

Hyun, JG; Barrett, TA. Oral Tolerance Therapy in Inflammatory Bowel Disease. *Am J Gastroenterol*, 2006;101:569–571.

Ito, K; Urisu, A. Diagnosis of Food Allergy Based on Oral Food Challenge Test. *Allergology International*, 2009;58:467-474.

Kelsall, BL; Leon, F. Involvement of intestinal dendritic cells in oral tolerance, immunity to pathogens, and inflammatory bowel disease. *Immunol Rev*, 2005; Aug;206:132-48.

Kirjavainen, PV; Arvola, T; Salminen SJ; Isolauri, E. Aberrant composition of gut microbiota of allergic infants: a target of bifidobacterial therapy at weaning? *Gut*, 2002;51:51–55.

Kondo, Y; Urisu, A. Oral Allergy Syndrome. *Allergology International*, 2009;58:485-491.

Kurihara, K. Immunotherapy for Food Allergy. *Allergology International*, 2010;59 in press.

Lee, JW; Epardaud, M; Sun, J; Becker, JE; Cheng, AC; Yonekura, AR; Heath, JK; Turley, SJ. Peripheral antigen display by lymph node stroma promotes T cell tolerance to intestinal self. *Nat Immunol*, 2007;Feb;8(2):181-90.

Li, XM; Brown, L. Efficacy and mechanisms of action of traditional Chinese medicines for treating asthma and allergy. *J Allergy Clin Immunol*, 2009; 123(2): 297–308.

Liu, K; Waskow, C; Liu, X; Yao, K; Hoh, J; Nussenzweig, M. Origin of dendritic cells in peripheral lymphoid organs of mice. *Nature Immunology*, 2007; VOL 8(6): 578-583

Mansueto, P; Montalto, G; Pacor, ML; Esposito-Pellitteri, M; Ditta, V; Bianco, CL; Leto-Barone, Stefania MG; Lorenzo, D. Food allergy in gastroenterologic diseases: Review of literature. *World J Gastroenterol*, 2006 December 28; 12(48): 7744-7752.

Min, SY; Park, KS; Cho, ML; Kang, JW; Cho, YG; Hwang, SY; Park, MJ; Yoon, CH; Min, JK; Lee, SH; Park, SH; Kim, HY. Antigen-induced, tolerogenic $CD11c^+$,$CD11b^+$ dendritic cells are abundant in Peyer's patches during the induction of oral tolerance to type II collagen and suppress experimental collagen-induced arthritis. *Arthritis Rheum,* 2006; Mar;54(3):887-98.

Moreno, FJ. Gastrointestinal digestion of food allergens: Effect on their allergenicity. *Biomedicine & Pharmacotherapy*, 2007; 61:50-60.

Park, MJ; Min, SY; Park, KS; Cho, YG; Cho, ML; Jung, YO; Park, HS; Chang, SH; Cho, SG; Min, JK; Park, SH; Kim, HY. Indoleamine 2,3-dioxygenase-expressing dendritic cells are involved in the generation of CD4+CD25+ regulatory T cells in Peyer's patches in an orally tolerized, collagen-induced arthritis mouse model. *Arthritis Res The,* 2008;10-11.

Paschoal, PO; Campos, SMN; Pedruzzi, MMB; Garrido, V; Bisso, M; Antunes, DMF; Nobrega, AF; Teixeira, G. Food allergy/hypersensitivity: Antigenicity or timing? *Immunobiology*, 2009; 214: 269–278.

Rancé, F. Novel *Approaches in Treating Food Allergy Using Allergens*. Microbial–Host Interaction: Tolerance versus Allergy. Nestlé Nutr Inst Workshop Ser Pediatr Program, 2009vol 64, pp 157–167, Nestec Ltd., Vevey/S. Karger AG, Basel, ©.

Roncarolo, MG; Battaglia, M. Regulatory T-cell immunotherapy for tolerance to self antigens and alloantigens in humans. *Nat Rev Immunol*, 2007; Aug;7(8):585-98.

Simpson, CR; Newton, J; Hippisley-Cox, J; Sheikh, A. Incidence and prevalence of multiple allergic disorders recorded in a national primary care database *J R Soc Med*, 2008: 101: 558–563.

Strachan, DP. Family size, infection and atopy: the first decade of the 'hygiene hypothesis'. *Thorax*, 2000;**55** (Suppl. 1):S2–10.

Teixeira, G; Antunes, D; Castro Júnior, A; Costa, J; Paschoal, PO; Campos, S; Pedruzzi, M; Araújo, V; Andrade, LA; Moreno, S; Nobrega, AF; Cardoso, GP. Induction of an Antigen Specific Gut Inflammatory Reaction in Mice and Rats: A Model for Human Inflammatory Bowel Disease. *Brazilian Archieves of Biology and Technology*, 2009;52(3):601-609.

Wells, HG. "Studies on the chemistry of anaphylaxis. III - Experiments with isolated proteins, experimentally those of hen's egg." *J. Infect. Dis,* 1911;8: 147-156.

Worbs, T; Bode, U; Yan, S; Hoff mann, MW; Hintzen, G; Bernhardt, G; Förster, R; Pabst, O. Oral tolerance originates in the intestinal immune system and relies on antigen carriage by dendritic cells. *The Journal of experimental medicine*, 2006Vol. 203, No. 3, March 20, 519–527.

Zeiger, RS. Food Allergen Avoidance in the Prevention of Food Allergy in Infants and Children. *Pediatrics*, 2003;111:1662-1671.

In: Food Allergies: Symptoms, Diagnosis, and Treatment
Editor: Patricia M. Rodgers
ISBN: 978-1-61728-748-0

Chapter 5

In Search of a More Comprehensive Allergy Diagnostic: Assessment of the Total-Body IgE Pool

***Eleonora Dehlink*[*1,2] *and Edda Fiebiger*[≠1]**

[1]Division of Gastroenterology and Nutrition, Children's Hospital Boston, Harvard Medical School, Boston, MA
[2]Department of Pediatrics and Adolescent Medicine, Medical University of Vienna, Vienna, Austria

Abstract

Allergic disorders have been a rising health problem in Western Countries over the last three decades. The majority of allergic disorders are elicited by IgE-dependent activation of the immune system; therefore, monitoring of serum IgE is commonly used for diagnosis of allergic conditions. Importantly, a significant number of patients present with allergic symptoms in the absence of elevated serum IgE. Here, we propose that total-body IgE cannot be correctly assessed by looking at serum IgE alone. In the absence of elevated serum IgE, tissue-resident IgE or IgE bound to peripheral blood cells might be critically involved in the elicitation of allergic symptoms. In this comment, we discuss options to expand diagnostic measures to an assessment of total-body IgE rather than serum IgE levels alone. Such additional diagnostic approaches might be particularly useful for evaluating the allergic status of patients with low serum IgE.

Immunoglobulin E (IgE)-mediated activation of mast cells and basophils is a hallmark of immediate-type allergic reactions. These effector cells of the allergic cascade release

* Co-Author: Eleonora Dehlink, MD, PhD, Medical University of Vienna, Department of Pediatrics and Adolescent Medicine, Waehringer Guertel 18-20, 1090 Vienna, Austria, Tel: +43-1-40400-3188, Fax: + 43-1-40400-3189, email: eleonora.dehlink@meduniwien.ac.at

≠ Corresponding Author: Edda Fiebiger, PhD, The Children's Hospital, 300 Longwood Avenue, Enders 724, Boston, MA 02115, Tel: +1-617-919-2548, Fax: +1-617-730-0498, email: edda.fiebiger@childrens.harvard.edu preformed intracellular mediators that are responsible for the classical symptoms of immediate-type allergy, such as allergic rhinitis, asthma, and anaphylaxis. IgE-mediated activation of the immune system is also thought to be responsible for delayed-type allergic responses, which are of the TH2-immune phenotype with IL-4, IL-5 and IL-13 as the prototypical cytokines [1, 2]. Therefore, elevated serum IgE is commonly used as a diagnostic marker for allergic diseases [3]. However, a significant number of patients present with allergic symptoms in the absence of elevated serum IgE. In this comment, we discuss the possibility that an assessment of total-body IgE rather than serum IgE levels alone might be a useful approach to improve the diagnostic evaluation of the allergic status of patients.

Patients suffering from type 1 allergies usually present with elevated total and allergen-specific serum IgE levels. While the amount of the circulating IgE generally correlates with the severity of allergies [4-6], allergic symptoms are frequently reported in patients without elevated serum IgE [7, 8]. This type of patient is represented in allergic diseases like asthma, rhinitis, and atopic dermatitis. Such symptoms of allergy are referred to as "intrinsic" or "non-allergic" forms of allergic diseases. Commonly, non-IgE-mediated immune mechanisms whose nature is not well understood are proposed as the underlying pathology [8]. We argue here that serum IgE is not necessarily an accurate readout for total-body IgE. Therefore, an individual's IgE-sensitization level might not be reflected correctly in the measurement of soluble IgE found in the serum. We also contend that additional pools of IgE exist that escape the classical diagnostic approach, in which only the levels of serum IgE alone are evaluated.

IgE bound to IgE-receptors on tissue-resident immune cells is one such additional IgE pool. The ability of the tissue-IgE pool to activate the immune system after local allergen exposure is tested by the skin prick test [9]. This test uses the classical wheal-and-flare reaction elicited by IgE-loaded immune cells as a readout. Skin prick testing thus demonstrates that triggering of the allergic cascade via tissue specific IgE is possible. The test confirms that normal serum IgE levels can mask tissue-specific allergies The value of skin prick testing is considered to be limited in patients with skin conditions like severe atopic eczema or patients who take medications that affect mast cell degranulation, such as antihistamines or steroids [10]. Nonetheless, the valuable information obtained by skin prick testing supports our argument that additional IgE measures could improve the assessment of the allergic status of a patient.

A significant portion of the tissue-IgE pool might be generated locally Local IgE production by tissue-resident B cell blasts could elicit tissue-restricted allergic reactions without increasing serum IgE. The locally produced IgE would bind to nearby tissue IgE-receptors and therefore never reach the circulation. Vicario et al. convincingly demonstrate that IgE-producing B cells accumulate in esophageal tissue of patients with eosinophilc esophagitis [11], an inflammatory condition of the esophagus that appears to be tightly linked with allergies [12]. Vicario et al. argue that the local production of IgE might result in sensitization and activation of tissue-resident mast cells and thereby critically contribute to disease pathogenesis. Importantly, these local IgE-producing B cells were found irrespective of the allergic status of the patients. Therefore, it is fair to conclude that local tissue IgE production would be a valuable marker in the subgroup of patients with eosiniophilic esophagitis who do not show elevated serum IgE levels. While up to 30% of eosinophilic esophagitis cases are described as non-IgE mediated, the actual number might be much smaller if tissue-IgE levels were used as an additional diagnostic marker. Standardized measurements of local IgE production would involve quantification of germline transcripts of

IgE in B cells at the mRNA level [11]. While certainly appealing, this approach does not seem feasible for large patient cohorts on a standardized basis for technical as well as financial reasons.

Serum IgE is described as having a fairly short half-life when compared to other immunoglobulins [13]. Cell surface-expressed IgE-receptors on peripheral blood cells could trap IgE and protect it from degradation. For example, monomeric interaction of IgE with the high affinity IgE-receptor FcεRI stabilizes the cell-surface expression of the receptor [14]. This mechanism is unique to IgE and is thought to be responsible for the observation of elevated numbers of IgE-loaded FcεRI-positive cells in tissue and peripheral blood cells of patients with allergies. Consequently, elevated IgE serum levels correlate with increased surface expression of FcεRI [15-17]. FcεRI consists of a ligand binding immunoglobulin domain-containing protein (α-chain) that binds the Fc-part of IgE, and signaling subunits that induce cellular activation (β- and γ-chains) [18]. Allergen-dependent crosslinking of IgE bound to FcεRI is a key event in allergic immune reactions. Humans express a tetrameric FcεRI ($Fc\varepsilon RI\alpha\beta\gamma_2$) on mast cells and basophils and a trimeric form ($Fc\varepsilon RI\alpha\gamma_2$) on antigen presenting cells [18, 19]. Due to the exceptionally high affinity of FcεRI for IgE (10^{10} M^{-1}) [20, 21], this receptor is considered the prominent IgE binding structure in humans *in vivo* [3, 18, 22]. Human IgE also operates via a second cell surface IgE-receptor: CD23, the low affinity IgE-receptor, which is expressed on B cells [3], monocytes [16] and dendritic cells [23, 24]. As a member of the C-type lectin superfamily, the CD23-IgE binding sites are composed of three lectin-type head domains [3]. In contrast to the high affinity receptor FcεRI, CD23 surface expression does not seem to be regulated by IgE [16]. Therefore, it is unlikely that IgE-binding to CD23 provides much diagnostic value.

We propose here that a considerable amount of IgE is bound to the surface of immune cells, mainly via FcεRI. We further argue that this cell-bound IgE pool has thus far escaped conventional allergy diagnostics despite being of high pathophysiological importance because increased levels of IgE-loaded FcεRI render immune cells more sensitive to allergen stimulation [24, 25]. Like immune-competent cells in the skin, peripheral blood cells that are loaded with allergen-specific IgE can be considered 'sensitized.' These cells are waiting to react to minor amounts of allergen, but this level of sensitization cannot be accounted for by standard measurements of serum IgE. It is thus conceivable that cell-bound IgE may be an under-investigated but relevant marker for allergic sensitization in the absence of elevated serum IgE.

Based on these arguments, we propose to include IgE bound to peripheral blood cells as an additional marker to complement conventional allergy diagnostics. Using multi-color flow cytometry analysis, Liang et al. presented an algorithm to calculate total IgE by combining serum- and cell-bound IgE levels [26]. The authors calculate arbitrary units of IgE-loaded peripheral blood B cells, basophils, and eosinophils by multiplying the percentage of CD23+IgE+ and FcεRI+IgE+ whole blood leukocytes and the mean fluorescence intensity of IgE on the respective cell population. Additionally, a formula to calculate units of cell-bound allergen-specific IgE by multiplying the ratio of allergen-specific IgE and total serum IgE by arbitrary units of cell-bound IgE is presented. Those arbitrary units of cell-bound total and allergen-specific IgE correlated with levels of free serum IgE. However, Liang et al. also discovered a patient with high cell-bound IgE despite normal serum IgE. The authors conclude that this individual might be mistaken as "low risk" due to low serum IgE, while cell-bound IgE could easily trigger an allergic reaction. We recently extended this observation to a pediatric cohort and reached similar conclusions. Analyzing serum and whole blood samples from 48 pediatric patients for total IgE, IgE-receptors, and cell-bound IgE showed a considerable subgroup of children who carried IgE at the surface of peripheral blood cells while serum IgE levels were not elevated (Dehlink et al., submitted for publication). Our results and the study of Liang and colleagues provide two independent lines of investigation that support the conclusion that cell surface-bound IgE could provide an important diagnostic marker to assess the sensitization level of immune cells. As a next important step, cell-bound IgE as a diagnostic marker needs to be confirmed in a prospective cohort study and placed in the context of clinical symptoms of allergy. It will be important to correlate allergic symptoms and positive skin prick tests in patients with low serum IgE and high cell-bound IgE. Sensitivity, specificity, positive- and negative predictive values of cell-bound IgE as a novel diagnostic parameter also have to be evaluated in thoroughly characterized study populations.

One might argue that flow cytometric analysis of IgE on peripheral blood cells is an incomplete approach to estimate total-body IgE. This method certainly disregards IgE-loaded immune effector cells in tissues, the primary site of most allergic reactions. Yet non-invasive measurement of tissue IgE-levels is extremely challenging, as discussed above. In contrast, the evaluation of surface-bound IgE levels on blood cells seems possible for diagnosis on a large scale since flow cytometry is commonly used for diagnostic purposes today. Most likely, a detailed analysis of the cell types that carry IgE in the periphery is not necessary for diagnostics. In the long run, one could even consider including measurements of IgE-bearing cells in mucus, nasal fluids, and bronchial or esophageal aspirates for certain types of allergies.

In summary, we argue that the IgE-pool is composed of three main fractions which are all involved in the elicitation of allergic symptoms: soluble serum IgE, IgE-bound to allergic effector cells in tissues, and a pool of IgE bound to the cell surface of peripheral blood cells. The latter IgE pool currently is not assessed with allergy diagnostics although it has high pathophysiologic relevance since immune cells can carry cell surface-bound IgE to sites of allergen contact, such as mucous membranes, and cause allergic symptoms in patients with low serum IgE. We thus conclude that the inclusion of flow cytometric measurements of surface-bound IgE as an additional laboratory parameter might improve the diagnosis of patients that present with allergies in the absence of elevated serum IgE.

ACKNOWLEDGEMENTS

This work was supported by a grant from The Gerber Foundation (to E.F.) and an Early Scientific Career Award from the Thrasher Research Fund (to E.D.).

REFERENCES

[1] Finkelman FD, Hogan SP, Hershey GK, Rothenberg ME, Wills-Karp M, Importance of cytokines in murine allergic airway disease and human asthma. *J Immunol* 2010;184: 1663-1674.

[2] Hamid Q, Tulic M, Immunobiology of asthma. *Annu Rev Physiol* 2009;71: 489-507.

[3] Gould HJ, Sutton BJ, IgE in allergy and asthma today. *Nat Rev Immunol* 2008;8: 205-217.

[4] Benhamou AH, Zamora SA, Eigenmann PA, Correlation between specific immunoglobulin E levels and the severity of reactions in egg allergic patients. *Pediatr Allergy Immunol* 2008;19: 173-179.

[5] Celik-Bilgili S, Mehl A, Verstege A, Staden U, Nocon M, Beyer K, Niggemann B, The predictive value of specific immunoglobulin E levels in serum for the outcome of oral food challenges. *Clin Exp Allergy* 2005;35: 268-273.

[6] Rolinck-Werninghaus C, Keil T, Kopp M, Zielen S, Schauer U, von Berg A, Wahn U, Hamelmann E, Specific IgE serum concentration is associated with symptom severity in children with seasonal allergic rhinitis. *Allergy* 2008;63: 1339-1344.

[7] Chehade M, IgE and non-IgE-mediated food allergy: treatment in 2007. *Curr Opin Allergy Clin Immunol* 2007;7: 264-268.

[8] Novak N, Bieber T, Allergic and nonallergic forms of atopic diseases. *J Allergy Clin Immunol* 2003;112: 252-262.

[9] Oppenheimer J, Nelson HS, Skin testing. *Annu Allergy Asthma Immunol* 2006;96: S6-12.

[10] Ownby DR, Allergy testing: in vivo versus in vitro. *Pediatr Clin North Am* 1988;35: 995-1009.

[11] Vicario M, Blanchard C, Stringer KF, Collins MH, Mingler MK, Ahrens A, Putnam PE, Abonia JP, Santos J, Rothenberg ME, Local B cells and IgE production in the oesophageal mucosa in eosinophilic oesophagitis. *Gut* 2010;59: 12-20.

[12] Rothenberg ME, Biology and treatment of eosinophilic esophagitis. *Gastroenterology* 2009;137: 1238-1249.

[13] Infuhr D, Crameri R, Lamers R, Achatz G, Molecular and cellular targets of anti-IgE antibodies. *Allergy* 2005;60: 977-985.

[14] Kubota T, Mukai K, Minegishi Y, Karasuyama H, Different stabilities of the structurally related receptors for IgE and IgG on the cell surface are determined by length of the stalk region in their alpha-chains. *J Immunol* 2006;176: 7008-7014.

[15] Maurer D, Fiebiger E, Reininger B, Wolff-Winiski B, Jouvin MH, Kilgus O, Kinet JP, Stingl G, Expression of functional high affinity immunoglobulin E receptors (Fc epsilon RI) on monocytes of atopic individuals. *J Exp Med* 1994;179: 745-750.

[16] Saini SS, Klion AD, Holland SM, Hamilton RG, Bochner BS, Macglashan DW, Jr., The relationship between serum IgE and surface levels of FcepsilonR on human leukocytes in various diseases: correlation of expression with FcepsilonRI on basophils but not on monocytes or eosinophils. *J Allergy Clin Immunol* 2000;106: 514-520.

[17] Sihra BS, Kon OM, Grant JA, Kay AB, Expression of high-affinity IgE receptors (Fc epsilon RI) on peripheral blood basophils, monocytes, and eosinophils in atopic and

nonatopic subjects: relationship to total serum IgE concentrations. *J Allergy Clin Immunol* 1997;99: 699-706.

[18] Kraft S, Kinet JP, New developments in FcepsilonRI regulation, function and inhibition. *Nat Rev Immunol* 2007;7: 365-378.

[19] Call ME, Wucherpfennig KW, Common themes in the assembly and architecture of activating immune receptors. *Nat Rev Immunol* 2007;7: 841-850.

[20] Garman SC, Kinet JP, Jardetzky TS, Crystal structure of the human high-affinity IgE receptor. *Cell* 1998;95: 951-961.

[21] Kinet JP, The high-affinity IgE receptor (Fc epsilon RI): from physiology to pathology. *Annu Rev Immunol* 1999;17: 931-972.

[22] Novak N, Kraft S, Bieber T, IgE receptors. *Curr Opin Immunol* 2001;13: 721-726.

[23] Bieber T, Fc epsilon RII/CD23 on epidermal Langerhans' cells. *Res Immunol* 1992;143: 445-447.

[24] Wollenberg A, Haberstok J, Teichmann B, Wen SP, Bieber T, Demonstration of the low-affinity IgE receptor Fc epsilonRII/CD23 in psoriatic epidermis: inflammatory dendritic epidermal cells (IDEC) but not Langerhans cells are the relevant CD1a-positive cell population. *Arch Dermatol Res* 1998;290: 517-521.

[25] Klubal R, Osterhoff B, Wang B, Kinet JP, Maurer D, Stingl G, The high-affinity receptor for IgE is the predominant IgE-binding structure in lesional skin of atopic dermatitis patients. *J Invest Dermatol* 1997;108: 336-342.

[26] Liang Y, Ganley-Leal LM, A simple method for measuring human cell-bound IgE levels in whole blood. *J Immunol Methods* 2009.

In: Food Allergies: Symptoms, Diagnosis, and Treatment
Editors: Patricia M. Rodgers
ISBN: 978-1-61728-748-0

Chapter 6

Development of an Anaphylaxis Order Set to Improve Emergency Department Anaphylaxis Management

Ronna L. Campbell, Lekshmi Vaidyanathan, Abhijit R. Kanthala and Wyatt W. Decker
Department of Emergency Medicine, Mayo Clinic, Rochester, Minnesota

Introduction

Anaphylaxis is a serious allergic reaction that is rapid in onset and may cause death.[1] The management of anaphylactic reactions occurs most commonly in the emergency department.[2, 3] Furthermore, food-related allergic reactions have been shown to be the leading cause of anaphylactic reactions treated in the emergency department.[4] A systematic algorithm for the diagnosis and management of anaphylaxis, especially food-related reactions, would allow emergency medicine practitioners to better recognize and manage anaphylaxis in the emergency department.

Epidemiology

Food-related allergic reactions are estimated to result in approximately 30,000 emergency department visits each year and 150–200 deaths.[4] Although the overall incidence of anaphylaxis is not precisely known, a recent population-based study over a 10-year period showed an incidence of 49.8 per 100,000 person-years.[5] Ingested foods accounted for 33.2% of the cases of anaphylaxis. This rate is significantly higher than previously reported estimates of the incidence of anaphylaxis.[6] Furthermore, a modest increase in the incidence of anaphylaxis was detected during this 10-year study, suggesting that the incidence of anaphylaxis may be increasing. The increased incidence is particularly pronounced in the first 2 decades of life.[7] Before the age of 15 years males are more commonly affected and after 15 years females are more likely to be affected. In children and young adults, foods are the most common trigger. In middle-aged and older adults, medications, stinging insect venoms and idiopathic anaphylaxis are more likely causes.[7]

NIAID/FAAN Clinical Criteria for the Diagnosis of Anaphylaxis
Anaphylaxis is highly likely when any one of the following 3 criteria is fulfilled:
1. Acute onset of an illness (minutes to several hours) with involvement of the skin, mucosal tissue, or both (eg, generalized hives, pruritus or flushing, swollen lips-tongue-uvula)
AND AT LEAST ONE OF THE FOLLOWING
a. Respiratory compromise (eg, dyspnea, wheeze-bronchospasm, stridor, reduced PEF, hypoxemia)
b. Reduced BP or associated symptoms of end-organ dysfunction (eg, hypotonia [collapse], syncope, incontinence)
2. Two or more of the following that occur rapidly after exposure to a likely allergen for that patient (minutes to several hours):
a. Involvement of the skin-mucosal tissue (eg, generalized hives, itch-flush, swollen lips-tongue-uvula)
b. Respiratory compromise (eg, dyspnea, wheeze-bronchospasm, stridor, reduced PEF, hypoxemia)
c. Reduced BP or associated symptoms (eg, hypotonia [collapse], syncope, incontinence)
d. Persistent gastrointestinal symptoms (eg, crampy abdominal pain, vomiting)
3. Reduced BP after exposure to known allergen for that patient (minutes to several hours):
a. Infants and children: low systolic BP (age specific) or greater than 30% decrease in systolic BP*
b. Adults: systolic BP of less than 90 mm Hg or greater than 30% decrease from that person's baseline
PEF: Peak expiratory flow
BP: blood pressure
*Low systolic blood pressure for children is defined as
< 70 mm Hg for children 1 month to 1 year
< (70 mm Hg + [2 x age]) from 1 to 10 years
< 90 mm Hg from 11 to 17 years
Used with permission.

Figure 1. NIAID/FAAN Clinical Criteria for the diagnosis of Anaphylaxis.

DIAGNOSIS

Emergency physicians are on the front line of medical care for patients suffering from anaphylaxis. However, studies have documented inconsistent emergency care and low compliance with guidelines on the management of anaphylaxis.[3, 8, 9] A comprehensive approach to the care of patients presenting to the emergency department with anaphylaxis is needed.

A major impediment to the consistent management of anaphylaxis has been the lack of universally accepted diagnostic criteria for anaphylaxis which often results in the failure to recognize anaphylaxis. A study by Klein and Yocum found that many patients who are diagnosed as having an allergic reaction in the emergency department were subsequently, on allergist review, considered to have experienced an anaphylactic episode.[10] This need for diagnostic criteria based on signs and symptoms was addressed at the Second Symposium on the Definition and Management of Anaphylaxis and diagnostic criteria were proposed to aid in the recognition of an anaphylactic reaction (Figure 1).[1] However, these criteria have not yet been prospectively validated or widely adapted into clinical practice and many emergency practitioners may not be familiar with these criteria. A study of perception of the frequency of anaphylaxis by allergists versus non-allergists by Simon et al. showed that 44.3% of the allergists thought that anaphylaxis was common and 55.4% thought it was rare. Among non-allergists, only 16.4% thought it was common and 82.2% considered the diagnosis rare.[11] This highlights the need for further physician education on the diagnostis of anaphylaxis.

Management

Epinephrine is the treatment of choice for patients experiencing anaphylaxis [1,12] and recent studies suggest that early treatment with epinephrine may decrease the risk of biphasic reactions.[13] The alpha-1 adrenergic effects of epinephrine cause vasoconstriction and can prevent and relieve upper airway edema and hypotension. Many patients suffering from anaphylaxis are not treated with epinephrine in the emergency department.[3,8,9] The factors contributing to this are not definitively known, however, unfamiliarity with the dosing of epinephrine for anaphylaxis treatment or fear of complications secondary to inappropriate dosing may be contributing to the low rate of treatment with epinephrine. Alternatively, it has been noted anecdotally that many patients who present to the emergency department with anaphylaxis are hemodynamically stable, and are already clinically improving on arrival and therefore would be unlikely to benefit from administration of epinephrine.

Anaphylaxis management guidelines proposed by the Second Symposium on the Definition and Management of Anaphylaxis recommend that all patients with a history of anaphylaxis to an allergen that they may encounter in a nonmedical setting should be given a prescription for self-injectable epinephrine.[1] They should also be referred to an allergist for follow-up.[1] However, a study evaluating patients presenting to the emergency department with food allergies found that less than 25% of patients with anaphylaxis were prescribed self-injectable epinephrine when discharged from the emergency department and even fewer were referred to an allergist.[8]

In addition to receiving a prescription for self-injectable epinephrine and referral to an allergist for follow up, guidelines also recommend that patients with anaphylaxis be observed for approximately 4-6 hours following the reaction due to the risk of a biphasic reaction.[1] The SAFE system was designed as a tool to improve anaphylaxis management and promote a safe discharge from the emergency department.[14] This system emphasizes that patients: 1) be advised of their risk of a biphasic reaction and instructed to seek immediate emergency care should this occur, 2) be assisted in identifying the allergen and avoiding it in the future, 3) be advised to follow-up with their primary physician or allergist and, 4) be provided with self-injectable epinephrine, instructed how to use it and the importance of carrying it at all times.

SYSTEMS BASED PRACTICE

An expert review on the emergency department management of food allergies by Clark and Camargo has called for the creation of systems that would disseminate anaphylaxis diagnosis and management guidelines and aid in the emergency department implementation of these recommendations.[15] These authors have suggested that an algorithm for the diagnosis and management of anaphylaxis, especially food-related reactions, would allow emergency medicine practitioners to more rapidly recognize and treat allergic reactions in the emergency department.

In our institution, a tertiary care medical center, with an annual emergency department volume of approximately 80,000 patients, we developed an Emergency Department Anaphylaxis Management Order Set. The order set was developed to optimize the diagnosis, management, observation and safe dismissal of these patients presenting to an emergency department.

The National Institute of Allergy and Infectious Disease and Food Allergy and Anaphylaxis Network (NIAID/FAAN) diagnostic criteria are highlighted on the order set to ensure accurate recognition of this condition. The order set also includes dosing for both emergency medical treatment as well as medications to be administered, if needed, over the subsequent 4-6 hours of observation. Drugs highlighted include epinephrine (intramuscular and intravenous infusion administration), bronchodilators, H1 receptor blockers, H2 receptor blockers and steroids. Appropriate adult dosage is included on the order set to avoid dosing errors.

The NIAID/FAAN Second Symposium on the Definition and Management of Anpahylaxis Summary Report recommends that patients be observed following an anaphylactic reaction based on the severity of the initial reaction, reliability of the patient, and access to care.[1] A recommended length of time is for observation is 4 to 6 hours in most patients, with prolonged observation times or hospital admission for severe or refractory symptoms.[16] The order set when used for observation of these patients in the emergency department observation unit helps ensure guideline compliance and simultaneously maintains the flow of the emergency department and decreases the need for hospital admission.

The order set helps promote a safe discharge from the emergency department as it includes a recommendation for a self-injectable epinephrine prescription as well as patient anaphylaxis education. Topics covered during education include the use of self-injectable epinephrine, the risk of a biphasic reaction and importance of allergen avoidance. An automated allergist referral is generated on discharge to ensure optimal follow up especially after the initial episode.

This protocol was designed to address the multifaceted aspects of anaphylaxis management and can be easily modified for implementation in other emergency departments and urgent care settings. Salient features of the order set are highlighted in figure 3.

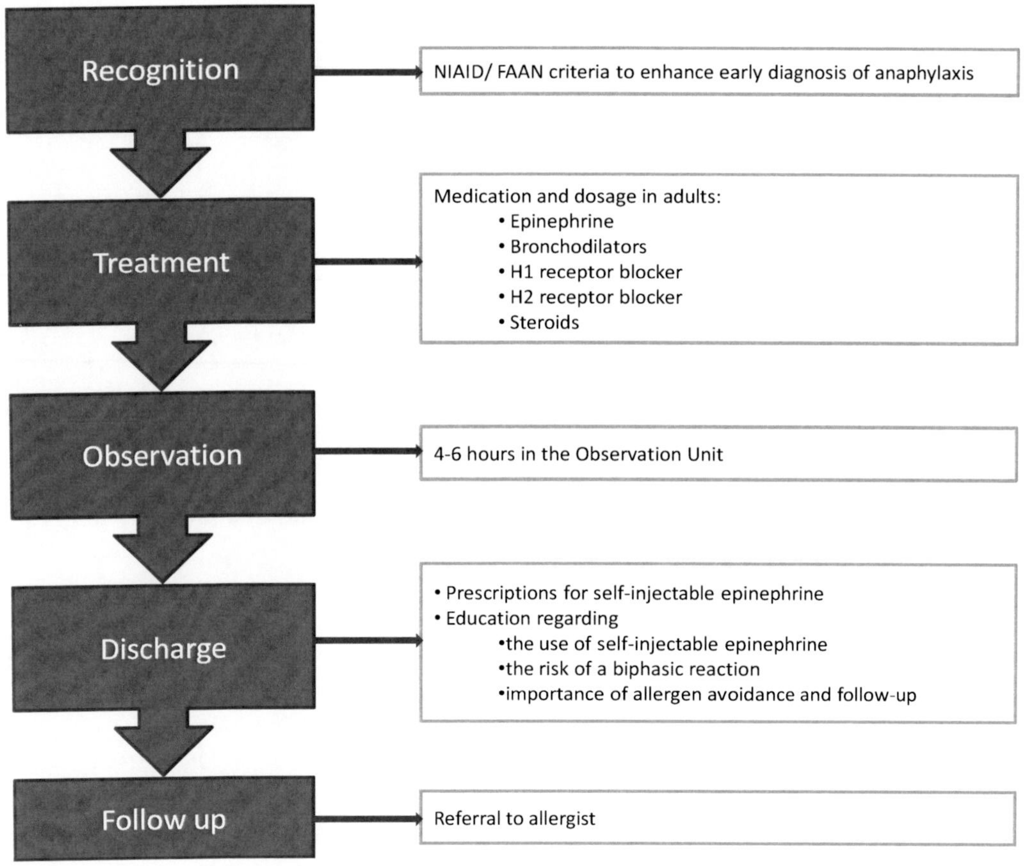

Figure 3. Salient features of the Emergency Department Anaphylaxis Management Order Set.

CONCLUSION

Emergency department concordance with anaphylaxis treatment guidelines continues to be low. An integrated algorithm for the emergency department management of anaphylaxis, such as the one discussed here, is essential for improved emergency department management of anaphylaxis.

REFERENCES

[1] Sampson, H.A., et al., Second symposium on the definition and management of anaphylaxis: summary report--Second National Institute of Allergy and Infectious Disease/Food Allergy and Anaphylaxis Network symposium.[reprint in Ann Emerg Med. 2006 Apr;47(4):373-80; PMID: 16546624]. *Journal of Allergy & Clinical Immunology*, 2006. 117(2): p. 391-7.

[2] Bohlke, K., et al., Epidemiology of anaphylaxis among children and adolescents enrolled in a health maintenance organization. *Journal of Allergy & Clinical Immunology*, 2004. 113(3): p. 536-42.

[3] Campbell, R.L., et al., Prescriptions for self-injectable epinephrine and follow-up referral in emergency department patients presenting with anaphylaxis. *Annals of Allergy, Asthma, & Immunology*, 2008. 101(6): p. 631-6.

[4] Sampson, H.A., Anaphylaxis and emergency treatment. *Pediatrics*, 2003. 111(6 Pt 3): p. 1601-8.

[5] Decker, W.W., et al., The etiology and incidence of anaphylaxis in Rochester, Minnesota: a report from the Rochester Epidemiology Project.[see comment]. *Journal of Allergy & Clinical Immunology*, 2008. 122(6): p. 1161-5.

[6] Yocum, M.W., et al., Epidemiology of anaphylaxis in Olmsted County: A population-based study.[see comment]. *Journal of Allergy & Clinical Immunology,* 1999. 104(2 Pt 1): p. 452-6.

[7] Simons FE. Anaphylaxis: Recent advances in assessment and treatment. *J Allergy Clin Immunol*, 2009. 124(4):625-36.

[8] Clark, S., et al., Multicenter study of emergency department visits for food allergies. *Journal of Allergy & Clinical Immunology,* 2004. 113(2): p. 347-52.

[9] Clark, S., et al., Multicenter study of emergency department visits for insect sting allergies. *Journal of Allergy & Clinical Immunology*, 2005. 116(3): p. 643-9.

[10] Klein, J.S. and M.W. Yocum, Underreporting of anaphylaxis in a community emergency room. *Journal of Allergy & Clinical Immunology,* 1995. 95(2): p. 637-8.

[11] Simons FE, Frew AJ, Ansotegui IJ, Bochner BS, Golden DB, Finkelman FD, Leung DY, Lotvall J, Marone G, Metcalfe DD, Müller U, Rosenwasser LJ, Sampson HA, Schwartz LB, van Hage M, Walls AF. Risk assessment in anaphylaxis: current and future approaches. *J Allergy Clin Immunol*, 2007. 120(1 Suppl): S2-24.

[12] Brown, S.G., et al., Insect sting anaphylaxis; prospective evaluation of treatment with intravenous adrenaline and volume resuscitation.[see comment]. *Emergency Medicine Journal*, 2004. 21(2): p. 149-54.

[13] Lieberman, P., Biphasic anaphylactic reactions.[see comment]. *Annals of Allergy, Asthma, & Immunology*. 95(3): p. 217-26; quiz 226.

[14] Lieberman, P., et al., SAFE: a multidisciplinary approach to anaphylaxis education in the emergency department. *Annals of Allergy, Asthma, & Immunology*, 2007. 98(6): p. 519-23.

[15] Clark, S. and C.A. Camargo, Jr., Emergency management of food allergy: systems perspective. *Current Opinion in Allergy & Clinical Immunology*, 2005. 5(3): p. 293-8.

[16] Sharma R, Sinha R, Menon PS, Sirohi D. Management Protocol for Anaphylaxis. *J Oral Maxillofac Surg*. 2009 Dec 23. [Epub ahead of print]

In: Food Allergies: Symptoms, Diagnosis, and Treatment
Editor: Patricia M. Rodgers
ISBN: 978-1-61728-748-0

Chapter 7

CLINICAL MANIFESTATIONS OF FOOD ALLERGY*

***Alexander K.C. Leung*[1,**] *and Deepak Kamat*[2]**

[1] University of Calgary, Alberta Children's Hospital, Calgary, Alberta, Canada

[2] Carman and Ann Adams Department of Pediatrics, Wayne State University, Children's Hospital of Michigan, Detroit, Michigan, USA

ABSTRACT

Food allergy is defined as an adverse reaction because of an abnormal immunological response to food protein. The immune pathogenesis is, in the majority of cases, IgE-mediated although it may also be cell-mediated (non-IgE) or mixed IgE/cell-mediated. Food allergy affects as many as 2 to 8% of young children and the presentation can be highly variable. There is usually a clear temporal relationship between food exposure and the development of allergic symptoms. At times, symptoms may develop hours or days after food exposure making the diagnosis difficult.

Food allergy usually presents as multi-system involvement, most commonly gastrointestinal symptoms which occur with a frequency of 50 to 80% of cases. These are followed by cutaneous symptoms and respiratory symptoms, occurring in 20 to 40%, and 4 to 25% of cases, respectively. Gastrointestinal manifestations include oral allergy syndrome, gastrointestinal anaphylaxis, allergic eosinophilic esophagitis, allergic eosinophilic gastroenteropathy, food protein-induced enteropathy, food protein-induced enterocolitis syndrome, food protein-induced proctocolitis, gluten-sensitive enteropathy, infantile colic, irritable bowel syndrome, and constipation. Cutaneous manifestations are urticaria/angioedema, atopic dermatitis, contact dermatitis, and dermatitis herpetiformis. Rhinitis/rhinoconjunctivitis, asthma, Heiner syndrome, and serous otitis media are the respiratory manifestations of food allergy. Other manifestations include systemic anaphylaxis, food-dependent exercise-induced anaphylaxis, migraine, epilepsy, diabetes mellitus, nephrotic syndrome, nocturnal enuresis, anemia, thrombocytopenia, vasculitis,

* A version of this chapter was also published in *Food Allergies: New Research*, edited by Carrie M. Chesterton, published by Nova Science Publishers. It was submitted for appropriate modifications in an effort to encourage wider dissemination of research.

** Correspondence to: Dr. Alexander K.C. Leung, MBBS, FRCPC, FRCP(UK&Irel), FRCPCH, FAAP, Clinical Professor of Pediatrics, The University of Calgary, #200, 233 – 16th Avenue NW, Calgary, Alberta, T2M 0H5 Canada. Telefax: (403) 230-3322; e-mail: aleung@ucalgary.ca and arthropathy/arthritis. This chapter discusses the various clinical manifestations of food allergy.

Keywords: food allergy, clinical manifestations

Table 1. Clinical Manifestations of Food Allergy

Gastrointestinal manifestations
Oral allergy syndrome Gastrointestinal anaphylaxis Allergic eosinophilic esophagitis Allergic eosinophilic gastroenteropathy Food protein-induced enteropathy Food protein-induced enterocolitis syndrome Food protein-induced proctocolitis Gluten-sensitive enteropathy Infantile colic Irritable bowel syndrome Recurrent abdominal pain Constipation
Cutaneous manifestations
Urticaria/angioedema Atopic dermatitis Contact dermatitis Dermatitis herpetiformis
Respiratory manifestations
Rhinitis/rhinoconjunctivitis Chronic sinusitis Asthma Heiner syndrome Serous otitis media Ménière's disease
Generalized manifestations
Systemic anaphylaxis Food-dependent exercise-induced anaphylaxis Hyperactivity
Neurologic manifestations
Migraine Epilepsy
Endocrine manifestation
Diabetes mellitus
Renal manifestations
Nephrotic syndrome Nocturnal enuresis
Hematologic manifestations
Anemia Thrombocytopenia
Cardiovascular manifestation
Vasculitis
Rheumatic manifestation
Arthropathy/arthritis

Gastrointestinal Manifestations

Oral Allergy Syndrome

Oral allergy syndrome (pollen-food allergy syndrome) is a complex of symptoms induced by exposure of the oral and pharyngeal mucosa to plant protein allergens [13,14]. Patients are usually sensitized to an aeroallergen initially [15]. The IgE antibodies to the aeroallergen cause the oral allergy syndrome [16]. Botanical cross-reactivity as a result of shared epitopes between pollen and causative fruits and vegetables has been suggested as a possible mechanism of local mast cell activation [17]. The oral allergy syndrome is considered a form of contact urticaria that is confined mainly to the oropharynx [2]. Symptoms include rapid onset of itching, tingling, burning, and/or angioedema of the lips, tongue, palate, and throat within minutes of ingestion of fresh fruit and vegetable [14]. Symptoms usually resolve rapidly. Occasionally, the clinical course is more dramatic with potentially fatal pharyngeal swelling or progression towards a generalized anaphylactic reaction [10,18]. The syndrome generally occurs in patients with inhalant allergy to birch, mugwort, or ragweed pollen and is associated with the ingestion of various fresh fruits (e.g., bananas, melons, citrus fruits) and raw vegetables (e.g. carrots, tomatoes, celery) [19-22]. It is uncommon to have several fruits and vegetables that cause the oral allergy syndrome in one patient [23]. However, allergy to ragweed may cross-react when exposed to fresh melon and banana [24]. Oral allergy syndrome is more prevalent in adults than in children [25]. Most patients have some degree of allergic conjunctivitis or allergic rhinitis because the IgE antibodies to an aeroallergen cross-react with the fruit or vegetable proteins [15,26]. It is interesting to note that if the offending fruit or vegetable is cooked, then the patient does not usually experience any symptom as the food allergens are generally destroyed by heating [4,15]. Patients who remain sensitive to cooked fruit or vegetable may be sensitive to proteins that do not cross-react with pollens and do not actually have oral allergy syndrome [21,27]. Although these patients react to food typically associated with oral allergy syndrome, the absence of pollenosis and presence of symptoms beyond the oropharynx suggest conventional food allergy rather than oral allergy syndrome [21].

Gastrointestinal Anaphylaxis

Gastrointestinal anaphylaxis is an IgE-mediated gastrointestinal hypersensitivity that often accompanies other systemic manifestations of food allergy [28,29]. This may be manifested as nausea, vomiting, abdominal pain, flatulence, abdominal distension, or diarrhea [2]. The reaction usually occurs within minutes to 2 hours of food ingestion [30]. Repeated ingestion of a food allergen may induce partial desensitization of mast cells in the gastrointestinal tract resulting in milder symptoms [2,18].

Allergic eosinophilic esophagitis is usually T-cell-mediated rather than IgE-mediated, and caused by allergens in the diet and, less commonly, in the air [32,34,36-38]. Allergic eosinophilic esophagitis occurs mainly in children and young adults [39-41]. This condition is being more frequently diagnosed over the past decade. It appears that the increase in prevalence is real and is not due to an increased awareness of this condition among physicians. The condition is more common in males and those with a family or personal history of atopy or proven food allergy [33,42,43]. Allergic eosinophilic esophagitis may present with irritability, sleep disturbance, food refusal, vomiting/ regurgitation, dysphagia, abdominal pain, substernal chest pain, occult blood loss, anemia, and failure to thrive [21,25,31,44,45]. Dauer et al. retrospectively reviewed the records of 71 children with biopsy-proven allergic eosinophilic esophagitis and found that the most common symptom was dysphagia, being present in 36 (51%) patients [31]. Eighteen (50%) of the 36 patients with dysphagia experienced at least one episode of food impaction. Other common symptoms include vomiting (31%) and abdominal pain (24%). The symptoms of recurrent vomiting /regurgitation may mimic those of gastroesophageal reflux but are refractory to anti-reflux treatment [25,45,46]. These symptoms do respond to dietary avoidance of food allergens [47]. Typically, affected patients have a negative pH probe study [48].

Allergic Eosinophilic Gastroenteropathy

Allergic eosinophilic gastroenteritis is characterized by infiltration of the gastrointestinal tract with eosinophils, peripheral eosinophilia, and absence of vasculitis [13,49,50]. The eosinophilic infiltrates may be quite patchy and may involve the mucosa, muscular layer, or serosal layer of the stomach or small intestine [24]. In addition to an IgE-mediated mechanism, cell-mediated immunity may also be operative [51]. T-cells specifically sensitized to antigens may release lymphokines capable of attracting eosinophils to the gastrointestinal tissue.

Although allergic eosinophilic gastroenteropathy may affect all ages, the disease is more common in individuals in the third through fifth decades [49]. Patients with mucosal involvement usually have postprandial nausea, vomiting, abdominal pain, watery diarrhea with or without blood, iron deficiency anemia, occasionally steatorrhea, and weight loss in adults or failure to thrive in children [44,52,53]. Patients with muscular involvement may have symptoms and signs of gastric outlet or intestinal obstruction, depending on the site of bowel involvement [24]. The serosal form is characterized by ascites, abdominal pain, and abdominal distension and is extremely rare in children [24,54].

Food Protein-Induced Enteropathy

Food protein-induced enteropathy is characterized by protracted diarrhea and vomiting with onset usually in infancy. This may result in malabsorption, protein-losing enteropathy, and failure to thrive [21,30]. The disorder is caused by a T-cell-mediated response most commonly to cow's milk protein [24]. Intestinal biopsy typically reveals a patchy villous atrophy, increased crypt length, and prominent mononuclear round cell infiltrates [8].

Food Protein-Induced Enterocolitis Syndrome

Food protein-induced enterocolitis syndrome is a cell-mediated hypersensitivity disease which occurs mainly in infants under 3 months of age [4]. The condition usually resolves by 2 years of age but may, rarely, persist into late childhood [25]. Although cow's milk and soy protein are most often responsible [21,33,54], other food antigens have occasionally been implicated, including food protein antigens passed in the maternal breast milk [5,28,55,56]. Classic symptoms are protracted vomiting and diarrhea with progression to dehydration and shock in 20% of patients [30,44,57]. Some infants may have irritability, lethargy, anemia, transient methemoglobinemia, abdominal distension, protein-losing enteropathy, and failure to thrive [21,24,57-59]. Stools generally contain occult blood, polymorphonuclear neutrophils, eosinophils, and Charcot-Leyden crystals [2]. Presumably, stimulation of T-cells by food allergens with secretion of tumor necrosis factor-α may play a role in the pathophysiology of this disorder [30,57,60]. A relative lack of expression of transforming growth factor-β may also have a role to play [57,60]. Skin tests for the offending antigen are usually negative [25]. Radioallergosorbent (RAST) assay, which detects specific IgE antibody, may also be negative in these patients. Jejunal biopsy specimens usually reveal villus atrophy and increased numbers of lymphocytes, eosinophils, and mast cells [61]. Colonoscopy and biopsy show inflammatory colitis and eosinophilic infiltration [55]. Symptoms usually resolve in 72 hours after the offending food substance has been removed from the diet.

Food Protein-Induced Proctocolitis

As with food protein-induced enterocolitis syndrome, food protein-induced proctocolitis is a T-cell mediated disorder. The disorder usually occurs in the first few months of life and is most often secondary to milk protein or soy protein hypersensitivity [44,54,61]. Approximately 60% of cases occur in breastfed infants [5]. Unlike food protein-induced enterocolitis syndrome, infants with food protein-induced proctocolitis generally appear healthy and have normal weight gain. These infants usually have occult or gross blood and sometimes mucus in their stools but they do not have diarrhea [30,62,63]. In general, hematochezia resolves within 72 hours of appropriate food-allergen avoidance [30]. In breastfed infants, elimination of food-allergen from the maternal diet may result in resolution of hematochezia. Colonic biopsy samples reveal mucosal edema, erythema, friability, ulceration, nodular lymphoid hyperplasia and eosinophilic infiltration [44,53,64]. Skin tests for the offending agents as well as RAST assays are usually negative in these patients.

Gluten-Sensitive Enteropathy

Gluten-sensitive enteropathy (celiac disease) is a disorder in which small-bowel mucosal damage is the result of a permanent sensitivity to gliadin, the alcohol-soluble portion of gluten, present in wheat, barley, and rye. Patients with gluten-sensitive enteropathy typically present with diarrhea/steatorrhea, abdominal distension, muscle wasting, and failure to thrive [1]. Other clinical manifestations include irritability, anorexia, vomiting, abdominal pain, oral ulcers, digital clubbing, delayed puberty, and infertility [65,66]. Occasionally, patients with gluten-sensitive enteropathy may be asymptomatic [67]. The presence of anti-gliadin, anti-endomysial, and anti-tissue transglutaminase antibodies of the IgA isotype and anti-gliadin antibodies of the IgG isotype support the diagnosis [21]. However, anti-gliadin antibody of

IgG subtype has been known to be positive in conditions such as cow's milk protein allergy, inflammatory bowel disease, and cystic fibrosis and therefore has poor specificity. In addition, patients with IgA deficiency may not have antibodies of IgA subtype in spite of suffering from gluten-sensitive enteropathy. It is recommended that the diagnosis of gluten-sensitive enteropathy be confirmed by intestinal biopsy before instituting dietary changes. Characteristically, biopsy of the jejunum shows villus atrophy, marked increase in crypt-villous ratio, and extensive cellular infiltrates [44]. Both cellular and complement-mediated cytotoxicity and lymphokine-induced damage have been implicated in the pathogenesis of the condition [47]. There is a genetic predisposition to the disease. There is a predominance of certain HLA types (B8, DQ2, DW3) in patients with gluten-sensitive enteropathy [1,2,68]. Environmental factors may influence expression of the genetic predisposition.

Infantile Colic

There is increasing evidence that cow's milk proteins may play an important role in the pathogenesis of infantile colic [69-75]. Approximately 25% of infants with moderate or severe colic have allergy to cow's milk protein [76,77]. Lothe and Lindberg showed that colic disappeared in 24 of 27 infants when they were given a cow's milk-free diet [73]. These infants were entered into a double-blind placebo-controlled crossover trial of whey protein. Eighteen infants receiving the whey protein capsules reacted with colic, two infants received placebo reacted with colic, and four infants did not react at all.

Iacono et al. put 70 cow's milk formula-fed infants with severe colic on soy-milk formula [71]. In 50 infants, there was a remission of symptoms when cow's milk protein was eliminated from their diet. Two successive challenges caused the return of symptoms in all these 50 infants. Follow-ups, after an average period of 18 months, showed that in 22 of 50 (44%) of the infants who had cow's milk protein-related colic and 1 of 20 (5%) of those with non-cow's milk protein-related colic developed an overt form of alimentary intolerance. Lucassen et al randomly selected 43 healthy infants with colic to receive whey hydrolysate formula or standard formula [74]. They found a decrease in the duration of crying in those infants fed with whey hydrolysate formula.

Jakobsson et al. studied the effectiveness of 2 formulae with extensively hydrolysed casein in 22 infants with severe colic [78]. One infant was considered as treatment failure and six infants as protocol failures. The remaining 15 infants showed a significant decrease in the lengths of time they cried as well as a decrease in the intensity of their crying on both formulae. When the infants were challenged in a double-blind design, 11 infants reacted with an increase in crying time to cow's milk protein or bovine whey protein.

Hill et al. studied the effect of diet change in 38 bottle-fed and 77 breast-fed colicky infants in a double-blind, randomized, placebo-controlled trial [70]. Bottle-fed infants were assigned to either casein hydrolysate or cow's milk formula. All mothers of breast-fed infants were started on an artificial color-free, preservative-free, additive-free diet and were randomized to receive either an active low allergen (milk free) diet or a control diet. Hill et al. showed that infants on the active diet had their distress reduced by 39% compared with 16% for those on the control diet.

Jakobsson and Lindberg put 66 mothers of 66 breast-fed infants with infantile colic on a cow's milk-free diet [79]. The colic disappeared in 35 infants; it reappeared after reintroduction of cow's milk into the mother's diet in 23 of the 35 infants. A double-blind crossover trial with cow's milk whey protein was performed on 16 of these 23 mothers and infants. Six infants had to be taken out of the study for various reasons. Of the remaining 10 infants, nine displayed signs of colic after their mothers had taken the whey-filled capsules.

Maternal ingestion of eggs, chocolate, citrus fruits, nuts, as well as certain seafood whilst breastfeeding may result in infantile colic [72,80-82]. Hill et al. randomized mothers of 107 term breastfed infants younger than 6 weeks of age with colic to follow a low-allergen diet with elimination of dairy products, soy, wheat, eggs, peanuts, tree nuts, and fish (n=53) and a control group (n=54) whose diet contained the known allergen [83]. Forty seven mothers in the treatment group and 43 mothers in the control group completed the study. Infants were identified as responders if there was at least 25% reduction in duration of crying/fussing on days 8 and 9. The authors showed that 74% of infants in the treatment group versus 37% of infants in the control group were responders (p=<0.001).

Irritable Bowel Syndrome

The pathogenesis of irritable colon syndrome is likely heterogeneous. Food allergy has been implicated in the pathogenesis of a subset of patients with irritable bowel syndrome [84,85]. The association of irritable bowel syndrome with specific IL-10 genotypes supports involvement of the immune system in its pathogenesis [58,86,87]. It has been shown that patients with irritable bowel syndrome have a greater area of intestinal mucosa occupied by mast cells than do healthy control individuals [88]. A study of dietary eliminations in patients with irritable bowel syndrome found a significant reduction in symptom score in those patients whose exclusions were guided by raised IgG antibodies to dietary antigens than did patients on a sham diet based on irrelevant antigens [89]. Reintroduction of eliminated foods resulted in aggravation of symptoms in patients whose dietary exclusions were guided by raised IgG antibodies to dietary antigens. Irritable bowel syndrome might result from an interplay between immunological dysfunction, impaired gut barrier functions, susceptible genes and other environmental factors [90]. It has been hypothesized that food antigens induce mast cells to secrete mediators that regulate gastrointestinal motility and pain perception through gastrointestinal neural system [84].

Recurrent Abdominal Pain

Recurrent abdominal pain is usually defined as three or more bouts of abdominal pain, severe enough to interfere with a child's normal activities, occurring over a period of not less than three months during the year preceding the examination [91,92]. Onset often occurs between five and 10 years of age. Typically, the pain is vague, poorly localized or periumbilical and may be crampy or sharp. Episodes of pain tend to cluster, alternating with pain-free periods of variable length [92]. Most episodes last for less than an hour. On cessation of the pain, the child is up and about as if nothing had happened. In the majority of cases, the cause is functional [91,92]. Organic causes account for 5 to 10% of cases [91,92]. Kokkonen et al. studied 84 children with recurrent abdominal pain [93]. Food allergy was diagnosed in 28 (33%) children based on an open elimination challenge test. The study was criticized because a formal diagnosis would require a double-blind placebo-controlled food challenge [94]. Further studies using double-blind placebo-controlled food challenges are necessary before food allergy can be established as a cause of recurrent abdominal pain in children.

Constipation

The vast majority of constipation in children is functional [95,96]. Constipation resulting from IgE sensitization to cow's milk has been described [97]. Loening-Baucke reviewed the records of 4,157 children between 0 to 24 months of age seen in general pediatric clinics for health maintenance and acute care visits [96]. Of the 185 children with constipation, food allergy was responsible for constipation in only 2 (1%) of these children [96]. In contrast, Iacono et al studied 27 consecutive infants with chronic "idiopathic" constipation and noted improvement or resolution of symptoms in 21(78%) of these infants after a 4-week period of a cow's milk-free diet [97]. These infants had a relapse of symptoms on cow's milk challenge. Iacono et al subsequently performed a randomized cross-over trial of a cow's milk-based diet versus a soy milk-based diet in 65 children with chronic constipation [98]. Forty-four (68%) of the 65 children had increased bowel movements and improvement of fecal score while receiving the soy milk. None of the children who received cow's milk had a response. In all 44 children with a response, the response was confirmed with a double-blind challenge with cow's milk. Daher et al studied 25 children with chronic constipation [99]. In seven (28%) patients, the constipation disappeared while they were following a diet free of cow's milk protein and reappeared within 48 to 72 hours after challenge with cow's milk. In two patients, a rectal biopsy revealed allergic colitis with eosinophilic infiltration and they therefore did not undergo the challenge. High serum levels of total IgE were observed in five (71%) of the seven patients who showed a clinical improvement. Two (29%) patients had a positive skin test and two (29%) had detectable levels of specific IgE. Carroccio et al treated 52 children with chronic constipation unresponsive to common treatment by exclusion of milk alone, or by an extensive oligoallergenic diet if unresponsive [100]. Twenty four patients were found to be suffering from cow's milk intolerance and six from multiple food intolerance. These patients had a normal stool frequency on elimination diet with recurrence of constipation on food challenge. These patients showed a significantly higher frequency of mucosal erosions, number of intraepithelial lymphocytes and eosinophils, and number of eosinophils in the lamina propria. The remaining 22 patients did not respond to the elimination diet. Murch identified 30 children with constipation who responded to the exclusion diet with resolution of symptom; six of these children were allergic to multiple antigens [58]. Rectal biopsy of the affected patients showed eosinophilic proctitis [58]. Carroccio et al performed a Medline search for articles published between 1970 and June 2006, using the key words "chronic constipation or constipation" and "food intolerance or allergy". The authors identified 33 papers but only 19 of them were related to the topic. Analysis of these papers showed a relationship between constipation and food allergy in a subgroup of pediatric patients with "idiopathic" constipation unresponsive to laxative treatment. Additional studies are necessary to substantiate the specific associations and to clarify the pathogenic mechanisms involved.

Cutaneous Manifestations

Urticaria/Angioedema

Acute urticaria and, to a lesser extent, angioedema are among the most common manifestations of food allergic reactions in children [29,44,52]. They tend to occur more commonly in younger patients and in atopic patients [101]. Symptoms result from activation of IgE-bearing cells by circulating food allergens absorbed through the gastrointestinal tract. The foods most commonly incriminated include eggs, milk, peanuts, and nuts [102]. In several studies, urticaria/angioedema occurred in 10 to 15% of infants with challenge-proven milk allergy [103,104]. In a study of 554 adults with urticaria, food allergy was demonstrated as the cause in only 1.4% of cases [105].

Even contact with foods may also cause acute urticaria [104,106,107]. Allergic contact urticaria can be seen in children who are sensitized to environmental allergens such as food or latex allergy [108]. There is a potential for cross-reactivity with various foods in individuals with latex allergy [108]. Food allergy is rarely the cause of chronic urticaria, unless the offending food is eaten almost every day [28,44,52,101].

Atopic Dermatitis

Atopic dermatitis is a multifactorial disease, and food allergy plays an immunopathogenic role in 30 to 50% of young children who had moderate to severe atopic dermatitis [5,109-111]. Burks et al. evaluated 46 patients who had atopic dermatitis from food hypersensitivity substantiated with double-blind placebo-controlled food challenges [112]. Sixty five food challenges were performed; 27 (42%) were interpreted as positive in 15 (33%) patients. Sampson et al. studied 350 patients with severe atopic dermatitis for possible food hypersensitivity [28,113,114]. Food allergy was diagnosed by double-blind placebo-controlled food challenges. Cutaneous reactions developed in 75% of the positive challenges within minutes to two hours, but only 30% of the positive responses were isolated cutaneous symptoms alone [28]. Most of the skin manifestations consisted of a markedly pruritic, erythematous rash that developed in sites with a predilection for atopic dermatitis.

In a well-designed prospective study of 113 patients with atopic dermatitis, marked improvement was noted in those who were maintained on an allergen elimination diet when compared with a similar group of patients who did not have food allergy or who did not adhere to the elimination diet [113]. Breuer et al. performed 106 double-blind placebo-controlled food challenges to cow's milk, egg, wheat, and soy on 64 children who had atopic dermatitis [115]. Twenty-eight (57%) of the 49 positive reactions resulted in late eczematous reactions either as isolated events or in combination with immediate reactions. Hill et al. evaluated 487 infants who had skin prick tests to cow's milk, egg, and peanut, and who had a family history of atopic dermatitis, asthma, or immediate food allergy in a parent or sibling [116]. One hundred and forty-one (28.9%) of these infants had atopic dermatitis by the age of 12 months. These authors found that as the severity of atopic dermatitis increased, so did the prevalence of IgE-mediated food allergy and also the frequency of adverse food allergy reactions. The relative risk of an infant who had atopic dermatitis to develop an IgE-mediated food allergy was 5.9 for the most severely affected group. The most frequently implicated foods include eggs, cow's milk, tree nut, peanut, soy, wheat, seafood, citrus fruits, and chocolate [117]. Approximately 30 to 40% of children lose their food hypersensitivity after one to two years of allergen avoidance and 80 to 85% outgrow their food allergies by 10 years of age [81,117]. Hypersensitivity to peanut, tree nut, and shellfish is more persistent [117].

The pathogenesis of atopic dermatitis likely involves both immediate and late-phase effects of IgE-mediated food hypersensitivity reactions as well as cell-mediated reactions [28,29,52,106]. The immediate or early phase of the reaction results from IgE-mediated cutaneous mast cell activation [29,114]. The late phase is characterized by a mixed cellular infiltrate (eosinophils, neutrophils, lymphocytes, and basophils) at six to eight hours and thereafter by a mononuclear round cell infiltrate indistinguishable from that seen in eczematous skin [113,118,119]. The pattern of cytokine expression is predominantly that of the Th2 type, namely, interleukin-4, -5 and -13 [101,102]. A single ingestion of food allergen may not provoke an eczematous lesion, but chronic ingestion of a food allergen can result in the classic changes of atopic dermatitis [109]. Children who have atopic dermatitis and documented food allergy might develop typical eczematous lesions while the disease is active, but might develop urticaria with ingestion of a food allergen when the atopic dermatitis is in remission [111]. On the other hand, atopic dermatitis is also seen in patients with X-linked agammaglobulinemia, suggesting that, at least in some cases, atopic dermatitis is not IgE-mediated [120]. Testing for cow's milk allergy, Hill et al. identified a delayed eczematous reaction in 17 of 135 children with atopic dermatitis [121]. Ten of the 17 children had negative prick test to cow's milk allergen, suggesting a non-IgE mediated pathogenesis. Lio suggests that there are at least two types of "food allergy" in patients with atopic dermatitis: the IgE-mediated immediate reactions and the cell-mediated eczematous reactions [120].

Contact Dermatitis

Contact dermatitis may be related to an immune-mediated reaction to food or a direct toxic effect of the food coming into contact with the skin [102,122]. Food-induced contact dermatitis is often seen among food handlers, especially those who handle raw shellfish and eggs [102,123,124]. Allergic contact cheilitis has been reported from the chewing of garlic [125] and from the contact of geraniol, a food additive contained in certain foods [126].

Dermatitis Herpetiformis

Gluten-sensitive enteropathy is found in 75 to 95% of patients with dermatitis herpetiformis [106,127]. Dermatitis herpetiformis is a cutaneous cell-mediated response to gliadin which is present in wheat, rye, and barley [44,102]. The disorder is characterized by a chronic, intensely pruritic, papulovesicular rash, symmetrically distributed over the extensor surfaces of the extremities and buttocks [8,102]. Approximately 80 to 90% of patients have the HLA-B8 haplotype, and more than 90% have the HLA-Dw3 haplotype [29,128]. Skin biopsy generally reveals granular and linear deposits of IgA, C3, as well as infiltrates with polymorphonuclear leukocytes. Immunoglobulin A deposits may activate complement through the alternative pathway and cause inflammation [29]. An IgE-mediated hypersensitivity reaction does not contribute to the pathogenesis. IgA antibodies to smooth muscle endomysium have been reported in patients with dermatitis herpetiformis-associated gluten-sensitive enteropathy [106]. Also, antibodies to tissue transglutaminase and epidermal transglutaminase are present in patients with dermatitis herpetiformis, suggesting that epidermal transglutaminase is the autoantigen in dermatitis herpetiformis [102].

Respiratory Manifestations

Rhinitis/ Rhinoconjunctivitis

Food-induced allergic rhinitis/rhinoconjunctivitis is more frequently observed in children than in adults [110,129]. Rhinitis/rhinoconjunctivitis following inhalation of food dusts or vapor is not uncommon in patients with food allergy [10]. Rhinitis/rhinoconjunctivitis typically occurs in association with other clinical manifestations such as cutaneous and/or gastrointestinal symptoms during acute allergic reactions to foods [19,130]. Rhinitis/ rhinoconjunctivitis as the sole manifestation of food allergy is quite uncommon [28,54,124,129]. Allergic rhinitis may be manifested as nasal congestion, sneezing, and rhinorrhea [117]. Allergic conjunctivitis is characterized by periocular erythema, ocular injection, pruritus, and tearing. It seems likely that ingested allergens can activate nasal mast cells in addition to mast cells elsewhere in the body [29].

Chronic Sinusitis

Allergy to food allergens has been suggested to be a rare cause of chronic sinusitis [131]. Food allergy should be suspected in refractory cases of chronic sinusitis in which no apparent cause can be found, especially in atopic individuals with perennial symptoms [108,131].

Asthma

Asthma from food allergy is a mixed IgE- and cell-mediated response due to the involvement of IgE antibodies, mast cells, eosinophils, and T-lymphocytes [21]. The condition occurs more often in children than in adults [132,133]. In several studies, 2 to 6% of children with asthma were found to have wheezing provoked by blinded food challenges [129,133-135]. Asthmatic children have a 14-fold higher risk of developing a severe allergic reaction to food compared with children without asthma [133,136].

In some children, food allergy may increase airway reactivity so that other triggers or environmental factors can more readily precipitate an asthmatic attack [137,138]. Even vapors containing proteins emitted from cooking food can induce asthmatic attacks [124,132,139,140]. Inhalational exposures to foods, particular in the workplace, account for approximately 1% of asthmatic attacks in the adult population [124,138]. Baker's asthma caused by inhalation of flour or mold-derived enzymes used as flour additives is a good example [44]. Affected individuals have asthmatic attacks in association with exposure to aerosolized wheat proteins and have positive skin prick tests or serum specific IgE to wheat proteins [135,138]. Likewise, peanut dust in airplanes can provoke allergic reactions in susceptible individuals [141]. Allergenic proteins may also reach the respiratory tract via the circulation or they may act via inflammatory mediators released from the skin or gastrointestinal tract [138].

Food-induced asthmatic reactions, when they occur in conjunction with other organ systems, generally indicate a more severe disease manifestation [132,142,143]. In a survey of six fatal and seven near fatal anaphylactic reactions after food ingestion, all patients had asthma and respiratory symptoms as part of their clinical manifestations [109]. Food allergy in early infancy increases the risk for developing asthma in later life [133,144,145]. This applies also to children who have outgrown their food allergies [142].

Heiner Syndrome

Primary pulmonary hemosiderosis with hypersensitivity to cow's milk (Heiner syndrome) is a rare condition that usually occurs in young children. The syndrome is characterized by chronic cough, wheezing, hemoptysis, pulmonary infiltrates, hemosiderosis, gastrointestinal blood loss, iron deficiency anemia, and failure to thrive [129,146]. Presumably, the syndrome results from aspiration of milk into the lungs with subsequent development of IgG cow's milk antibodies and an immune complex Arthus-type reaction in the alveoli [68,147]. If the vasculitis is severe, alveolar bleeding and pulmonary hemosiderosis may result [147]. Affected children usually have high titers of precipitins to multiple constituents of cow's milk and positive results on intradermal skin tests to various cows' milk proteins [146]. Dietary elimination of cow's milk results in symptomatic improvement, and reintroduction of cow's milk results in recurrence of symptoms. It has been postulated that antigen-antibody complexes and cell-mediated hypersensitivity play a pathogenic role in this syndrome based on the presence of elevated serum levels of milk-specific IgG antibodies and the in vitro proliferative response of the patient's lymphocytes to milk antigen [29].

Serous Otitis Media

Serous otitis media, defined as non-purulent collection of fluid in the middle ear, is a multifactorial disease [148]. Food allergy may play a role in the pathogenesis in a subgroup of children with serous otitis media [149-151]. It has been hypothesized that allergic inflammation in the nasal mucosa may cause Eustachian tube dysfunction which may result in serous otitis media [130,150]. IgG complexes with cow's milk protein might also contribute to the middle ear inflammation [152]. In the study by Aydoğan et al., food allergy was detected in 25 (44.6%) of 56 patients with serous otitis media [148]. In patients with food allergy, serous otitis media was detected in 7 (25%) of 28 patients. In the control group of 28 patients, food allergy was diagnosed in 5 (18%) patients and serous otitis media in one (3%) patient. The incidence of food allergy in serous otitis media group was statistically significant when compared to the normal group ($p<0.05$). The risk of otitis media in children having food allergy was 3.7 times higher than the control ($p<0.05$). Bernstein et al evaluated 100 patients aged 2 to18 years with recurrent serous otitis media for IgE-mediated hypersensitivity [149]. Thirty five of these patients had allergic rhinitis. Total IgE was increased in the middle ear fluid in 16 of the 35 patients with allergic rhinitis and in only 2 of the 65 patients in the non-allergic group. In 8 of these 16 patients (23% of the allergic group), levels of IgE per milligram of protein were higher in the middle ear effusion than in the corresponding serum, thus suggesting local production of IgE by the middle ear mucosa in these patients. In a subset of infants with recurrent serous otitis media, IgG complexes with food antigen may contribute to middle ear inflammation and serous otitis media [130,152]. Nsouli et al. evaluated 104 unselected children with recurrent serous otitis media for food allergy [151]. There was a significant statistical association, by chi-square analysis, between food allergy and recurrent serous otitis media in 81 (78%) of the 104 patients. An elimination diet led to a significant amelioration of serous otitis media in 70 (86%) of 81 patients. An open challenge diet with the suspected offending food(s) provoked a recurrence of serous otitis media in 66 (94%) of 70 patients. Further studies with double-blind placebo-controlled food challenge are necessary to confirm these findings.

Ménière's Disease

Ménière's disease is characterized by recurrent vertigo, fluctuating hearing loss, aural fullness or pressure, and tinnitus [153,154]. Derebery et al did a mail-survey on 1490 patients with Ménière's disease [153]. Of 734 respondents with Ménière's disease, 296 (40.3%) had or suspected food allergies and 272 (37%) had confirmatory skin or in vitro tests for allergy. These prevalence rates were significantly higher than those found in the control group of patients ($n=172$) with otologic problems other than Ménière's disease, of which 43 (25%) had or suspected food allergies and 38 (22.2%) had confirmatory skin or in vitro tests for allergy (differences all significant at $p\leq 0.005$). Keleş et al. studied 46 patients aged between 26 and 68 years and 46 age-matched controls. The authors found that total serum IgE levels were above the normal levels in 19 (41.3%) of the patients with Ménière's disease and 9 (19.5%) of the controls [154]. A history of allergy was found in 31 (67.3%) of the patients with Ménière's disease and 16 (34.7%) of the controls. When the specific IgE levels were measured (all seasons, tree, fungus, fruit, egg white, cow's milk, wheat flour, corn flour, beef, and rice), the number of patients having all the panels negative was eight (17.9%) in patients with Ménière's disease and 31 (67.3%) in the controls. Cow's milk allergy was the most common identifiable cause of Ménière's disease. It has been hypothesized that immune complexes circulating in the blood might hinder the filtering ability of the endolymphatic sac [154].

GENERALIZED MANIFESTATIONS

Systemic Anaphylaxis

Systemic anaphylaxis is an uncommon but potentially fatal manifestation of food allergy [109]. Systemic anaphylaxis usually occurs within minutes, but occasionally hours after the ingestion of an offending food [155]. Peanuts, nuts, eggs, and seafood are responsible for the majority of these reactions [65,156]. Systemic anaphylaxis results when antigen binds to allergen-specific IgE on mast cells and basophils with sudden release of potent biologically active inflammatory mediators affecting multiple target organs [45]. The mediators include histamine, heparin, and tryptase [7]. Early symptoms may include pruritus, "metallic" taste in the mouth, sensation of tightness in the throat, flushing, urticaria, dizziness, nausea, vomiting, abdominal pain, angioedema, and wheezing [157]. This may rapidly progress to laryngeal edema, dyspnea, stridor, diaphoresis, cyanosis, chest pain, hypotension, cardiac dysrhythmias, and shock [52,158]. The degree of anaphylactic reactions varies and may be manifested in a partial form [12]. In general, the more rapidly anaphylaxis occurs after exposure to an offending agent, the more likely the anaphylactic reaction is to be severe and potentially life-threatening [156]. Anaphylactic reactions to foods can be biphasic with an early and late phase separated by one to eight hours or there may be multiple recurrences separated by asymptomatic periods lasting for hours [10,68]. Some very severe anaphylactic reactions are protracted and last continuously for many hours without remission [68]. Risk factors for severe anaphylactic reactions include history of a previous anaphylactic reaction, history of poorly controlled asthma, allergy to peanuts, nuts and shellfish, and use of ß-blockers or acetycholinesterase inhibitors [1,159]. Low levels of serum platelet-activating factor acetylhydrolase may be a marker for more severe food-induced anaphylaxis [159].

Food-Dependent Exercise-Induced Anaphylaxis

Anaphylaxis has been reported after the ingestion of foods in association with exercise [160-162]. Food-dependent exercise-induced anaphylaxis represents 7 to 9% of anaphylactic reactions [163,164]. The condition is twice as common in females and 60% of cases occur in individuals under the age of 30 years [157,159,163]. There is often a history of atopy [163]. One subset of patients may develop anaphylaxis in temporal proximity to ingestion of any type of food [44,157]. The other subset may develop anaphylaxis with exercise in conjunction with ingestion of a specific food [157]. The latter subset is more common than the former subset [157]. Foods associated with food-specific exercise-induced anaphylaxis include crustaceans, celery, grapes, tomato, wheat, buckwheat, chicken, and dairy products [44,165]. Rarely, two foods have to be eaten together to provoke an anaphylactic attack [167]. When each food is taken separately, food-dependent exercise-induced anaphylaxis does not occur [167]. Typical symptoms include urticaria, angioedema, dyspnea, and abdominal pain [168]. These may progress to hypotension and shock. Loss of consciousness is seen in approximately 30% of cases [168].

Although various exercises may lead to anaphylaxis in susceptible individuals, jogging is the exercise most frequently reported, followed by aerobics and walking [44,163,169].

Anaphylaxis usually occurs when exercise takes place within two to four hours of food ingestion [157]. Unlike exercise-induced anaphylaxis, anaphylactic symptoms develop only in the presence of both food ingestion and exercise [170]. Food-dependent exercise-induced anaphylaxis often presents with pruritus about the scalp before the symptoms become generalized [157].

The exact mechanism of food-dependent exercise-induced anaphylaxis is not known. There is evidence of IgE-mediated sensitization to the food allergen [163]. Skin testing may show an immediate flare-and-wheal reaction to the implicated food [162]. Blood flow differences to the gut, increased food allergen absorption, increased spontaneous leukocyte histamine release, lowered mast cell releasability threshold, and enhanced mast cell responsiveness to physical stimuli may have a role in the pathogenesis of this condition [44,162,169,171].

Hyperactivity

A few anecdotal reports have suggested a role of food allergy in some children with hyperactivity [172,173]. To date, controlled studies have not substantiated the efficacy of an elimination diet in the treatment of hyperactivity [174]. The placebo effect may account for the favorable results in some of the uncontrolled studies [174-176].

Neurologic Manifestations

Migraine

Several double-blind studies have shown that some patients with migraine had adverse reactions to certain foods, as shown by dietary exclusion and subsequent challenge [177-179]. There was no clearly proven immunologic effect of food components in many of these patients [12]. Migraine can be triggered by foods rich in tyramine, tryptamine, serotonin, and histamine, and this is based mainly on pharmacologic rather than immunologic effects [180,181]. According to the revised nomenclature for allergy published by the European Academy of Allergy and Clinical Immunology, these kinds of adverse reactions are classified as toxic reactions rather than food hypersensitivity [182]. The present consensus is that food allergy does not play a significant role in migraine [110].

Epilepsy

Several authors have proposed a possible role of food allergy in a subset of children with epilepsy [183-185]. Frediani et al. have noted a significantly higher proportion of allergic disorders in 72 epileptic patients versus 202 aged-matched controls [184]. Using skin prick tests, the percentage of epileptic children who tested positive for cow's milk protein (24/72) and especially for lactalbumin (16/72) and β-lactoglobulin (10/72) was significantly higher than the percentage of controls that tested positive for the same allergens: 7/202 for cow's milk protein, 4/202 for lactalbumin, and 2/202 for β-lactoglobulin. In patients with allergic disorders, there is an increase in the proportion of electroencephalographic anomalies, often in the form of occipital dysrhythmias [184]. Crayton et al. reported on a patient whose epileptic fits were triggered and increased in frequency by double-blind food challenges [183]. Frediani et al. reported on a nine-year-old boy whose epileptic symptoms disappeared as a result of an allergen-free diet with no anticonvulsant therapy [185].

Endocrine Manifestation

Diabetes Mellitus

Cow's milk has been implicated as a possible trigger of the autoimmune response that destroys pancreatic ß-cells in genetically susceptible individuals, thereby leading to diabetes mellitus [186-188]. Karjalainen et al. measured IgG antibovine serum albumin antibodies in the serum of 142 children with newly diagnosed insulin-dependent diabetes mellitus [188]. These children had elevated serum concentrations of IgG antibovine serum albumin antibodies that declined after diagnosis and reached normal levels in most patients within one to two years. These authors speculate that patients with insulin-dependent diabetes mellitus have immunity to cow's milk albumin, with antibodies to an albumin peptide that are capable of reacting with a β-cell-specific surface protein. Such antibodies could participate in the development of islet cell dysfunction. Cavallo et al. measured the in vitro peripheral T-lymphocyte response to β-casein in 47 patients with recent-onset insulin-dependent diabetes mellitus [186]. Twenty four of 47 (51.1%) patients with insulin-dependent diabetes mellitus versus 0 of 10 patients with autoimmune thyroid disease and 1 of 36 (2.8%) healthy people had a positive response to ß-casein. A positive response was defined as a stimulation index above the mean value plus 2 SD of healthy people. These authors suggest that exposure to cow's milk triggers a cellular and humoral anti- ß-casein immune response that may cross-react with a β-cell antigen and lead to destruction of the β-cell. A subsequent study, however, showed a lack of association between early exposure to cow's milk and β-cell autoimmunity [189]. Norris et al. screened 253 children aged nine months to seven years with first-degree relatives who had insulin-dependent diabetes mellitus for β-cell autoimmunity [189]. Eighteen cases of β-cell autoimmunity were detected at baseline. These children were compared with 153 unrelated autoantibody-negative children selected from the cohort as controls. There were no differences in the proportion of cases and controls that were exposed to cow's milk or foods containing cow's milk by 3 months or 6 months of age. Further studies are necessary to clarity this important issue.

Renal Manifestations

Nephrotic Syndrome

Food allergy may play a role in the pathogenesis of nephrotic syndrome in a selected group of children [190-193]. Sandberg et al. reported 6 children with steroid-responsive nephrotic syndrome [190]. In the relapse period, a milk-free diet led to remission without steroid therapy. In the remission period, challenge with cow's milk resulted in a relapse in 4 patients. Sieniawska et al. evaluated the role of cow's milk in 17 children with steroid-resistant nephrotic syndrome [193]. Cows' milk was excluded from the diet for at least 14 days without changing the previously ineffective prednisone dosage. Six patients went into remission three to eight days after the elimination of cow's milk. After a period of two to three weeks of remission, cow's milk challenge was positive in three of the six patients. The group of responders to a milk-free diet was characterized by young age, feeding with cow's milk or unmodified powdered milk formulas in the neonatal period, and coexistence of allergic symptoms. The authors suggest that cellular mechanisms may play a role in cow's milk-induced steroid-resistant nephrotic syndrome as evidenced by the late-onset reaction to cow's milk challenge, positive leukocyte migration inhibition tests, absence of specific IgE antibodies, and negative skin test results. These studies, however, contain some design flaws and better objective studies are needed to prove the association between milk ingestion and nephrotic syndrome.

Nocturnal Enuresis

Several authors have noted that food allergy might play a role in nocturnal enuresis [194-196]. Mungan et al. studied an allergy panel that included total IgE, 10 examples of inhalant-specific IgE, 10 examples of food-specific IgE, eosinophilic cationic protein and Phadiotop on 37 children with nocturnal enuresis and 18 children without nocturnal enuresis as a control [94]. The authors did not find statistically significant differences between the two groups in terms of levels of total IgE, the 10 examples of inhalant-specific IgE and Phadiotop. However, two (soybean and hazelnut) of the 10 food-specific IgE and eosinophilic cationic protein level did differ significantly between the two groups. Further studies are necessary before a causal relationship can be established.

Hematologic Manifestations

Anemia

Iron deficiency anemia may develop in children with cow's milk allergy secondary to gastrointestinal blood loss. This may be caused by milk-induced enterocolitis syndrome [54], milk-induced colitis, allergic eosinophilic gastroenteropathy [52], and Heiner syndrome [146].

Thrombocytopenia

A few anecdotal reports suggest that thrombocytopenia may be caused by food allergy [197-199]. Whitefield and Barr reported a girl with the syndrome of thrombocytopenia and absent radius who showed marked gastrointestinal disturbance with clinical evidence of cow's milk allergy and in whom there appeared to be a direct correlation between cow's milk exposure, gastrointestinal upset, and thrombocytopenia [197]. Jones reported a newborn male infant with idiopathic thrombocytopenic purpura in whom withdrawal of a milk formula produced an improvement in the platelet count and reintroduction of the milk formula led to hematologic relapse on two occasions [198]. It has been suggested that a type II cytotoxic reaction may account for the thrombocytopenia seen after the ingestion of milk [199].

CARDIOVASCULAR MANIFESTATION

Vasculitis

Food-induced vasculitis has been described [200,201]. In the majority of cases, it is mediated by type III immunologic reaction (Arthus type) in which the antigen combines with its specific IgG and complement to form circulating complexes [200]. The circulating complexes deposit in the small blood vessels and initiate vasculitis. Occasionally, food-induced vasculitis may be IgE-mediated. Businco et al. reported two patients with leucocytoclastic vasculitis confirmed by skin biopsy [200]. The first patient had cutaneous vasculitis with large joint involvement, caused by cow's milk and egg as confirmed by blind food challenge. The second patient had cutaneous and mucous membrane vasculitis with large joint involvement caused by chocolate. Lunardi et al. described five patients with allergy and cutaneous vasculitis of 1 to 13 years' duration [201]. Double-blind food challenges identified the offending agent to be a food in two patients, an additive in another two patients, and both food and additive in the fifth patient.

RHEUMATIC MANIFESTATION

Arthropathy/Arthritis

A few anecdotal reports suggest that arthropathy/arthritis may be the result of food hypersensitivity [202-204]. Parke et al. described a 38-year-old woman who had progressive rheumatoid arthritis for 11 years [205]. Her rheumatoid arthritis improved within three weeks of changing to a milk-free diet and deteriorated within 24 hours with a milk challenge. Golding reported three patients with food-induced synovitis [206]. van de Larr et al. described six patients with rheumatoid arthritis which responded to a diet limited to an elemental formula [207]. Double-blind placebo-controlled trial confirmed a relationship with specific food in four of the six patients. Long-term benefit from avoidance of the specific foods, however, was noted only in two patients. Panush monitored 97 patients with inflammatory arthritis and found that no more than 5% of the patients with rheumatic disease had immunologic sensitivity to foods [204]. Denman et al. have not been able to detect any consistent correlation between controlled dietary challenges and exacerbations of inflammatory arthritis [208]. In those cases in which inflammatory arthritis responds to dietary manipulation, it is possible that dietary restriction non-specifically moderates the inflammatory manifestations of the disease or the placebo effect may be responsible [208].

Karatay et al. have shown that individualized diet challenges consisting of allergenic foods may regulate tumor necrosis factor-α and interleukin-1β levels in selected patients with rheumatoid arthritis [209]. Tumor necrosis factor-α and interleukin-1β are cytokines which promote inflammation and may play an important role in the development of rheumatoid arthritis [209].

Conclusions

The clinical manifestations of food allergy can be protean. There is usually a clear temporal relationship between the allergic reaction and prior exposure to food. At times, recognition of the allergic symptoms can be difficult as they may develop hours or days after food ingestion and the presentation could be atypical or unusual. In addition, the offending agent might not be the main food that was ingested [210]. Awareness of the various clinical manifestations of food allergy is important so that appropriate investigations can be planned and treatment initiated.

References

[1] Burks, W; Ballmer-Weber, BK. Food allergy. *Mol. Nutr. Food Res.* 2006;50:595-603.

[2] Scurlock, AM; Lee, LA; Burks, AW. Food allergy in children. *Immunol. Allergy Clin. North Am.* 2005;25:369-388.

[3] Hyams JS. Food allergy (food hypersensitivity). In: Kleigman, RM; Behram, RE; Jenson, HB; et al. (eds). *Nelson Textbook of Pediatrics*. Philadelphia: Saunders. 2007; pp.1585-1587.

[4] Pirson, F. Food allergy: a challenge for the clinician. *Acta Gastroenterol. Belg.* 2006;69:38-42.

[5] Sampson, HA; Leung, DY. Adverse reactions to foods. In: Kleigman, RM; Behram, RE; Jenson, HB; et al. (eds). *Nelson Textbook of Pediatrics*. Philadelphia: Saunders. 2007; pp. 986-990.

[6] Bangash, SA; Bahna, SL. Pediatric food allergy update. *Curr. Allergy Asthma Rep.* 2005;5:437-444.

[7] Keet, CA; Wood RA. Food allergy and anaphylaxis. *Immunol. Allergy Clin. North Am.* 2007;27:193-212.

[8] Mansueto, P; Montalto, G; Pacor, ML; et al. Food allergy in gastroenterologic diseases: review of literature. *World J. Gastroenterol.* 2006;12:7744-7752.

[9] Sicherer, SH; Sampson, HA. Food allergy. *J. Allergy Clin. Immunol.* 2006;117:S470-S475.

[10] Asero, R; Ballmer-Weber, BK; Beyer, K; et al. IgE-mediated food allergy diagnosis: current status and new perspectives. *Mol. Nutr. Food Res.* 2007;51:135-147.

[11] Minford, AMB; MacDonald, A; Littleword, JM. Food intolerance and food allergy in children: A review of 68 cases. *Arch. Dis. Child.* 1982;57:742-747.

[12] Stern, M. Allergic enteropathy. In: Walker, WA; Durie, PR; Hamilton, JR; et al. (eds). *Pediatric Gastrointestinal Disease*. St Louis: Mosby. 1996; pp. 677-692.

[13] Burks, AW; Sampson, HA. Diagnostic approaches to the patient with suspected food allergy. *J. Pediatr.* 1992;121:S64-S71.

[14] Sugita, K; Kabashima, K; Nakashima, D; et al. Oral allergy syndrome caused by raw fish in a Japanese sushi bar worker. *Contact dermatitis*. 2007;56:369-370.

[15] Nash, S; Burks, AW. Oral allergy syndrome. *Curr. Allergy Asthma Rep*. 2007;7:1-2.

[16] Purohit-Sheth, TS; Carr, WW. Oral allergy syndrome (pollen-food allergy syndrome). *Allergy Asthma Proc*. 2005;26:229-230.

[17] Seidman, E. Food allergic disorders of the gastrointestinal tract. In: Roy, CC; Silverman, A; Allagille, D. (eds). *Pediatric Clinical Gastroenterology*. St Louis: Mosby. 1995; pp. 374-384.

[18] Sampson, HA. Food allergy – accurately identifying clinical reactivity. *Allergy*. 2005;60:19-24.

[19] Aiuti, F ; Paganelli, R. Food allergy and gastrointestinal diseases. *Ann. Allergy*. 1983;51:275-280.

[20] Amlot, PL; Kemeny, DM; Zachary, C; et al. Oral allergy syndrome: symptoms of IgE mediated hypersensitivity to foods. *Clin. Allergy*. 1987;17:33-42.

[21] Lee, LA; Buirks, AW. Food allergies: prevalence, molecular characterization, and treatment/prevention strategies. *Annu. Rev. Nutr*. 2006;26;539-565.

[22] Ortolani, C; Ispano, M; Pastorello, EA; et al. Comparison of results of skin prick tests (with fresh foods and commercial food extracts) and RAST in 100 patients with oral allergy syndrome. *J. Allergy Clin. Immunol.* 1989;83:683-690.

[23] Hallett, R; Teuber, SS. Food allergies and sensitivities. *Nutr. Clin. Care*. 2004;7:122-129.

[24] Garcia-Careaga, M; Kerner, JA, Jr. Gastrointestinal manifestations of food allergies in pediatric patients. *Nutr. Clin. Pract*. 2005;20:526-535.

[25] Spergel, JM; Pawlowski, NA. Food allergy: mechanisms, diagnosis, and management in children. *Pediatr. Clin. North Am*. 2002;49:73-96.

[26] Strobel, S; Hourihane, OB. Gastrointestinal allergy: clinical symptoms and immunological mechanisms. *Pediatr. Allergy Immunol*. 2001;12(Suppl 14):43-46.

[27] Pastorello, EA; Robino, AM. Clinical role of lipid transfer proteins in food allergy. *Mol. Nutr. Food Res*. 2004;48:356-362.

[28] Hoffman, KM; Sampson, HA. Evaluation and management of patients with adverse food reactions. In: Bierman, CW; Pearlman, DS, Shapiro, GG; et al. (eds). *Allergy, Asthma, and Immunology from Infancy to Adulthood*. Philadelphia: WB Saunders. 1996; pp. 665-686.

[29] Burks, AW; Sampson, H. Food allergies in children. *Curr. Probl. Pediatr*. 1993;23:230-252.

[30] Sicherer, SH. Clinical aspects of gastrointestinal food allergy in childhood. *Pediatrics*. 2003;111:1609-1616.

[31] Dauer, EH; Freese, DK; El-Youssef, M; et al. Clinical characteristics of eosinophilic esophagitis in children. *Ann. Otol. Rhinol. Laryngol*. 2005;114:827-833.

[32] Furuta, GT; Straumann, A. Review article: the pathogensis and management of eosinophilic oesophagitis. *Aliment. Pharmacol. Ther*. 2006;24:173-182.

[33] Heine, RG. Pathophysiology, diagnosis and treatment of food protein-induced gastrointestinal diseases. *Curr. Opin. Allergy Clin. Immunol*. 2004;4:221-229.

[34] Spergel, JM. Eosinophilic esophagitis in adults and children: evidence for a food allergy component in many patients. *Curr. Opin. Allergy Clin. Immunol.* 2007;7:274-278.

[35] Furuta, T; Liacouras CA; Collins, MH; et al. Eosinophilic esophagitis in children and adults: a systemic review and consensus recommendations for diagnosis and treatment. *Gastroenterology.* 2007;133:1342-1363.

[36] Noel, RJ; Rothenberg, ME. Eosinophilic esophagitis. *Curr. Opin. Pediatr.* 2005;17:690-694.

[37] Martin-Muńoz, MF; Lucendo, AJ; Navarro, M, et al. Food allergies and eosinophilic esophagitis – two case studies. *Digestion*. 2006;74:49-54.

[38] Pentiuk, SP; Miller, CK; Kaul, A. Eosinophilic esophagitis in infants and toddlers. *Dysphagia*. 2007;22:44-48.

[39] Cheung, KM; Oliver, MR; Cameron, DJ, et al. Esophageal eosinophilia in children with dysphagia. *J. Pediatr. Gastroenterol. Nutr.* 2003;37:498-503.

[40] Croese, J; Fairley, SK; Masson, JW; et al. Clinical and endoscopic features of eosinophilic esophagitis in adults. *Gastrointest. Endosc.* 2003;58:516-522.

[41] Fox, VL; Nurko, S; Furuta, GT; et al. Eosinophilic esophagitis: it's not just kid's stuff. *Gastrointest. Endosc.* 2002;56:260-270.

[42] Liacouras, CA. Eosinophilic esophagitis in children and adults. *J. Pediatr. Gastroenterol. Nutr.* 2003;37:S23-S28.

[43] Remírez, JA; Escudero, R; Cáceres, O; et al. Eosinophilic esophagitis. *Allergol. Immunopathol. (Madr).* 2006;34:79-81.

[44] American College of Allergy, Asthma, & Immunology. Food allergy: a practice parameter. *Ann. Allergy Asthma Immunol.* 2006;96(Suppl 2):S1-S68.

[45] Sampson, HA; Leung, DY. Anaphylaxis. In: Kleigman, RM; Behram, RE; Jenson, HB; et al. (eds). *Nelson Textbook of Pediatrics*. Philadelphia: Saunders. 2007; pp. 983-985.

[46] Kaczmarski, SJ. Gastroesophageal reflux in children and adolescents. Clinical aspects with special respect to food hypersensitivity. *Adv. Med. Sci.* 2006;51:327-335.

[47] Kelly, KJ; Lazenby, AJ; Rowe, PC; et al. Eosinophilic esophagitis attributed to gastroesophageal reflux: improvement with an amino acid-based formula. *Gastroenterology.* 1995;109:1503-1512.

[48] Nowak-Wegrzyn, A. Food allergy to proteins. *Nestlé Nutr. Workshop Ser. Pediatr. Program.* 2007;59:17-35.

[49] Gonsalves, N. Food allergies and eosinophilic gastrointestinal illness. *Gastroenterol. Clin. North Am.* 2007;36:75-91.

[50] Klein, NC; Hargrove, RI; Sleisenger, MH; et al. Eosinophilic gastroenteritis. Medicine (Baltimore). 1970;49:299-319.

[51] Cello, JPE. Eosinophilic gastroenteritis: a complex disease entity. *Am. J. Med.* 1979;67:1097-1104.

[52] Brigino, E; Bahna, SL. Clinical features of food allergy in infants. *Clin. Rev. Allergy Immunol.* 1995;13:329-345.

[53] Proujansky, R; Winter, HS; Walker, WA. Gastrointestinal syndromes associated with food sensitivity. *Adv. Pediatr.* 1988;35:219-238.

[54] Bock, SA; Sampson, HA. Food allergy in infancy. *Pediatr. Clin. North Am.* 1994;41:1047-1067.

[55] Lake, AM. Dietary protein enterocolitis. *Curr. Allergy Rep.* 2001;1:76-79.

[56] Zapatero Remón, L; Alonso Lebrero, E; Martin Fernández, E; et al. Food protein-induced enterocolitis syndrome caused by fish. *Allergol. Immunopathol. (Madr).* 2005;33:312-316.

[57] Nowak-Wegrzyn, A; Sampson, HA; Wood, RA; et al. Food protein-induced enterocolitis syndrome caused by solid food proteins. *Pediatrics.* 2003;111:829-835.

[58] Murch, S. Allergy and intestinal dysmotility – evidence of genuine causal linkage? *Curr. Opin. Gastroenterol.* 2006;22:664-668.

[59] Yimyaem, P; Chongsrisawat, V; Vivatvakin, B, et al. Gastrointestinal manifestations of cow's milk protein allergy during the first year of life. *J. Med. Assoc. Thai.* 2003;86:116-123.

[60] Hojsak, I; Kljaić-Turkalj, M; Mišak. Z; et al. Rice protein-induced enterocolitis syndrome. *Clin. Nutr.* 2006;25:533-536.

[61] Sampson, HA. Food allergies. In: Oski, FA; DeAngelis, CD; Feigin, RD. (eds). *Principles and Practice of Pediatrics.* Philadelphia: JB Lippincott. 1994; pp. 227-232.

[62] Hirose, R; Yamada, T; Hayashida, Y. Massive bloody stools in two neonates caused by cow's milk allergy. *Pediatr. Surg. Int.* 2006;22:935-938.

[63] Swart, JF; Ultee, K. Rectal bleeding in a preterm infant as a symptom of allergic colitis. *Eur. J. Pediatr.* 2003;162:55-56.

[64] Stern, M. Gastrointestinal allergy. In: Walker, WA; Durie, PR; Hamilton, JR; et al. (eds). *Pediatric Gastrointestinal Disease.* St Louis: Mosby. 1991; pp. 557-574.

[65] Sampson, HA. Food allergies. In: McMillan, JA; Feigin, RD; DeAngelis, C; et al. *Oski's Pediatrics: Principles & Practice.* Philadelphia: Lippincott Williams & Wilkins. 2006; pp. 2417-2423.

[66] Troncone, R; Bhatnagar, S; Butzner, D; et al. Celiac disease and other immunologically mediated disorders of the gastrointestinal tract: Working Group Report of the Second World Congress of Pediatric Gastroenterology, Hepatology, and Nutrition. *J. Pediatr. Gastroenterol. Nutr.* 2004;39:S601-S610.

[67] Dewar, DH; Ciclitira, PJ. Clinical features and diagnosis of celiac disease. *Gastroenterology.* 2005;128:S19-S24.

[68] Anderson, JA. Food allergy and intolerance. In: Lieberman, P; Anderson, JA. (ed). *Current Clinical Practice: Allergic Diseases: Diagnosis and Treatment.* 3rd edition. Totowa: Humana Press, 2007, pp. 271-294.

[69] Estep, DC; Kulczycki, A, Jr. Treatment of infant colic with amino acid-based infant formula: a preliminary study. *Acta Paediatr.* 2000;89:22-27.

[70] Hill, DJ; Hudson, IL; Sheffield, LJ; et al. A low allergen diet is a significant intervention in infantile colic: results of a community-based study. *J. Allergy Clin. Immunol.* 1995;96:886-892.

[71] Iacono, G; Carroccio, A; Montalto, G; et al. Severe infantile colic and food intolerance: a long-term prospective study. *J. Pediatr. Gastroenterol. Nutr.* 1991;12:332-335.

[72] Leung, AK; Lemay, JF. Infantile colic: a review. *J. R. Soc. Health.* 2004;124:162-166.

[73] Lothe, L; Lindberg, T. Cow's milk whey protein elicits symptoms of infantile colic in colicky formula-fed infants: a double-blind crossover study. *Pediatrics.* 1989;83:262-266.

[74] Lucassen, PL; Assendelft, WJ; Gubbels, JW; et al. Infantile colic: crying time reduction with a whey hydrolysate: a double-blind, randomized, placebo-controlled trial. *Pediatrics.* 2000;106:1349-1354.

[75] Savino, F. Focus on infantile colic. *Acta Paediatr.* 2007;96:1259-1264.
[76] Hill, DJ; Hosking, CS. Infantile colic and food hypersensitivity. *J. Pediatr. Gastroenterol. Nutr.* 2000;30:S67-S76.
[77] Kalliomäki, M; Lappala, P; Korvenranta, H; et al. Extent of fussing and colic type crying preceding atopic disease. *Arch. Dis. Child.* 2001;84:349-350.
[78] Jakobsson, I; Lothe, L; Ley, D; et al. Effectiveness of casein hydrolysate feedings in infants with colic. *Acta Paediatr.* 2000; 89:18-21.
[79] Jakobbson, I; Lindberg, T. Cow's milk proteins cause infantile colic in breast-fed infants: a double-blind crossover study. *Pediatrics.* 1983;71:268-271.
[80] Hewson, P; Oberklaid, F; Menahem, S. Infant colic, distress, and crying. *Clin. Pediatr.* 1987;26:69-75.
[81] Leung, AK. Food allergy: a clinical approach. *Adv. Pediatr.* 1998;45:145-177.
[82] Nutrition Committee, Canadian Paediatric Society. Dietary manipulations for infantile colic. *Paediatr. Child Health.* 2003;8:449-452.
[83] Hill, DJ; Roy, N; Heine, RG; et al. Effect of a low-allergen maternal diet on colic among breastfed infants: a randomized, controlled trial. *Pediatrics.* 2005;116:e709-e715.
[84] Kalliomäki, MA. Food allergy and irritable bowel syndrome. *Curr. Opin. Gastroenterol.* 2005;21:708-711.
[85] Park, MI; Camilleri, M. Is there a role of food allergy in irritable bowel syndrome and functional dyspepsia? A systemic review. *Neurogastroenterol. Motil.* 2006;18:595-607.
[86] Gonsalkorale, WM; Perrey, C; Pravica, V; et al. Interleukin 10 genotypes in irritable bowel syndrome: evidence for an inflammatory component? *Gut.* 2003;52:91-93.
[87] van der Veek, PP; van den Berg, M; de Kroon, YE; et al. Role of tumor necrosis factor-α and interleukin-10 gene polymorphisms in irritable bowel syndrome. *Am. J. Gastroenterol.* 2005;100:2510-2516.
[88] Barbara, G; Stanghellini, V; de Giorgio, R; et al. Activated mast cells in proximity to colonic nerves correlate with abdominal pain in irritable bowel syndrome. *Gastroenterology.* 2004;126:693-702.
[89] Atkinson, W; Sheldon, TA; Shaath, N; et al. Food elimination based on IgG antibodies in irritable bowel syndrome: a randomized controlled trial. *Gut.* 2004;53:1459-1464.
[90] Isolauri, E; Rautava, S; Kalliomäki, M. Food allergy in irritable bowel syndrome: new facts and old fallacies. *Gut.* 2004;53:1391-1393.
[91] Leung, AK; Wong, BE; Cho, HY, et al. Recurrent abdominal pain in childhood. *Singapore Pediatr. J.* 1996;38:44-48.
[92] Leung, AK; Lemay, JF; Barker, C. Recurrent abdominal pain in children. *Can. J. Diagn.* 2002;19(5):68-80.
[93] Kokkonen, J; Ruuska, T; Karttunen, T; et al. Mucosal pathology of the foregut associating with food allergy and recurrent abdominal pains in children. *Acta Paediatr.* 2001;90:16-21.
[94] Husby, S; Host, A. Recurrent abdominal pain, food allergy and endoscopy. *Acta Paediatr.* 2001;90:3-4.
[95] Leung, AK; Chan, PY; Cho, HY. Constipation in children. *Am. Fam. Physician.* 1996;54:611-627.
[96] Loening-Baucke, V. Prevalence, symptoms and outcome of constipation in infants and toddlers. *J. Pediatr.* 2005;146:359-363.

[97] Iacono, G; Carroccio, A; Cavataio, F; et al. Chronic constipation as a symptom of cow milk allergy. *J. Pediatr.* 1995;126:34-39.

[98] Iacono, G; Cavataio, F; Montalto,G; et al. Intolerance of cow's milk and chronic constipation in children. *N. Engl. J. Med.* 1998;339:1100-1104.

[99] Daher, S; Tahan, S; Solé, D; et al. Cow's milk protein intolerance and chronic constipation in children. *Pediatr. Allergy Immunol.* 2001;1:339-342.

[100] Carroccio, A; Scalici, C; Maresi, E; et al. Chronic constipation and food intolerance: a model of proctitis causing constipation. *Scand. J. Gastroenterol.* 2005;40:33-42.

[101] Burks, W. Skin manifestations of food allergy. *Pediatrics.* 2003;111:1617-1624.

[102] Fasano, MB. Dermatologic food allergy. *Pediatr. Ann.* 2006;35:727-731.

[103] Host, A; Halken, S. A prospective study of cow milk allergy in Danish infants during the first 3 years of life. *Allergy.* 1990;45:587-596.

[104] Hill, DJ; Firer, MA; Shelton, MJ; et al. Manifestations of milk allergy in infants: clinical and immunologic findings. *J. Pediatr.* 1986;109:270-276.

[105] Champion, RH; Roberts, SO; Carpenter RG; et al: Urticaria and angioedema: a review of 554 patients. *Br. J. Dermatol.* 1969;81:588-597.

[106] Lemanske, RF Jr; Sampson, HA. Adverse reactions to foods and their relationships to skin diseases in children. *Adv. Pediatr.* 1988;35: 89-218.

[107] Winston, GB; Lewis, CW. Contract dermatitis. *Int. J. Dermatol.* 1982;21:573-578.

[108] Pastar, Z; Lipozencic, J. Adverse reactions to food and clinical expressions of food allergy. *SKINmed.* 2006;5:119-125.

[109] Sampson, HA. The immunopathogenic role of food hypersensitivity in atopic dermatitis. *Acta Derm. Venereol.* 1992;176:S34-S37.

[110] Gontzes, P; Bahna, SL. Food allergy for the primary care physician. *Primary Care.* 1987;14:547-558.

[111] Leung, AK; Hon, KL; Robson, WL. Atopic dermatitis. *Adv. Pediatr.* 2007;54:241-273.

[112] Burks, AW; Mallroy, SB; Williams, LW; et al. Atopic dermatitis: clinical relevance of food hypersensitivity reactions. *J. Pediatr.* 1988;113:447-451.

[113] Sampson, HA; McCaskill, CC. Food hypersensitivity and atopic dermatitis: evaluation of 113 patients. *J. Pediatr.* 1985;107:669-675.

[114] Sampson, HA; Mendelson, L; Rosen, JP. Fatal and near-fatal anaphylactic reactions to food in children and adolescents. *N. Engl. J. Med.* 1992;327:380-384.

[115] Breuer, K; Heratizadeh, A; Wulf, A, et al. Late eczematous reactions to food in children with atopic dermatitis. *Clin. Exp. Allergy.* 2004;34:817-824.

[116] Hill, DJ; Hosking, CS. Food allergy and atopic dermatitis in infancy: an epidemiology study. *Pediatr. Allergy Immunol.* 2004;15:421-427.

[117] Leung, AK; Bowen, TJ. Seasonal allergic rhinitis and food allergy. In: Bergman, AB. (ed). *Twenty Common Problems in Pediatrics.* New York: McGraw-Hill, 2001, pp. 219-233.

[118] Dolovich, J; Hargreave, FE; Chalmers, R; et al. Late cutaneous allergic responses in isolated IgE-dependent reactions. *J. Allergy Clin. Immunol.* 1973;52:38-46.

[119] Solley, GO; Gleich, GJ; Jordan, RE; et al. The late phase of the immediate wheal and flare skin reactions: its dependence on IgE antibodies. *J. Clin. Invest.* 1976;58:408-420.

[120] Lio, PA. Atopic dermatitis and food allergies: true, true and related? *Arch. Dis. Child. Educ. Pract. Ed.* 2007;92:ep56-ep60.

[121] Hill, DJ; Duke, AM; Hosking, CS; et al. Clinical manifestations of cow's milk allergy in childhood. II. The diagnostic value of skin tests and RAST. *Clin. Allergy.* 1988;18:481-490.
[122] Brancaccio, RR; Alvarez, MS. Contact allergy to food. *Dermatol. Ther.* 2004;17:302-313.
[123] Judd, L. A descriptive study of occupational skin disease. *N. Z. Med. J.* 1994;107: 147-149.
[124] Sampson, HA. Update on food allergy. *J. Allergy Clin. Immunol.* 2004;113:805-819.
[125] Ekeowa-Anderson, AL. Allergic contact cheilitis to garlic. *Contact Dermatitis.* 2007;56:174-175.
[126] Tamagawa-Mineoka, R; Katoh, N; Kishimoto, S. Allergic contact cheilitis due to geraniol in food. *Contact Dermatitis.* 2007;56:242-243.
[127] Hall, RP. Dermatitis herpetiformis. *J. Invest. Dermatol.* 1992;99:873-881.
[128] Solheim, BG; Ek, J; Thune, PO; et al. HLA antigens in dermatitis herpetiformis and coeliac disease. *Tissue Antigens.* 1976;7:57-59.
[129] El-Gamal, YM; Hossny, EM. Respiratory food allergy. *Pediatr. Ann.* 2006;35:733-740.
[130] James, JM. Respiratory manifestations of food allergy. *Pediatrics.* 2003;111:1625-1630.
[131] Ortolani, C. Atlas on mechanisms in adverse reactions to food. *Allergy.* 1995;50:5-81.
[132] James, JM; Crespo, JF. Allergic reactions to foods by inhalation. *Curr. Allergy Asthma Rep.* 2007;7:167-174.
[133] Ozol, D; Mete, E. Asthma and food allergy. *Curr. Opin. Pulm. Med.* 2008;14:9-12.
[134] Onorato, J; Merland, N; Terral, C; et al: Placebo-controlled double-blind food challenge in asthma. *J. Allergy Clin. Immunol.* 1986;78:1139-1146.
[135] Roberts, G; Lack, G. Food allergy and asthma – what is the link? *Paediatr. Respir. Rev.* 2003;4:205-212.
[136] Rance, F; Micheau, P; Marchac, V; et al. Food allergy and asthma in children. *Rev. Pneumol. Clin.* 2003;59:109-113.
[137] James, JM; Eggleston, PA; Sampson, HA. Food allergy increases airway reactivity. *Am. J. Crit. Care Respir. Med.* 1994;149:59-64.
[138] Roberts, G; Lack, G. Relevance of inhalational exposure to food allergens. *Curr. Opin. Allergy Clin. Immunol.* 2003;3:211-215.
[139] Crespo, JF; Pascual, C; Dominguez, C; et al. Allergic reactions associated with airborne fish particles in IgE-mediated fish hypersensitive patients. *Allergy.* 1995; 50:257-261.
[140] Roberts, G; Golder, N; Lack, G. Bronchial challenges with aerosolized food in asthmatic, food-allergic children. *Allergy.* 2002;57:713-717.
[141] Sicherer, SH; Furlong, TJ; DeSimone, J; et al. Self-reported allergic reactions to peanuts on commercial airlines. *J. Allergy Clin. Immunol.* 1999;104:186-189.
[142] Simpson, AB; Glutting, J; Yousef, E. Food allergy and asthma morbidity in children. *Pediatr. Pulmonol.* 2007;42:489-495.
[143] Wang, J; Visness, CM; Sampson, HA. Food allergen sensitization in inner-city children with asthma. *J. Allergy. Clin. Immunol.* 2005;115:1076-1080.
[144] Gustafsson, D; Sjöberg, O; Foucard, T. Sensitization to food and airborne allergens in children with atopic dermatitis followed up to 7 years of age. *Pediatr. Allergy Immunol.* 2003;14:448-452.

[145] Kotaniemi-Syrjanen, A; Reijonen, T; Romppanen, J. Allergen-specific immunoglobulin E antibodies in wheezing infants: the risk for asthma in later childhood. *Pediatrics.* 2003;111:e255-e261.

[146] Heiner, DC; Sears, JW. Chronic respiratory disease associated with multiple circulating precipitins to cow's milk. *Am. J. Dis. Child.* 1960;100:500-502.

[147] Bahna, SL. Adverse food reactions by skin contact. *Allergy*. 2004;59(Suppl 78):66-70.

[148] Aydoğan, B; Kiroğlu, M; Altintas, D; et al. The role of food allergy in otitis media with effusion. *Otolaryngol. Head Neck Surg*. 2004;130:747-750.

[149] Bernstein, JM; Lee, J; Conboy, K; et al. Further observations on the role of IgE-mediated hypersensitivity in recurrent otitis media with effusion. *Otolaryngol. Head Neck Surg.* 1985;93:611-615.

[150] Luyasu, S; Morisset, M; Guenard, L; et al. Acute recurrent otalgia and food allergy: a case report and review of the literature. *Eur. Ann. Allergy Clin. Immunol*. 2005;37:60-62.

[151] Nsouli, TM; Nsouli, SM; Linde, RE; et al. Role of food allergy in serous otitis media. *Ann. Allergy.* 1994;73:215-219.

[152] Juntti, H; Tikkanen, S; Kokkonen, J; et al. Cow's milk allergy is associated with recurrent otitis media during childhood. *Acta Otolaryngol*. 1999;119:867-873.

[153] Derebery, MJ; Berliner, KI. Prevalence of allergy in Meniere's disease. *Otolaryngol. Head Neck Surg*. 2000;123:69-75.

[154] Keleş, E; Gödekmerdan, A; Kalidağ, T; et al. Ménière's disease and allergy: allergens and cytokines. *J. Laryngol. Otol*. 2004;118:688-693.

[155] Golbert, TM; Patterson, R; Pruzansky, JJ. Systemic allergic reactions to ingested antigens. *J. Allergy.* 1969;44:96-107.

[156] Joint Task Force on Practice Parameters; American Academy of Allergy, Asthma and Immunology; American College of Allergy, Asthma and Immunology; Joint Council of Allergy, Asthma and Immunology. The diagnosis and management of anaphylaxis: an updated practice parameter. *J. Allergy Clin. Immunol*. 2005;115:S483-S523.

[157] Sampson, HA. Anaphylaxis and emergency treatment. *Pediatrics*. 2003;111: 1601-1608.

[158] Brown, SG. Cardiovascular aspects of anaphylaxis: implications for treatment and diagnosis. *Curr. Opin. Allergy Clin. Immunol*. 2005;5:359-364.

[159] Wang, J; Sampson, HA. Food anaphylaxis. *Clin. Exp. Allergy*. 2007;37:651-660.

[160] Maulitz, RM; Pratt, DS; Schocket, AL. Exercise-induced anaphylactic reactions to shellfish. *J. Allergy Clin. Immunol.* 1979;63:433-434.

[161] Sheffer, AL; Austen, KF. Exercise-induced anaphylaxis. *J. Allergy Clin. Immunol.* 1980;66:106-111.

[162] Kidd, JM III; Cohen, SH; Sosman, AJ; et al. Food-dependent exercise-induced anaphylaxis. *J. Allergy Clin. Immunol.* 1983;71:407-411.

[163] Beaudouin, E; Renaudin, JM; Morisset, M; et al. Food-dependent exercise-induced anaphylaxis – update and current data. *Eur. Ann. Allergy Clin. Immunol*. 2006;38:45-51.

[164] Castells, MC; Horan, RF; Sheffer, AL. Exercise-induced anaphylaxis (EIA). *Clin. Rev. Allergy Immunol.* 1999;17:413-424.

[165] Noma, T; Yoshizawa, I; Ogawa, N; et al. Fatal buckwheat dependent exercise induced anaphylaxis. *Asian Pacific J. Allergy Immunol*. 2001;19:283-286.

[166] Senna, G; Mistrello, G; Roncarolo, D; et al. Exercise-induced anaphylaxis to grape. *Allergy*. 2001;56:1235.
[167] Dohi, M; Suko, M; Sugiyama, H; et al. 3 cases of food-dependent exercise-induced anaphylaxis in which aspirin intake exacerbated anaphylactic symptoms. *Arerugi*. 1990;39:1598-1604.
[168] Morita, E; Kunie, K; Matsuo, H. Food-dependent exercise-induced anaphylaxis. *J. Dermatol. Sci.* 2007;47:109-117.
[169] Anderson, JA. The clinical spectrum of food allergy in adults. *Clin. Exp. Allergy*. 1991;21:S304-S315.
[170] Silverstein, SR; Frommer, DA; Dobozin, B; et al. Celery-dependent exercise-induced anaphylaxis. *J. Emerg. Med.* 1986;4:195-199.
[171] Buchbinder, EM; Bloch, KJ; Moss, J; et al. Food-dependent, exercise-induced anaphylaxis. *JAMA*. 1983;250:2973-2974.
[172] Feingold, BF. Food additives and child development. *Hosp. Pract.* 1973;8:11-21.
[173] Feingold, BF. Hyperkinesis and learning disabilities linked to artificial food flavors and colors. *Am. J. Nurs.* 1975;75:797-803.
[174] Leung, AK; Robson, WL; Fagan, JE; et al. Attention-deficit hyperactivity disorder: getting control of impulsive behavior. *Postgrad. Med.* 1994;95:153-160.
[175] Leung, AK; Lemay, JF. Attention deficit hyperactivity disorder: an update. *Adv. Ther.* 2003;20:303-318.
[176] Varley, CK. Diet and the behavior of children with attention deficit disorder. *J. Am. Acad. Child Psychiatry*. 1984;23:182-185.
[177] Monro, J; Carini, C; Brostoff, J. Migraine is a food-allergic disease. *Lancet*. 1984;1:719-721.
[178] Mansfield, LE; Vaughan, TR; Waller, SF; et al. Food allergy and adult migraine: double-blind and mediator confirmation of an allergic etiology. *Ann. Allergy*. 1985;55:126-129.
[179] Egger, J; Carter, CM; Soothill, JF; et al. Oligoantigenic diet treatment of children with epilepsy and migraine. *J. Pediatr.* 1989;114:51-58.
[180] Fotherby, KJ; Hunter, JO. Symptoms of food allergy. *Clin. Gastroenterol.* 1985;14:615-629.
[181] Pearson, DJ; McKee, A. Food allergy. *Adv. Nutr. Res.* 1985;7:1-37.
[182] Johansson, SG; Hourihane, JO; Bousquet, J; et al. A revised nomenclature for allergy. An EAACI position statement from the EAACI nomenclature task force. *Allergy*. 2001;56:813-824.
[183] Crayton, JW; Stone, T; Stein, G. Epilepsy precipitated by food sensitivity: report of a case with double-blind placebo-controlled assessment. *Clin. Electroencephalographol.* 1981;12:192-198.
[184] Frediani, T; Lucarelli, S; Pelliccia, A; et al. Allergy and childhood epilepsy: a close relationship? *Acta Neurol. Scand.* 2001;104:349-352.
[185] Frediani, T; Pelliccia, A; Aprile, A; et al. Partial idiopathic epilepsy: recovery after allergen-free diet. *Pediatr. Med. Chir.* 2004;26:196-197.
[186] Cavallo, MG; Fava, D; Monetini, L; et al. Cell-mediated immune response to ß casein in recent-onset insulin-dependent diabetes: implications for disease pathogenesis. *Lancet*. 1996;348:926-928.
[187] Harrison, LC. Cow's milk and IDDM. *Lancet*. 1996;348:905-906.

[188] Karjalainen, J; Martin, JM; Knip, M; et al. A bovine albumin peptide as a possible trigger of insulin-dependent diabetes mellitus. *N. Engl. J. Med.* 1992;327:302-307.
[189] Norris, JM; Beaty, B; Klingensmith, G et al. Lack of association between early exposure to cow's milk protein and ß-cell autoimmunity: diabetes autoimmunity study in the young (DAISY). *JAMA.* 1996;276:609-614.
[190] Sandberg, DH; McIntosh, RM; Bernstein, CW; et al. Severe steroid-responsive nephrosis associated with hypersensitivity. *Lancet.* 1997;1:388-391.
[191] Genova, R; Sanfilippo, M; Rossi, ME; et al. Food allergy in steroid-resistant nephrotic syndrome. *Lancet.* 1987;1:1315-1316.
[192] Laurent, J; Rostoker, G; Robera, R; et al. Is adult idiopathic nephrotic syndrome food allergy? Value of oligoantigenic diets. *Nephron.* 1987;47:7-11.
[193] Sieniawska, M; Szymanik-Grzelak, H; Kowalewska, M; et al. The role of cow's milk protein intolerance in steroid-resistant nephrotic syndrome. *Acta Paediatr.* 1992;81:1007-1012.
[194] Mungan, NA; Seckiner, I; Yesilli, C; et al. Nocturnal enuresis and allergy. *Scand. J. Urol. Nephrol.* 2005;39:237-241.
[195] Oei, HD; Pelikan-Filipek, M; Pelikan, Z; et al. Enuresis and encopresis as a reaction to food. *Ned. Tijdschr. Geneeskd.* 1989;133:1555-1557.
[196] Rawashdeh, YF; Hvistendahl, GM; Kamperis, K; et al. Demographics of enuresis patients attending a referral centre. *Scand. J. Urol. Nephrol.* 2002;36:348-353.
[197] Whitefield, MF; Barr, DGD. Cow's milk allergy in the syndrome of thrombocytopenia with absent radius. *Arch. Dis. Child.* 1976;51:337-343.
[198] Jones, RHT. Congenital thrombocytopenia and milk allergy. *Arch. Dis. Child.* 1977;52:744-745.
[199] Caffrey, EA; Sladen, GE; Isaacs, PET; et al. Thrombocytopenia caused by cow's milk. *Lancet.* 1981;2:316.
[200] Businco, L; Falconieri, P; Bellioni-Businco, B; et al. Severe food-induced vasculitis in two children. *Pediatr. Allergy Immunol.* 2002;12:68-71.
[201] Lunardi, C; Bambara, LM; Biasi, D; et al. Elimination diet in the treatment of selected patients with hypersensitivity vasculitis. *Clin. Exp .Rheum.* 1992;10:131-135.
[202] Panush, RS; Carter, RL; Katz, P; et al. Diet therapy for rheumatoid arthritis. *Arthritis Rheum.* 1983;26:462-471.
[203] Panush, RS; Stroud, RM; Webster, EM. Food-induced (allergic) arthritis: Inflammatory arthritis exacerbated by milk. *Arthritis Rheum.* 1986;29:220-226.
[204] Panush, RS. Food induced ("allergic") arthritis: clinical and serologic studies. *J. Rheumatol.* 1990;17:291-294.
[205] Parke, AL; Hughes, GR. Rheumatoid arthritis and food: a case study. *Br. Med. J.* 1981;282:2027-2029.
[206] Golding, DN. Is there an allergic synovitis? *J. R. Soc. Med.* 1990;83:312-314.
[207] van der Laar, MA; van der Korst, JK. Food intolerance in rheumatoid arthritis. I. A double blind, controlled trial of the clinical effects of elimination of milk allergens and azo dyes. *Ann. Rheum. Dis.* 1992;51:298-302.
[208] Denman, AM; Mitchell, B; Ansell, BM. Joint complaints and food allergic disorders. *Ann. Allergy.* 1983;51:260-263.

[209] Karatay, S; Erdem, T; Yildirim, K; et al. The effect of individualized diet challenges consisting of allergenic foods on TNF-α and IL-1β levels in patients with rheumatoid arthritis. *Rheumatology.* 2004;43:1429-1433.

[210] Bahna, SL. Unusual presentations of food allergy. *Ann. Allergy Asthma Immunol.* 2001;86:414-420.

In: Food Allergies: Symptoms, Diagnosis, and Treatment
Editors: Patricia M. Rodgers
ISBN: 978-1-61728-748-0

Chapter 8

Potential Effect of Combined High Pressure and Enzymatic Treatments on the Acceleration of Proteolysis and Reduction of Immunoreactivity of Dairy Proteins. Prevention and Treatment of Cow's Milk Allergy

Elena Peñas and Rosario Gómez*
Instituto del Frío, ICTAN (C.S.I.C), Spain

Abstract

The prevalence of cow's milk allergy (CMA) ranges from 0.5% to 7.5% in children in the first half year of life, although generally resolves by 3 years of age. However, it may be a precursor to other, and sometimes more serious, atopic diseases, asthma, and respiratory allergies. The prevention of cow's milk proteins sensitisation, early allergy and atopic dermatitis is therefore an important strategy in limiting atopic disease in later childhood and adulthood, and research efforts have been done into prevention strategies. Because infants may absorb more food allergen during their first year than later in life, the best strategy to prevent food sensitisation is to avoid the relevant allergenic proteins, with exclusive breast-feeding as a first option. The second option is the use of hypoallergenic (HA) hydrolysates based formulas during the first 6 months of life, mainly in none or partially breastfed infants from atopic families (at risk infants).

Since residual allergenicity has been reported in several commercial preparations developed from enzymatic hydrolysis of heat treated (HT) proteins, the use of high hydrostatic pressure (HHP) as an alternative to HT has generated increasing interest over the last decade, investigation widely developed by our group. The combined HHP and enzymatic treatments of proteins might be of interest to the dairy industry to produce new foods suitable for children having a milk allergy and also for those from atopic families (at risk infants).

---

* Corresponding author

The main objective of this review is to provide the reader with an up-to-date summary and analyse new trends which have emerged in the last few years in this developing area.

INTRODUCTION

Breast-feeding is the most suitable form of nutrition for neonates due to the specific content of nutrients and growth and defense factors of human milk (Hattevig et al., 1990; Neville et al., 1991; Wold and Adlerberth, 1998).When exclusive breast-feeding during the first months of life is not possible, mother's milk must be replaced or supplemented with infant formulas, which are often based on unhydrolysed cow´s milk. In predisposed infants, the ingestion of these formulas can induce immunological responses to cow's milk proteins (CMP) (Holt and Jones, 2000). This syndrome is known as cow's milk allergy (CMA); it is mainly an IgE mediated hypersensitivity reaction where multiple sensitisation to different CMP is observed in about 75% of milk allergic patients (Fritsché, 2003). The three-dimensional structure of proteins seems to be an important feature in cow´s milk protein allergenicity, although no definite relationship can be established between protein structure and allergenicity.

The prevalence of CMA ranges from 0.5% to 7.5% in children in the first half year of life (Høst et al., 1988), although generally resolves by 3 years of age. However, it may be a precursor to other, and sometimes more serious, atopic diseases, asthma, and respiratory allergies (Kulig et al., 1998; Exl et al., 2000). The prevention of CMP sensitisation, early allergy and atopic dermatitis is therefore an important strategy in limiting atopic disease in later childhood and adulthood, and research efforts have been done into prevention strategies (Exl, 2001). Because infants may absorb more food allergen during their first year than later in life, the best strategy to prevent food sensitisation is to avoid the relevant allergenic proteins (Dannaeus et al., 1978; Chandra et al., 1985; Hattevig et al., 1990), with exclusive breast-feeding as a first option. The second option is the use of hypoallergenic (HA) cow´s milk based formulas during the first 6 months of life, mainly in none or partially breastfed infants from atopic families (at risk infants).

Enzymatic hydrolysis and heat treatment (HT) are normally used to reduce the content of β-Lg and other intact proteins in milk and consequently, to reduce the antigenicity of milk proteins in the production of protein hydrolysates from cow´s milk to use in HA formulas (Nakamura et al., 1993; Siemensma et al., 1993). Heat treatment seems to affect conformational epitopes, but has only a moderate effect on allergenicity of milk proteins when it is used alone; however, its use prior to enzymatic hydrolysis improves the access of proteolytic enzymes to hidden peptidic cleavage bonds of proteins, and consequently removes the sequential epitopes depending on the temperature used (Lee, 1992). At temperatures below 60–65°C, only reversible modifications of pure β-Lg at neutral pH occur, and the hydrophobic protein core is unfolded and solvent exposed (Bonomi et al., 2003; Cairoli et al., 1994; Iametti et al., 1996), thus making the inner parts of protein accessible to enzymes. At higher temperature, dissociation of the β-Lg dimmer into monomers occurs, and soluble and relatively small aggregates are formed in heated solutions (Bonomi et al., 2003; Cairoli et al., 1994; Iametti et al., 1997). These aggregates might hide sites of attack from the action of proteases, some of which may be relevant to allergenic properties of the protein. The elimination of residual high-molecular weight peptides, proteins and enzymes used in the digestion by ultrafiltration after the hydrolysis process, contributes also to the reduction of antigenicity of the hydrolysates (Gorthler et al., 1995). However, residual allergenicity has been reported in several of these commercial preparations (Caffarelli et al., 2002; Calvo & Gómez, 2002; Oldaeus et al., 1991; Restani et al., 1995; Rosendal, A. & Barkholt, 2000; Van Berensteijn et al., 1995), which could be due to the inaccessibility of some epitopes to proteases even in the denatured protein.

The HA formulas can be classified into extensively (eHF) and partially/moderately hydrolysed formulas (pHF), depending on the degree of hydrolysis obtained (Aggett et al., 1993; Businco et al., 1993), but there is no unanimous agreement on this classification. Although molecular weight is an important classifier, studies have shown that products with hydrolysates of comparable molecular weight may have different preventive or treatment effects (Halken et al., 2001). eHF would present lower allergic potential than pHF and should be only used for infants with established CMA. However, the pHF with confirmed reduced allergenicity should be used for primary prevention of CMA in non-sensitised at-risk infants (Høst et al., 1999). A statement from the American Academy of Paediatrics (AAP) on the topic of HA infant formulas indicates for the first time that pHF may be of benefit in long-term protection to CMA. Such formulas are sufficiently reduced in allergenicity that they do not sensitise at-risk infants but still contain enough immunogenicity to deviate the immune system from hypo sensitivity against cow´s milk proteins (Fritsché, 2003).

For these reasons, in recent years, there has been growing interest in the development of a new range of hypoallergenic hydrolysates with limited hydrolysis. High hydrostatic pressure (HHP) technology could be a valuable alternative to thermal processing in their development, considering the conformational changes of proteins induced by this physical treatment as shown by several scientific papers. This non thermal technique for food processing has generated increasing interest over the last decade since it can compete with conventional heat treatment for the reduction of microbial populations, maintaining sensorial and nutritional properties of food (Préstamo et al., 2000), mineral balance (De la Fuente et al., 1998) and thermolabile nutrients such as vitamins (Kimura et al., 1994). However, relatively few data are available on the reduction of protein antigenicity by combination of enzymatic hydrolysis and HHP.

The main objective of this review is to provide the reader with an up-to-date summary and analyse new trends which have emerged in the last few years in this developing area.

1. Development of Hydrolysates

HHP treatment constitutes an effective approach for producing protein hydrolysates in a short time, since improved digestibility of proteins that can not be hydrolysed without difficulty at ambient pressure has been reported after pressuring them. Thus, the hydrolysis of β-Lactoglobulin (β-Lg) by pepsin increased considerably with pressures up to 300 MPa when only negligible digestion occurred at atmospheric pressure (Dufour et al., 1995; Stapelfeldt et al., 1996). The enhanced proteolysis of β-Lg under pressure conditions was also observed during chymotryptic (Chicon et al., 2006; Van Willige and Fitzgerald, 1995), trypsin (Dufour et al., 1995; Stapelfeldt et al., 1996; Maynard et al., 1998; Van Willige and Fitzgerald, 1995), and thermolysin hydrolysis (Okamoto et al., 1991; Dufour et al., 1995; Stapelfeldt et al., 1996). Moreover, selective hydrolysis of β-Lg by thermolysin in whey protein concentrates seems to occur under pressure, while α-lactalbumin (α-La) is resistant to the treatment (Hayashi et al., 1987). Increased hydrolysis of pressurised proteins has been attributed to the combination of several phenomenons, such as the unfolding of proteins induced by HHP that favours the accessibility of proteases to new cleavage sites in the proteins, increasing the susceptibility of proteins to enzymatic hydrolysis (Bonomi et al., 2003), better binding of enzymes to proteins and/or the activation of enzymes by HHP (Stapelfeldt et al., 1996; Maynard et al., 1998).

a

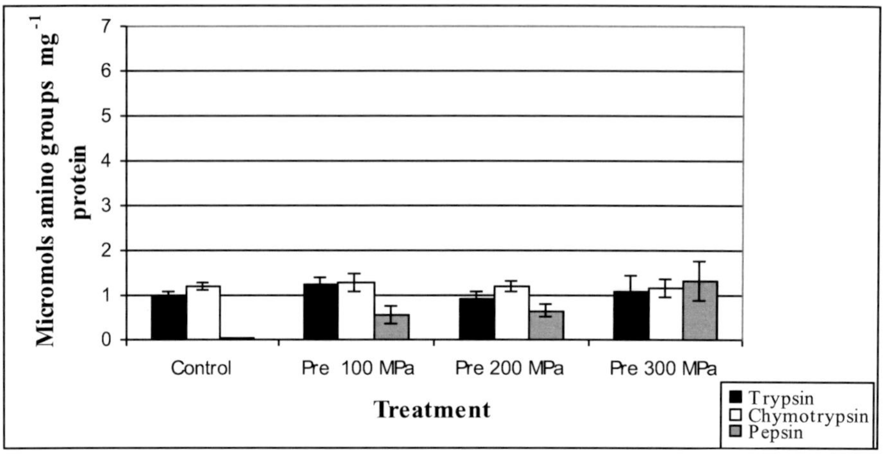

b

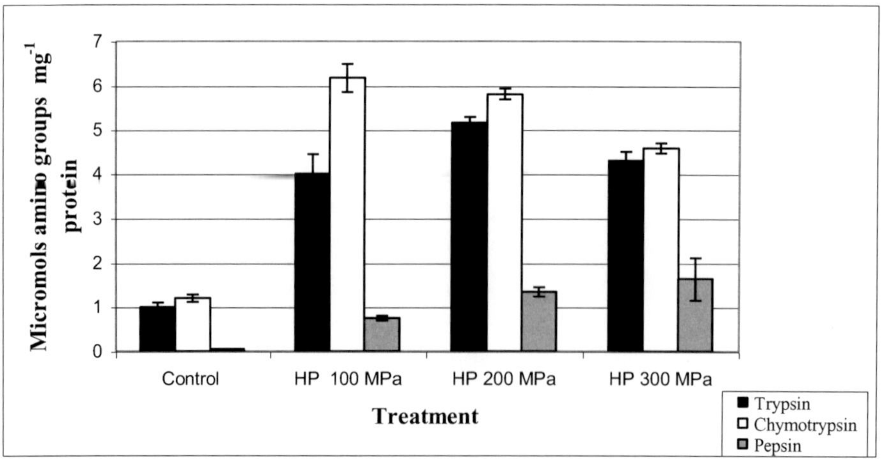

Figure 1. Degree of hydrolysis determined by *o*-phthaldialdehyde method during hydrolysis of dairy whey proteins by digestive enzymes. (a) high pressure treatment (100, 200 or 300 MPa, for 15 min at 37ºC) prior to hydrolysis with pepsin, chymotrypsin and trypsin; (b) hydrolysis performed during the high-pressure treatment (100, 200 or 300 MPa, for 15 min at 37ºC).

Our group studied the effect of HHP on the proteolysis of bovine whey (WP) by digestive enzymes (Peñas et al., 2006a). The extent of proteolysis by chymotrypsin and trypsin was significantly enhanced ($p \leq 0.05$) when the digestion took place at 100 and 200 MPa, respectively. However, no significant differences between control samples and those hydrolysed after HP treatment by both enzymes were found. On the other hand, HP treatment enhanced the proteolysis by pepsin, and the highest degree of hydrolysis by this enzyme was obtained at 300 MPa, but there were no significant differences between the application of pressure treatment prior to or during the enzymatic digestion (Figure 1).

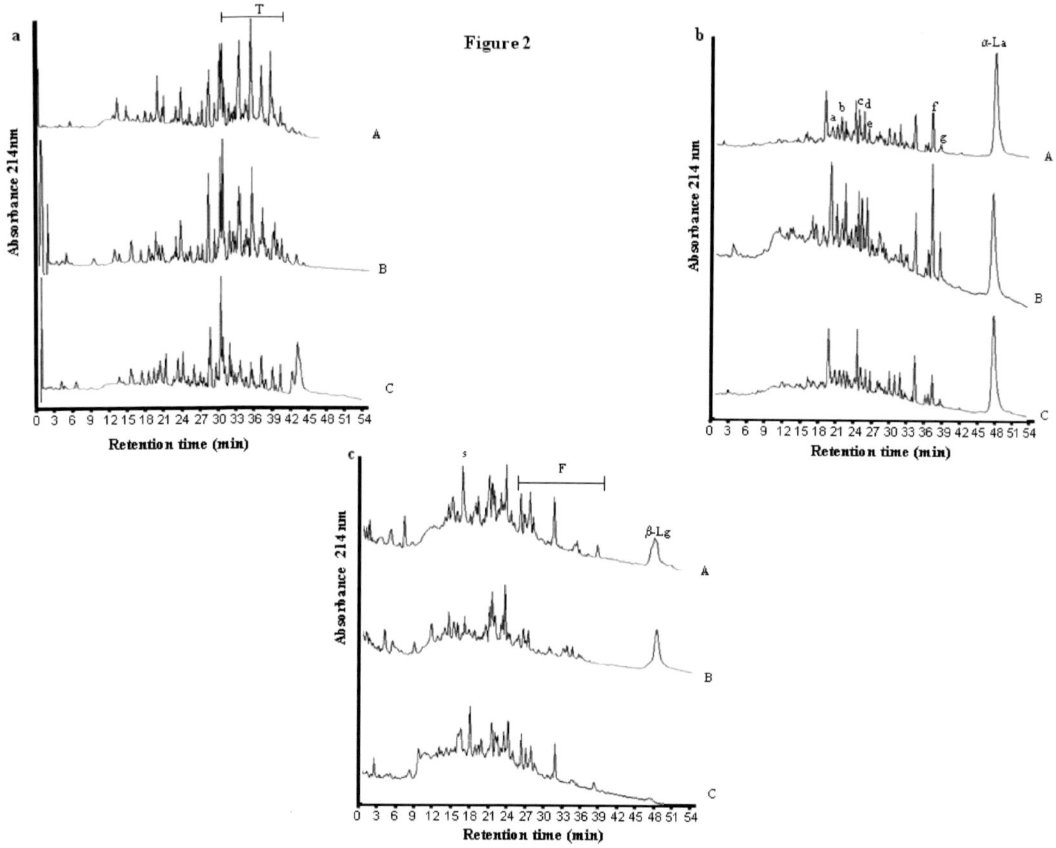

Figure 2. RP-HPLC profile of dairy whey hydrolysates obtained by digestive enzymes: trypsin (a), chymotrypsin (b) and pepsin (c). (A) Hydrolysis of untreated WP at atmospheric pressure (0.1 MPa). (B) Hydrolysis at atmospheric pressure of WP treated by HP. (C) Hydrolysis of WP under HP.

The chromatograms of the trypsin WP hydrolysis (Figure 2a) indicated complete hydrolysis of α-lactalbumin (retention time: RT of 47.60 min) and β-lactoglobulin (RT of 49.26 min) occurred at ambient pressure, resulting in the appearance of a large number of peptides (Figure 2a). The greatest pressure-induced difference was observed when the enzymatic digestion took place under pressure. These hydrolysates showed the lowest relative concentration of hydrolysis products with high hydrophobicity that eluted between 31.5 and 41.5 min (T fraction), but also presented hydrophobic peaks eluting between 42 and 45 min, which could correspond to aggregates of peptides (Figure 2a, C).

The chromatographic profile of chymotriptic hydrolysates showed the dissapaerance of the β-Lg peak in all digestions, while α-La seemed to be resistant to the chymotryptic action (Figure 2b). The whey pressurisation before chymotrypsin digestion seemed to favour the formation of peaks eluting at 20.5, 23.4, 38.5 and 39 min (a, b, f, g), while the application of pressure during proteolysis resulted in a progressive reduction of peaks c and d (25.5 and 26.2 min, respectively) and their possible conversion into peak e, eluting at 27.0 min.

Pepsin was active against α-La under all conditions tested, and no protein peak was observed in the digests (RT of 47.60) (Figure 2c). However, control hydrolysates and those obtained from pressurised whey proteins showed a significant amount of β-Lg (Figure 2c, A, B). In contrast, this protein was hydrolysed under 200 MPa (Figure 2c, C). Differences in peptide profile were only found in the digestion of pressurised whey proteins (Figure 2c B), showing a lower relative concentration of the peak eluting at 18.5 (s) and hydrophobic peaks eluting between 25 and 39 min (fraction F).

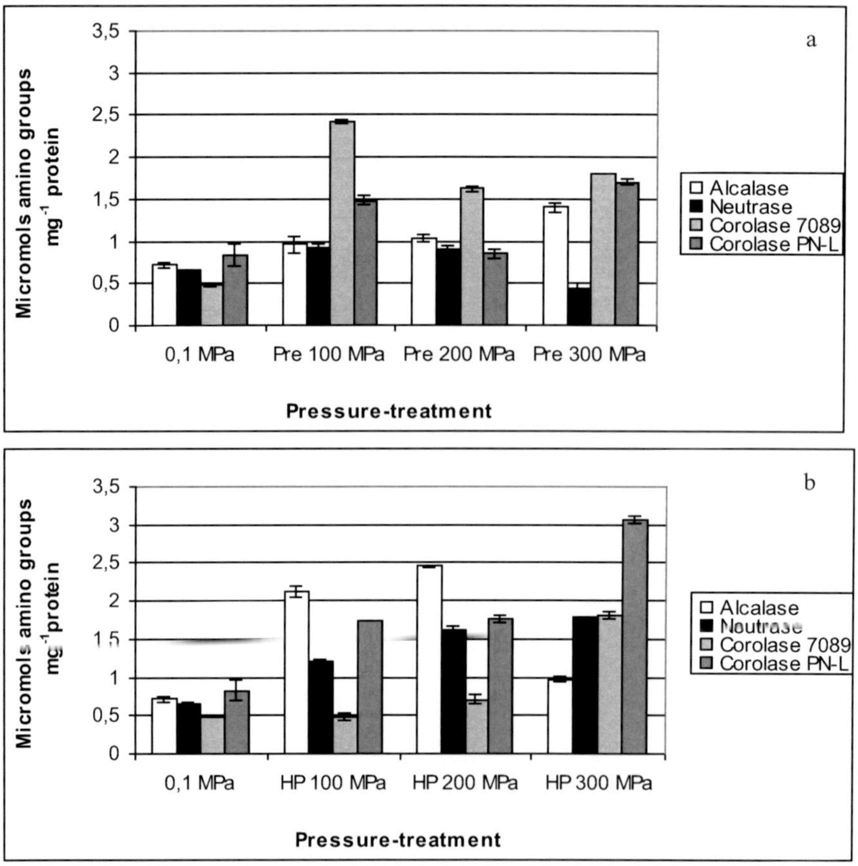

Figure 3. Degree of hydrolysis determined by *o*-phthaldialdehyde method during hydrolysis of bovine whey proteins by food grade proteases. (a) high pressure treatment (100, 200 or 300 MPa, for 15 min at 37°C) prior to hydrolysis with alcalase, neutrase, corolase 7089 and corolase PN-L. (b) hydrolysis performed during the high-pressure treatment (100, 200 or 300 MPa, for 15 min at 37°C).

In addtion to these studies with digestive enzymes, our group evaluated the influence of HHP on the enzymatic hydrolysis of bovine WP by four food grade proteases (alcalase, neutrase, corolase 7089 and corolase PN-L) (Peñas et al., 2006c). An important increase of the extent of hydrolysis was observed for all proteases assayed with the application of HHP treatment prior to (Figure 3a) or during enzymatic digestions (Figure 3b). The highest level of hydrolysis was obtained at 200 MPa for alcalase and at 300 MPa for neutrase and corolases 7089 and PNL.

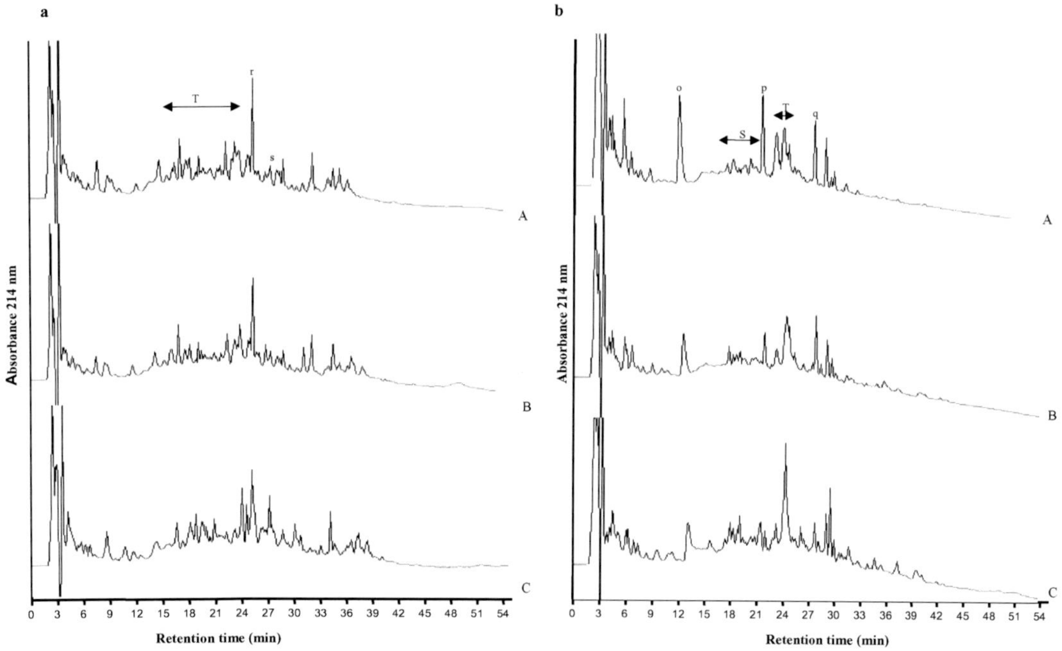

Figure 4. RP-HPLC profile of bovine whey hydrolysates obtained by food grade proteases: neutrase (a), corolase PN-L. (A) Hydrolysis of untreated WP at atmospheric pressure (0.1 MPa). (B) Hydrolysis at atmospheric pressure of WP treated by HP. (C) Hydrolysis of WP under HP.

The pressurisation of WP prior to or during its hydrolysis by Alcalase or Corolase 7089 did not lead to important changes in the peptide composition of the hydrolysates, as compared with the respective digestions of the untreated WP. For neutrase hydrolysates (Figure 4a), the pressure seemed to reduce the relative abundance of the peak eluting at 24.96 (peak r) and the effect was more pronounced in the digestions performed under HHP than in those conducted after the HP treatment. An increase of relative abundance of peak with retention time of 26.96 (peak s) and more hydrophilic peptides eluting at lower retention time (fraction T) was also observed in the hydrolysates obtained under 200 MPa as compared with control hydrolysate.

The effect of HHP on the quantitative peptide composition of corolase PN-L hydrolysates was also significant (Figure 4b), affecting mainly to the hydrophilic fractions (S, T) eluting between 17.01-21.02 and 23.16-25.16 min, respectively, as well as to the peptides o, p, q eluting at 12.34, 21.87 and 28 min, respectively. The pressure effect was stronger when it was applied during the enzymatic digestion (Figure 4b, C), showing these hydrolysates the highest relative proportion of S and T fractions and the lowest abundance of the peptides o and p as compared to control hydrolysates performed at atmospheric pressure (Figure 4b, A). Also, lower proportion of the hydrophobic peptide (peak q) eluting at 28 min was observed. These findings confirmed previous reports on differences in the relative abundance or nature of the peptides obtained under high pressure from the hydrolysates obtained at atmospheric pressure (Nakamura et al., 1993, Bonomi et al., 2003). On the other hand, these results suggest a possible positive effect of the HP treatment on the organoleptic characteristics of the hydrolysates obtained by Corolase PN-L, since a low content of hydrophobic peptides is related with high palatability (Clemente, 2000).

2. Reduction of Immunoreactivity of Dairy Proteins by Combined High Pressure and Enzymatic Treatments

It is well known that milk proteins are denatured by high pressure and these structural changes could modify the antigenic regions of milk proteins, leading to the transient exposure of formerly hidden epitopes, which are not accessible in the native protein. In accordance with that, several research groups suggested the possibility of combining enzimatic hydrolysis and high pressure to reduce the allergic potential of dairy proteins. Okamoto et al., (1991) reported that thermolysin hydrolysates treated at 200 MPa, 30°C, for 3 hours showed lower anti-β-Lg monoclonal antibodies (5 kinds) binding activity than the unpressurised hydrolysate. However, positive response on anti-α-La antibody was found in all pressurised hydrolysates, results related by the authors with the resistance of α-La to the pressure. Nakamura et al. (1993) described a reduction of the antigenicity of whey protein hydrolysates obtained by papain and proleather® enzymes after pressurisation up to 400 MPa, compared to unpressurised control samples hydrolysed at atmosheric pressure. Bonomi et al. (1999, 2003) reported reduced immunoreactivity of trypsin and chymotrypsin hydrolysates from β-Lg when performed at pressures up to 600 MPa. Zeece et al., (2008) found that HHP-treatment of β-Lg at 400-600 MPa for 10 min increased its subsequent hydrolysis by pepsin. Resultant peptides were identified and mapped, and segments (7-10 residues) were associated with allergic response in human patients, suggesting the authors the suitability of HHP technology for reducing of known allergens in foods.

Our group studied the antigenicity of dairy whey protein (WP) hydrolysates obtained by combination of HP and enzymatic digestion by using three digestive enzymes and five food grade proteases (alcalase, neutrase, corolases 7089 and PN-L or papain). We observed a reduction of the antigenicity of the hydrolysates obtained by combining 200 or 300 MPa and trypsin or pepsin, respectively, by using an ELISA test and a pool of seven sera from patients allergenic to bovine milk (Peñas et al., 2006a), compared to untreated bovine milk (Figure 5) and enzymatic treatment alone. However, no decrease of immunoreactivity after the combined treatment was found for chymotryptic hydrolysates developed at 100 MPa, results that could be attributed to the presence of residual α-lactalbumin in these hydrolysates. The immunoreactivity of WP hydrolysates obtained by food grade proteases was also analysed by using immunoblotting technique and murine anti β-Lg monoclonal antibodies (Peñas et al., 2006c). Low or no immunoreactivity associated with the presence of residual β-lactoglobulin was found in hydrolysates obtained from bovine WP at 300 MPa by the five food grade enzymes. The antigenic response corresponded mainly with polymeric forms of β-Lg in either neutrase digests (Figure 6b) and those obtained from WP treated at 100-200 MPa prior to its hydrolysis with alcalase and corolase 7089 (Figure 6 a and c), as well as in corolase PNL hydrolysates performed at 100 MPa (Figure 6 d). These results were confirmed by using sera from paediatric patients allergic to cow's milk proteins (results not shown).

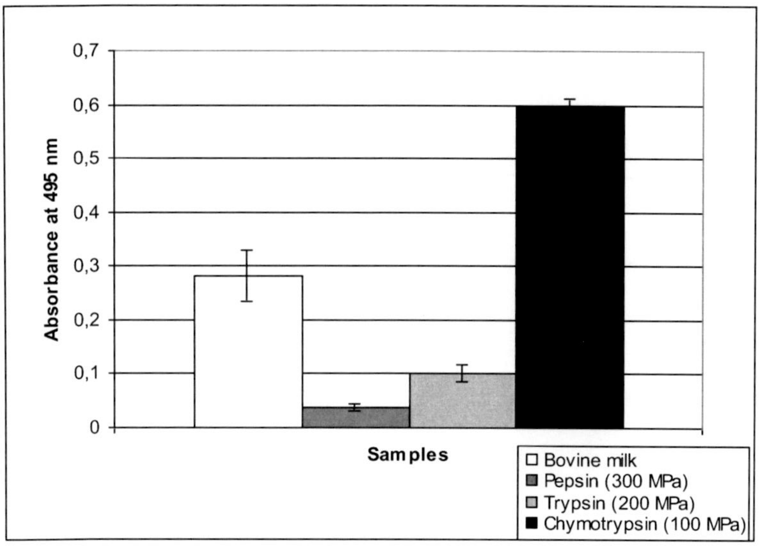

Figure 5. Residual immunochemical reactivity determined by an ELISA assay (expressed as absorbance units at 495 nm) of dairy whey hydrolysates using a pool of seven sera from allergic children to bovine milk.

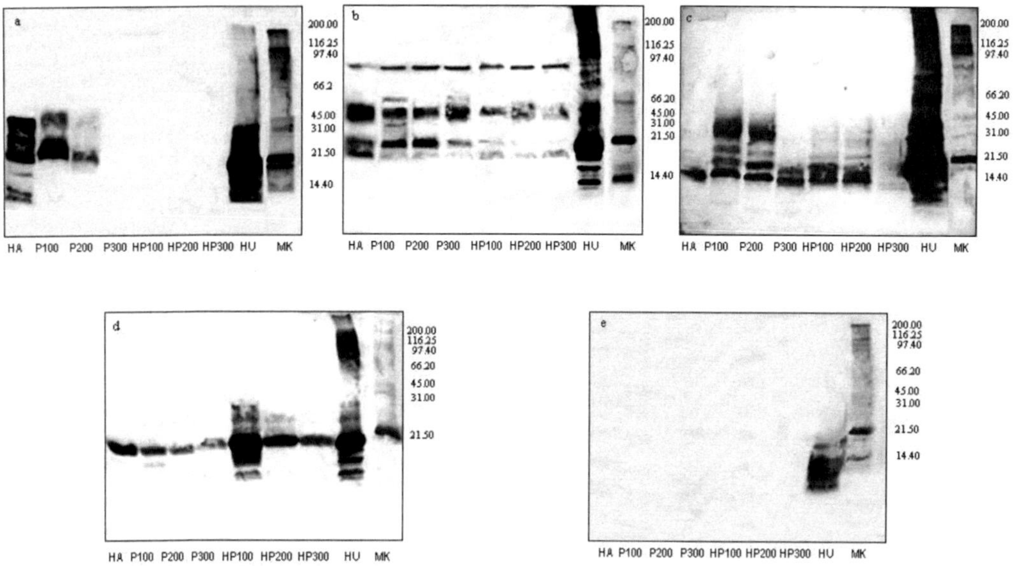

Figure 6. Immunoblotting of polypeptides obtained by hydrolysis of dairy whey proteins with Alcalase (a), Neutrase (b), Corolase 7089 (c), Corolase PN-L (d) and Papain (e) incubated with monoclonal anti β-lactoglobulin antibodies. MK: Molecular weight standard solution, HU: unhydrolysed bovine whey, HA: hydrolysis at atmospheric pressure (0.1 MPa), P100=:hydrolysis after pressurisation at 100 MPa, hydrolysis after pressurisation at 200 MPa, P300: hydrolysis after pressurization after 300 MPa, HP100: hydrolysis at 100 MPa, HP200: hydrolysis at 200 MPa, HP300: hydrolysis at 300 MPa.

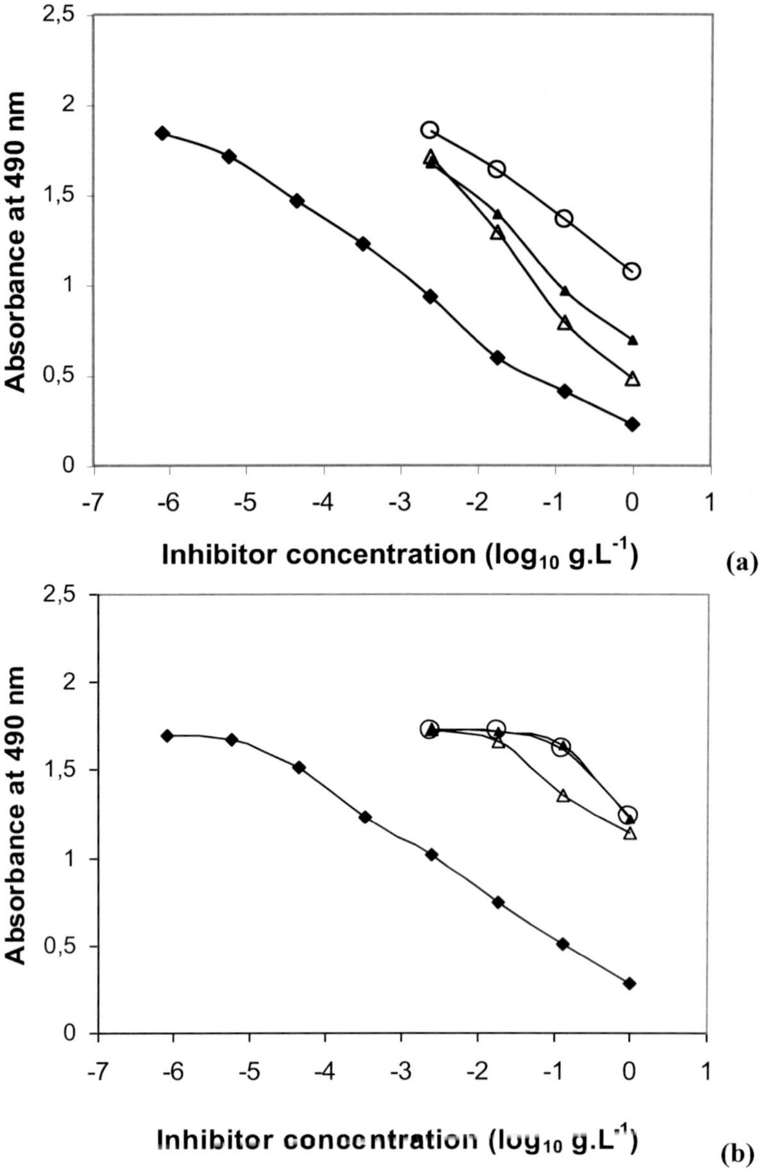

Figure 7. Inhibition of IgG binding to β-lactoglobulin in hydrolysates from bovine whey (WP) proteins by combining enzymatic and high pressure (HP) treatments. (a) Corolase PN-L, (b) Neutrase. ♦=ß-lactoglobulin standard; Δ=control; ▲= Hydrolysis of WP under100 MPa; ○= Hydrolysis of WP under 300 MPa.

The immunochemical reactivity of the hydrolysates obtained by corolase PN-L and neutrase that show different RP-HPLC peptide profile and maximum grade of hydrolysis were also evaluated by inhibition ELISA test using polyclonal rat anti-β-Lg antibodies (Figure 7). Corolase PN-L hydrolysates obtained under 300 and 100 MPa presented lower specific antibodies binding activity than the control hydrolysate, The lowest values were found in hydrolysates obtained at 300 MPa (Figure 7 a). The neutrase hydrolysates obtained under HHP retained also lower residual antigenicity than those obtained at atmospheric pressure, although these differences did not reach statistical significance. These results suggest that the reduction of antigenicity of hydrolysates by the combined enzymatic/HP treatments may be a compromise between the specificity of enzyme used to eliminate sequential epitopes (Van Beresteijn et al.,1995) and structural unfolding and denaturation of WP proteins induced by HP (Dumay et al., 1994), which could favour the exposure of conformational antigenic epitopes to proteases

CONCLUSION

High pressure and selected enzymes may be useful tools for obtaining protein hydrolysates with low antigenicity and limited hydrolysis in a short time to use them as nitrogen ingredient in hypoallergenic infant formulas. Dissociation of β-Lg into its subunits and the unfolding of the protein monomers under pressures up to 300 MPa have been reported. Thus, the reduction of antigenicity of hydrolysates by the combined enzymatic/HP treatments may be a compromise between the specificity of enzyme used to eliminate sequential epitopes and structural unfolding and denaturation of WP proteins induced by HP, which could favour the exposure of some conformational antigenic epitopes not accessible to proteases in the native protein.

REFERENCES

Aggett, P. J., Haschke, F., Heine, W., Hernell, O., Koletzko, B., Rey, J., Rubino, A., Schoch, G., Senterre, J.& Strobel, S. (1993). Committee of Nutrition. Comment on antigen-reduced infant formula. *Acta Paediatrica*, 82, 314-319.

Bonomi, F., Fiocchi, A., Frokjaer, A., Gaiaschi, A., Iametti, S., Poiesi, C., Rasmussen, P., Restani, P.& Rovere, P. (2003). Reduction of immunoreactivity of bovine β-lactoglobulin upon combined physical and proteolytic treatment. *Journal of Dairy Research,* 70, 51-59.

Bonomi, F., Iametti, S., Rasmussenm P., Restani P., & Rovere, P. (2000). Advances in the combined application of enzymatic and physical treatments for reducing food allergenicity. *High Pressure Research*, 19, 175-181.

Businco, L., Dreeborg, S., Einarsson, R., Giampetro, P.G., Host, A., Keller, K. M., Strobel, S. & Wahn, U. (1993), Hydrolysed cow's milk formulae. Allergenicity and use for treatment and prevention. *Pediatric Allergy and Immunology*, 4, 101-111.

Cairoli, S., Iametti, S. & Bonomi, F. (1994). Reversible and irreversible modifications of β-lactoglobulin upon heating. *Journal of Protein Chemistry,* 13, 347-354.

Caffarelli, C., Plebani, A., Poiesi, C., Petroccione, T., Spattini, A. & Cavagni, G. (2002). Determination of allergenicity to three cow's milk hydrolysates and an amino acid-derived formula in children with cow's milk allergy. *Clinical and Experimental Allergy,* 32, 74-79.

Calvo, M. M. & Gómez, R. (2002). Peptidic profile, molecular mass distribution and immunological properties of commercial hypoallergenic infant formulas. *Milchwissenschaft*, 57 (4), 187-190.

Chandra, R. K., Puri, S., & Cheesmam P. S. (1985). Predictive value of cord blood IgE in the development of atopic disease and the role of breastfeeding in its prevention. *Clinical Allergy*, 15, 517-522.

Chicon, R., Lopez-Fandiño, R., Quiros, A. & Belloque, J. 2006. Changes in chymotrypsin hydrolysis of beta-lactoglobulin A induced by high hydrostatic pressure. *Journal of Agricultural and Food Chemistry,* 54(6), 2333-2341.

Clemente, A. (2000). Enzymatic protein hydrolysates in human nutrition. *Trends in Food Science and Technology,* 11, 254-262.

Dannaeus, A., Johansson, S. G. O.& Foucard, T. (1978). Clinical and immunological aspects of food allergy in childhood II. Development of allergic symptoms and humoral immune response to food in infants of atopic mothers during the first 24 months of life. *Acta Paediatrica Scandinavica,* 67, 497-504.

De la Fuente, M., Olano, A., Casal, V. & Juarez, M. (1998). Effects of high pressure and heat treatment on the mineral balance of goats milk. *Journal of Dairy Research*, 66, 65-72.

Dufour, E., Hervé, G. & Haertle, T. (1995). Hydrolysis of β-lactoglobulin by thermolysin and pepsin under high hydrostatic pressure. *Biopolymers*, 35, 475-483.

Exl, B. M., Muller-Teicher, G. & Vandenplas, Y. (2000). Preventive possibilities within the context of cow's milk allergy. *Allergy and Clinical Immunology International*, 12, 68-76.

Exl B. M. (2001). A review of recent developments in the use of moderately hydrolyzed whey formulae in infant nutrition. *Nutrition Research*, 21 (1-2), 355-379.

Fritsché R. (2003). Animal models in food allergy: assessment of allergenicity and preventive activity of infant formulas. *Toxicology Letters*, 140-141, 303-309.

Gorthler, I., Urbank, R. & Forster, J. (1995). Characterization of antigens and allergens in hypoallergenic formulae. *European Journal of Pediarics,* 154, 289-294.

Halken, S., Skanstrup, H. K., Jacobsen, H. P., Estmann, A., Engberg, F.A., Hansen, L. G., Kalliomäki, M., Salminen, S., Anvilommi, H., Kero, P., Koskinen, P. & Isolauri, E. (2001). Probiotics in primary prevention of atopic disease: a randomised placebo-controlled trial. *Lancet*, 357, 1076-1079.

Hattevig, G., Kjelman, B., Sigurs, N., Grodzinsky, E., Hed, J. & Bjorksten, B. (1990). The effect of maternal avoidance of eggs, cow's milk, and fish during lactation on the development of IgE and IgA antibodies in infants. *Journal of Allergy and Clinical Immunology,* 85, 108-115.

Hayashi, R., Kawamura,Y.& Kunugi.S. (1987). Introduction of high pressure to food processing: preferential proteolysis of β-lactoglobulin in milk whey. *Journal of Food Science,* 52, 1107-1108.

Holt, P. G. & Jones, C. A. (2000). The development of the immune system during pregnancy and early life. *Allergy*, 55, 688-697.

Høst, A., Husby, S. & Østerbakkem, M. O. (1988). A prospective study of cow's milk allergy in exclusively breast-fed infants: incidence, pathogenic role of early inadvertent exposure to cow's milk formula, and characterization of bovine milk protein in human milk. *Acta Paediatrica Scandinavica*, 77, 663-670.

Høst, A., Kiletzko, B., Dreborg, S., Muraro, A., Wahn, U., Aggett, P., Bresson, J. L., Hernell, O., Lafeber, H., Michaelsen, K.F., Micheli, J. L., Rigo, J., Weaver, L., Heymans, H., Strobel, S. & Vandenplas, Y. (1999), Dietary products used in infants for treatment and prevention of food allergy. Joint statement of the European Society for Paediatric Allergology and Clinical Immunology (ESPACI). Committee on Hypoallergenic formulas and the European Society for Paediatric Gastroenterology, *Hepatology and Nutrition* (ESPGHAN) Committee on Nutrition. *Archives of disease in childhood*, 81, 80-84.

Iametti, S., Transidico, P., Bonomi, F., Vecchio, G., Pittia, P., Rovere, P. & Dall'Aglio, G. (1997). Molecular modifications of β-lactoglobulin upon exposure to high pressures. *Journal of Agricultural and Food Chemistry,* 45, 23-29.

Iametti, S., De Gregori, B., Vecchio, G. & Bonomi, F. (1996). Modifications occur at different structural levels during the heat denaturation of β-lactoglobulin. *European Journal of Biochemistry,* 237, 106-112.

Kimura, K., Ida, M., Yosida, Y., Ohki, K., Fukumoto, T. & Sakui, N. (1994). Comparison of keeping quality between pressure-processed jam and heat-processed jam: Changes in flavour components and nutrients during storage. *Bioscience, Biotechnology and Biochemistry*, 58(8), 1386-1391.

Kulig, M., Bergmann, R., Tacke, U., Wahn, U. & Guggenmoos-Holzman, I. (1998). Long lasting sinsitisation to food during the first two years precedes allergy airway disease. *Pediatric Allergy and Immunology*, 9, 61-67.

Lee, Y. H. (1992). Food-processing approaches to altering allergenic potential of milk-based formula. *Journal of Pediatrics*, 121, S47-S50.

Maynard, F., Weingand, A., Hau, J. & Lost, R. (1998). Effects of high-pressure treatment on the tryptic hydrolysis of bovine β-lactoglobulin AB. *International Dairy Journal,* 8, 125-133.

Nakamura, T., Sado, H. & Syukunobe, Y. (1993). Production of low antigenic whey protein hydrolysates by enzymatic hydrolysis and denaturation with high pressure. *Milchwissenschaft* 48(3), 141-144.

Neville, M. C., Allen, J. C., Archer, P. C., Casey, C. E., Seacat, J., Keller, R. P., Lutes, V., Rasbach, J. & Neifert, M. (1991). Studies in human lactation milk volume and nutrient composition during weaning and lactogenesis. *American Journal of Clinical Nutrition,* 54, 81-92.

Okamoto, M., Hayashi, R., Enomoto, A., Kaminoga, W. A. S. & Yamauchi, K. (1991) High-pressure proteolytic digestion of food proteins: selective elimination of β-lactoglobulin in bovine milk whey concentrate. *Agricultural and Biological Chemistry*, 55, 1253-1257.

Peñas, E., Préstamo, G., Baeza, M. L., Martínez-Molero, M. I. & Gómez, R. (2006a). Effects of combined high pressure and enzymatic treatments on the hydrolysis and immunoreactivity of dairy whey proteins. *International Dairy Journal,* 16, 831-839.

Peñas, E., Restani, P., Ballabio, C., Préstamo, G., Fiocchi, A. & Gómez, R. (2006b), Evaluation of the residual antigenicity of dairy whey hydrolysates obtained by combination of enzymatic hydrolysis and high-pressure treatment, *Journal of Food Protection*, 69, 1707-1712

Peñas, E., Snel, H., Floris, R., Préstamo, G. & Gómez, R. (2006c). High pressure can reduce the antigenicity of bovine whey protein hydrolysates. *International Dairy Journal,* 16, 969-975.

Préstamo, G., Lesmes, M., Otero, L. & Arroyo, G. (2000). Soybean vegetable protein (tofu) preserved with high pressure. *Journal of Agricultural and Food Chemistry,* 48, 2943-2947.

Oldaeus, G., Björkstén, B., Einarsson, R. & Kjellman, N. I. M. (1991). Antigenicity and allergenicity of cow milk hydrolysates intended for infant feeding. *Pediatric Allergy and Immunology,* 4, 156-164.

Restani, P., Velonà, T., Plebani, A., Ugazi, A.G., Poiesi, C., Muraro, A. & Galli, C. L. (1995). Evaluation by SDS-PAGE and immunoblotting of residual antigenicity in hydrolysed protein formulas. *Clinical and Experimental Allergy*, 25, 651-658.

Rosendal, A. & Barkholt, V. (2000). Detection of potentially allergic material in 12 hydrolyzed milk formulas. *Journal of Dairy Science,* 83, 2200-2210.

Siemensma, A.D., Weijer, W.J. & Bak, H.J. (1993). The importance of peptide lengths in hypoallergenic infant formulae. *Trends Food Science and Technology*, 4, 16-21.

Stapelfeldt, H., Petersen, P. G., Kristiansen, K.R., Qvist, K.B. & Skibsted, L. H. (1996). Effect of high hydrostatic pressure on the enzymatic hydrolysis of β-lactoglobulin B by trypsin, thermolysin and pepsin. *Journal of Dairy Research,* 63, 111-118.

Van Berensteijn, E. C. H., Meijer, J. G. M. & Schmidt, D. G. (1995). Residual allergenicity of hypoallergenici infant formulas and the occurrence of milk-specific IgE antibodies in patients with clinical allergy. *Journal of Allergy and Clinical Immunology*, 96 (3), 365-374.

Van Willige, R. W. G. & Fitzgerald, R. J. (1995). Tryptic and chymotryptic hydrolysis of β-lactoglobulin A, B, and AB at ambient and high pressure. *Milchwissenschaft*, 50, 183-186.

Wold, A. E. & Adlerberth, I. (1998). Does breast-feeding affect the infant's immune responsiveness? *Acta Paediatrica*, 87, 19-23.

Zeece, M., Huppertz, T. & Kelly, A. (2008). Effect of high pressure treatment on *in-vitro* digestibility of β-lactoglobulin. *Innovative Food Science and Emerging Technologies*, 9, 62-69.

In: Food Allergies: Symptoms, Diagnosis, and Treatment ISBN: 978-1-61728-748-0
Editor: Patricia M. Rodgers

Chapter 9

PREVENTION STRATEGIES FOR FOOD ALLERGY MIGHT INTERVENE WITH THE DEVELOPMENT OF ATOPIC DERMATITIS AND THE ATOPIC MARCH

***Betty C.A.M. van Esch*[1,2], *Linette E.M. Willemsen*[1], *Johan Garssen*[1,2] *and Léon M.J. Knippels*[1,2]**

[1] Pharmacology, Utrecht Institute Pharmaceutical Sciences , Faculty of Beta Sciences, Utrecht University, Utrecht, the Netherlands

[2]Immunology, Danone Research Centre for Specialised Nutrition, Wageningen, the Netherlands

SUMMARY

Food allergy, atopic dermatitis, rhinitis and allergic asthma are common atopic diseases in Western countries and their prevalence has been rising the past thirty years (1-3). Prevention of food allergy induced by the three major food allergens, hen's egg, cow's milk and peanut is considered important to prevent related diseases like atopic dermatitis, allergic rhinitis and allergic asthma later in life. There is a strong relation between food allergy and eczema in young children under the age of 1 year (4-6). The route of sensitization to food allergens is still not completely elucidated and might involve the skin or airways beside sensitization via the gastrointestinal tract. Breastfeeding is still considered the best way of preventing food sensitization. Prebiotic oligosaccharides and cytokines like IL10 and TGF_{β} which are abundantly present in human milk, might provide an immunological milieu that favors the induction of oral tolerance in the Th2 prone infant. However, if breastfeeding is not possible or sufficient, hydrolysed formulae are the second best option for children with a genetic predisposition to develop allergic diseases. Recent studies provide evidence that the induction of specific oral tolerance is preferred in preventing sensitization to food allergens early in life (7-10). For prevention of clinical symptoms in sensitized children, different approaches of specific immune modulation are currently investigated to desensitize or tolerize cow's milk allergic infants; subcutaneous immunotherapy (SIT), sublingual immunotherapy (SLIT) or oral immunotherapy (OIT). In the current chapter primary prevention of allergic disease or treatment strategies to prevent clinical symptoms in sensitized individuals are described. Furthermore, the use of animal models is discussed in relation to food allergy, atopic dermatitis and the predisposition to other allergies later in life (i.e. atopic march).

FOOD ALLERGY

Food allergy affects about 4-5 % of young children with hen's egg, cow's milk (2-3%) and peanut (>1 %) being the three most important diagnosed food allergies in children with incidences of emergency hospitalization after life-threatening food-induced anaphylaxis (11). Whilst it is established that there is a strong genetic compound to food hypersensitivity it is hypothesized that factors responsible for the increasing number of children suffering from allergic reactions may be found in changing environmental conditions, westernized life style, diet, air pollution, and the increased consumption of additives and preservatives in food. Moreover, food allergy might partly be associated with the immature gut and the Th2 prone young infant. The type of antigen, antigen dose and age at first exposure are all thought to play a crucial role in the subsequent immune response (12) and most likely results from either a failure in establishing oral tolerance or a breakdown in existing tolerance. The route of sensitization to food allergens is still not completely elucidated and might involve the skin or airways beside sensitization via the gastrointestinal tract. Recent findings show that many cases of hen's egg and cow's milk allergy persist later in life. Only 11 % of hen's egg and 18 % of cow's milk and peanut allergy resolved at the age of 4 years (13). However, in contrast to peanuts 80% of cow's milk and hen's egg allergy resolved at 16 years of age (14, 15).

Hypersensitivity reactions were classified into four different types by Coombes and Gell. Aeroallergens, food allergens, drugs and insect venoms are the major allergens encountered that are responsible for induction of type1-hypersensitivity reactions. This response may arise in individuals who have a propensity to exert an allergic response characterized by the production of allergen-specific IgE. Binding of IgE to the high affinity receptor FcεR1 on mast cells followed by subsequent cross-linking of the receptors by the allergen provokes degranulation and the release of mediators such as histamine, leukotriens and cytokines. About 60 % of food allergic patients have IgE-mediated allergic responses and IgE mediated allergy is an important indicator of susceptibility to develop atopic diseases like atopic dermatitis and allergic asthma later in life (16, 17). IgE mediated mast cell activation results in clinical symptoms involving the skin (urticaria, angiodema and atopic dermatitis), gastrointestinal tract (nausea, vomiting, abdominal pain, constipation and diarrhea), airways (cough, wheeze) and systemic symptoms within a few minutes to one hour after ingestion of the food which can potentially lead to a life threatening anaphylactic shock. It should be realized that in atopic diseases like food allergy, atopic dermatitis, rhinitis and asthma, a considerable number of patients exhibit clinical features without detectable local or systemic IgE. Mast cells are involved in the pathogenesis of IgE-mediated and non-allergic hypersensitivity responses. Several *in vivo* studies indicate that they are involved in allergic asthma and gastrointestinal allergy (18-21). Although antigen-specific mast cell activation results from cross-linking the high-affinity IgE receptor also other mechanisms can be involved in antigen specific activation in the absence of IgE antibodies. A novel potential mechanism for the elicitation of immediate hypersensitivity-like reactions via immunoglobulin free light chain (IgLC) has been described (22). Transfer of antigen-specific IgLC into naive mice sensitizes them to the respective antigen resulting in local mast cell activation upon challenge, leading to edema formation after skin challenge or acute bronchoconstriction after intranasal challenge (21-24). In a recent study, CD25 depletion in mice orally sensitized to whey proteins was found to alter the nature of the allergic response from IgE- to IgLC dependent (25). Human studies confirm a significant role for IgLC in allergic diseases like atopic dermatitis, allergic rhinitis and food allergy. Children with severe atopic dermatitis have higher concentrations of lambda and kappa IgLC in serum (26). Furthermore, in non-IgE mediated rhinitis patients both lambda and kappa IgLC concentrations were found to be enhanced in nasal secretions (27). A recent study showed that IgLC levels were enhanced in children with Double Blind Placebo Controlled Food Challenge (DBPCFC) diagnosed food allergy (26). Overall these data suggest that IgLC might be a promising new biomarker in the early diagnoses of allergic diseases like food allergy. More studies are needed to define the correlation between IgLC and allergic disease.

Atopic Dermatitis

The prevalence of atopic dermatitis is 10-20% in young children (1). There is a strong relation between food allergy and eczema in young children under the age of 1 year (4-6) although there is some debate on the association between food allergy and atopic dermatitis (28). It is estimated that in one third of the children suffering from atopic dermatitis the skin symptoms are triggered by sensitization to food (5, 6). Moreover, food allergens can exaggerate symptoms of atopic dermatitis by promoting Th2 activation in the skin as dendritic cells (DC) in the gastro intestinal tract are able to carry the allergen to the dermis where they may lead to degranulation of mast cells (29).

Impaired barrier function of the skin is considered to associate with atopic dermatitis (30) in which genetic predisposition may probably play an important role. The protein filaggrin is part of the inner layer of the skin forming the cornified envelope, a specialized structure playing an essential role in the skin barrier (31). Mutations of filaggrin genes are associated with skin diseases like, ichtyosis vulgaris and atopic dermatitis (32, 33). The expression of the protein filaggrin was reduced in the skin of atopic dermatitis patients which was linked to mutations in chromosome 1q20 located genes including filaggrin encoding for the structural proteins of the epidermis (34-36). It is clear that genetic (filaggrin nul/nul mutations and environmental factors like breastfeeding, allergen exposure or infections) may underlie the development of atopic dermatitis in early life and is often the first manifestation of atopy in a triad of events including rhinitis and allergic asthma (16) called the atopic march.

Atopic March

The atopic march is the natural history of atopic manifestations, characterized by a progression of clinical signs of atopic disease. In general, clinical signs of atopic dermatitis predate the development of asthma and allergic rhinitis, suggesting that atopic dermatitis is the "entry point" for subsequent allergic disease. Early sensitization to food might also be considered as one of the entry points. Sensitization to hen's egg or cow's milk (determined by skin prick testing) in genetically predisposed children was predictive of adult asthma (17, 37).

It is generally accepted that atopic dermatitis, when affecting children before two years of age, increases the risk of developing allergic asthma later in life (1). This can be explained by the observations that allergens (i.e. food and aero-allergens) taken up by the damaged skin results in new sensitizations which might underlie the development of food allergy and atopic dermatitis. Ultimately, this may lead to allergic rhinitis and allergic asthma later in life. Epicutaneous sensitization to food and aero-allergens is supported by clinical and animal studies (38, 39). Removal of the stratum corneum in mice followed by skin exposure to antigen led to eczema like symptoms and consequent airway hyper-responsiveness after allergen challenge (39). Moreover, topical creams containing peanut, applied to inflamed skin have been related to allergic responses in human (40). Skin sensitization is predominantly regulated by Langerhans cells causing a systemic immune response. Upon allergen binding to $Fc_{\varepsilon}R_1$ receptors, Langerhans cells migrate to the local lymph nodes were they can induce Th2 polarization. Subsequently, Th2 cells migrate through the circulatory system to various sites including nasal, lung and intestinal mucosa. Subsequent inhalation or oral exposure of allergens may result in clinical symptoms in lungs or the gastrointestinal tract.

The atopic march hypothesis is mainly based on cross-sectional studies (41-43). Only a few prospective studies showed the relation between atopic dermatitis early in life and the progression into asthma later in life (44, 45). However, concomitant wheezing reflecting early sensitization is an important predictive factor in this relation. In the German Multicenter Atopy Study (MAS; 1314 newborns of whom 499 are high risk infants) early wheezing was found to be the decisive factor in the association between atopic dermatitis and childhood asthma in infants (46). In contrast , a recent Australian study showed that atopic dermatitis early in life is associated with childhood asthma in boys even when early wheezing and early sensitization has been taken into account (45). Hence, besides the clear relation between atopic dermatitis and allergic disease later in life, early sensitization to inhalant or food allergens in high risk children may be an important factor in pursuing the atopic march (47, 48). It is fair to state that sensitization to food and inhalant-allergens either via the skin, respiratory system or the gastro-intestinal tract may contribute to clinical symptoms of food allergy, atopic dermatitis, allergic asthma and rhinitis.

Prevention of Food Allergy

Although the causal relationship between food allergy, atopic dermatitis, allergic rhinitis and asthma is still under discussion, prevention of the first and most common allergies early in life might be important to delay or even stop the development of atopic diseases later in life. The two major strategies to prevent sensitization to food allergens are avoidance of the allergic protein (i.e. epitope exclusion) or improving establishment of oral tolerance.

Breastfeeding

Breastfeeding is considered to be the golden standard and the best way of preventing sensitization and might help the establishment of oral tolerance in the Th2 prone young infants. It provides a unique combination of lipids, proteins, carbohydrates, vitamins and minerals. Furthermore, there are numerous bioactive compounds with immunological properties such as soluble IgA, antioxidants, oligosaccharides, probiotics, Toll-like receptor ligands, cytokines, hormones, fatty acids and many more. Each compound can individually, additionally or synergistically act on the immune system of the neonate. The breast milk content changes over time to ensure optimal passive and active protection and growth for the child (49-51). TGF_{β} and IL-10 present in human milk might play a role in diminishing the risk of allergic disease in infancy (52) as these cytokines are considered regulatory cytokines involved in tolerance induction. In addition, prebiotic oligosaccharides which are abundantly present in human milk may have many immunological properties and might facilitate tolerance induction (49, 53). However, breastfeeding cannot totally eliminate the risk of sensitization because of passage of some proteins through the gut barrier and as a consequence their release in human milk (54-56). Prebiotic fibers manufactured to resemble some of these human oligosaccharides are defined as "non-digestible food ingredients that beneficially affect the host by selectively stimulating the growth and/or activity of one or a limited number of bacterial species already resident in the colon, and thus attempt to improve host health" (57). These manufactured prebiotic oligosaccharides might improve infant formulae by generic immune modulation. They possess the capacity to induce a beneficial immunoglobulin profile in infants at risk for allergy (58) and diminish the incidence of atopic dermatitis in high risk children (59). In addition, symptoms of food allergy (60) and allergic asthma (61) are reduced in mice fed these specific oligosaccharides. Dietary intervention with these oligosaccharides may be a promising new approach by supporting the establishment of oral tolerance induction in young children. However, breastfeeding is still considered the golden standard and hydrolysed formulae are the second best option for children with a genetic predisposition to develop allergic diseases if breastfeeding is not possible or sufficient.

Avoidance versus Oral Tolerance

The complete avoidance of even very low amounts of known allergens is the most followed strategy in high risk children and avoidance of food and house dust mite allergens has shown promising results in preventing allergic asthma (62). Early introduction of solid food was considered a risk factor in the development of food allergies and was partly based on experiments in rodents (12, 63) leading to the recommendation that atopic mothers may wish to avoid dietary antigens such as hen's egg, fish and nuts during pregnancy and lactation. However, in contrast recent results indicate that avoidance of dietary compounds failed to prevent food allergy (9-10, 64) indicating that early introduction of solid food might play a significant role in avoiding sensitization to food allergens. This is supported by the fact that the prevalence of peanut allergy is significantly lower in countries were peanut is consumed at an early age (8, 65). Furthermore, fish consumption of newborns during the first year of life was found to reduce the risk of allergy (i.e. rhinitis, eczema) and sensitization to food and airborne allergens by the age of four years (66). Moreover, allergens given via the oral route are considered important inducers in the maturation of the immune system (67, 68), indicating that early oral exposure to food might be necessary to induce oral tolerance and might be beneficial above avoidance strategies (7).

Oral tolerance provides a unique defense mechanism to maintain the intestinal immune homeostasis. It enables the mucosal immune system to generate a protective inflammatory response against potential pathogens while remaining quiescent when harmless food proteins enter the intestine (69). At the intestinal mucosa a single layer of epithelium separates the inner milieu from the external environment. Intact food derived epitopes that escaped gastrointestinal degradation may be taken up in the intestine by regulatory DC's in Peyers patches or in the villous lamina propria and presented to naïve T-cells in the Peyer's patches or mesenteric lymph nodes resulting in a protective immune response (70, 71). Several subclasses of DC's with regulatory properties are present in the intestine and might therefore be important in oral tolerance induction to harmless food antigens and play a key role in preventing oral sensitization to dietary antigens by the induction of regulatory T-cells (72, 73). The conventional myeloid $CD11c^{+}CD11b^{+}$ DC's and the $CD11c^{+}B220^{+}$ plasmacytoid dendritic cells (pDC) from the Peyer's patches have unique regulatory functions and may contribute to oral tolerance induction (73, 74). They possess the capacity to suppress T-cell responses (75-77) most likely by inducing the differentiation of naive T-cells into regulatory T-cells (74, 78, 79). $CD103^{+}$ DC's that are predominantly present in the lamina propria take up antigen and migrate to the mesenteric lymph nodes (70-71, 80-82) where they drive the induction of regulatory T-cells (83). The site of mucosal antigen uptake by DC's and consequent presentation to T-cells remains elusive. Uptake of antigens in M-cells in Peyer's patches has been shown to be involved in oral tolerance induction as well (84-88) although mesenteric lymph nodes seem to be the major site for T-cell recognition (79, 89). Also the liver, as an intestinal site for antigen presentation, is considered to play a role in the induction of regulatory T-cells and subsequent tolerance induction (90, 91).

In general, when oral administered harmless food is taken up by intestinal mucosal DC's regulatory T-cells are generated that support oral tolerance induction. These regulatory T-cells encompass natural or inducible $CD4^{+}CD25^{+}Foxp3^{+}$, TGF-β producing Th3 and IL-10-producing Tr1 regulatory T-cells (69, 92, 93). It is believed that the induction of regulatory T-cells, acting via cell-cell contact or suppressive cytokines (e.g. IL10, TGF_{β}), are crucial in inducing or maintaining oral tolerance (94-97) although other mechanisms like anergy or clonal deletion of effector Th2-cells (high-dose tolerance) may have overlapping functionality.

Hydrolysed Formulae

Hydrolysed formulae are considered the second best option for children with a genetic predisposition to develop allergic diseases if breastfeeding is not possible or sufficient. Hypoallergenic formulae are commonly used to manage cow's milk allergy and are generally categorized into partial and extensively hydrolysed hypoallergenic formulae. Cow's milk subjected to enzymatic hydrolysis, heat treatment and/or ultra filtration, reduces the molecular weight and consequently the allergenicity of the proteins. Although there is general scientific and clinical agreement that triggering of the allergic reaction in cow's milk allergic infants can be avoided with extensive hydrolysed formulae or amino acid based formulae (e.g. epitope exclusion) debate on the most effective strategy to avoid initial sensitization remains intense (98).

Infants fed hydrolysed formulae have a reduced risk of developing cow's milk allergy compared to those fed cow's milk formulae (99). 10 Years of clinical studies show that both partial and extensive hydrolysed formulae are effective in preventing cow's milk allergy in high risk children (100-104). Clinical studies addressing the effectiveness of hydrolysed formulae in preventing cow's milk allergy were mainly designed as avoidance strategies to prevent sensitization and are limited in answering whether the beneficial effects are due to avoidance of the allergic epitopes or a result of oral tolerance induction. Partial rather than extensive hydrolysed formulae possesses the capacity to induce oral tolerance to the offended protein (88, 105-107). In a recent study using a mouse model for cow's milk allergy we showed, that feeding a partial but not an extensive whey hydrolysate prior to oral whey sensitization reduced the clinical symptoms upon challenge with whey in these animals. These effects coincided with enhanced numbers of intestinal regulatory T-cells and the protective effect was transferable to naïve recipient mice using the mesenteric lymph nodes of the donor mice (van Esch *et al*; submitted). It is clear that for safety reasons the potential sensitizing capacity of these hydrolysed formulae need to be assessed before they can be used in young children. Immunological *in vitro* assays are important tools for the efficacy and safety testing of hydrolysed formulae in prevention of clinical symptoms in already sensitized infants. *In vivo* animal models for cow's milk allergy have the additional advantage that they are useful to predict the efficacy and safety of hydrolysed formulae in humans in terms of primary prevention of cow's milk allergy or potential residual sensitizing properties of the hydrolysed formulae. A combination of both *in vitro* as well *in vivo* models should be considered for optimal safety and efficacy testing in terms of avoidance, tolerance induction or potential sensitizing capacity of hydrolysed formulae (108) (van Esch and Knipping *et al*, submitted).

Prevention of Clinical Symptoms in Food Allergy

In children already sensitized to the most common allergens present in cow's milk, hen's egg and peanuts the standard care is mainly based on strict avoidance strategies and pharmacotherapy for symptom relieve. For basic foods such as cow's milk, hen's egg and peanuts this might become more and more difficult because of the widespread use in processed food (109). Therefore, specific immune therapies aiming at restoring tolerance to harmless food proteins have been under intensive investigation the past decade. Different approaches of specific immune modulation are currently investigated which might lead to a specific long lasting immune suppression. The re-establishment of tolerance in sensitized children to the first and most common allergies in early life might even delay or stop the atopic march. Allergen immunotherapy redirects allergen-specific T-cell responses from a Th2 to a Th1 profile along with tolerance induction mediated by regulatory T-cells. There is a strong rationale for improving the efficacy of allergen-specific immunotherapy by reducing the incidence and severity of IgE mediated adverse reactions. Approaches to address this problem include the use of modified allergens, novel adjuvants and alternative routes of administration. It is known that the allergenicity of cooked or baked product is reduced although it remains important to evaluate the potential (residual) antigenicity/allergenicity of new or modified protein products in animal models (110). Allergen specific immune therapies include subcutaneous immunotherapy, sublingual immunotherapy and oral immunotherapy. These methods generally involve administering small yet increasing doses of antigen aimed to reduce clinical symptoms occurring during the natural exposure to the allergen itself. Treatment is performed in a controlled setting and in the case of sublingual and oral immunotherapy followed by regular home dosing of a maximum tolerated amount of antigen (111). Whether these different strategies for specific immune therapy redirect the immune response or induce a transient effect is still under discussion.

Subcutaneous Immunotherapy (SCIT)

The most effective curative treatment for IgE-mediated allergy is SCIT and has been proven effective in respiratory and bee venom allergy. The history of SCIT began almost one hundred years ago by the observation by Leonard Noon that the subcutaneous route of administration was effective in reducing clinical symptoms of hay-fever. Immune modulation by SCIT include the modulation of T and B cell responses and is accompanied by a significant decrease of allergen specific IgE and increase in allergen specific IgG antibodies, mainly IgG_4. Animal studies showed that these effects where dependent on IL-10 and may act via indoldiamine 2,3-deoxygenase (IDO) dependent metabolites (112-114). However, SCIT is not yet available for the management of food allergy because of the high risk of inducing anaphylaxis by accidental intake of the offending allergen (i.e. peanut) (115, 116). Several specific strategies to reduce the allergenicity of therapeutic preparations, while maintaining their therapeutic benefit, are being developed. Several studies examined the differential effects of reducing allergen size most particularly by producing peptides. Allergenic peptides are still able to stimulate the allergen-specific T cells, but due to reduced size peptides are unable to crosslink IgE on mast cells thereby avoiding the inducting of clinical reactions (117). This so called peptide immunotherapy has been investigated and seem effective in bee venom allergy (118) and allergic asthma (119, 120). Recently it has been shown that peptide immunotherapy reduced the allergic response in a mouse model of egg allergy (121). From this point of view, also cow's milk hydrolysates derived peptides might be an option for SCIT in cow's milk allergic infants. However, less invasive therapies might be preferred for the management of cow's milk and egg allergy in the young infant.

Sublingual Immunotherapy (SLIT)

The sublingual route for specific immunotherapy has been routinely used for more then ten years in Europe (122-123). The first randomized double blind placebo controlled clinical trial was published in 1986. Because of the less invasive character SLIT is considered a safe and well tolerated alternative for SCIT in young children (124, 125) although there is a minor risk of inducing anaphylaxis. Since the distribution of antigens administered is limited the adverse effects elicited by SLIT are very low (126). Animal models mimicking SLIT for the treatment of allergic diseases are currently being investigated and might give important insight in the mechanisms underlying SLIT. Three different subtypes of oral DC's have been identified in mice (127). $CD11b^+Cd11c^-$, $CD11b^+CD11c^+$ mucosal DC's, B220+ pDC's and a minor population of $CD207^+$ Langerhals cells. However, Langerhals cells represent the predominating DC population within the human oral mucosa and represent a more immature DC subpopulation which might underlie their tolerogenic properties in SLIT. Moreover, animal models are used to optimize treatment protocols of SLIT (128), improving efficacy using adjuvants, to facilitate the generation of regulatory T-cells or Th1 type responses (129-130), and muco-adhesive substances. The clinical efficacy of SLIT has been proven in the treatment of allergic rhinitis (pollen) and allergic asthma (house dust mite) in children (131-133). The most important concern to be elucidated in SLIT is the optimal dose of allergen to be used because effectiveness has been shown over a very large range of doses. In a recent randomized, placebo controlled study Pajno *et al.* reported that SLIT may provide an additional therapeutic tool for the treatment of house dust mite sensitized children with atopic dermatitis (122). The allergic form of atopic dermatitis affects the majority of the patients and occurs in the context of an IgE sensitization towards food or environmental allergens. Therefore, SLIT might be a potential strategy for preventing symptoms in food allergy. So far, at least one clinical study described the efficacy of SLIT for hazelnut allergy (134).

Oral Immunotherapy (OIT)

OIT aiming at the tolerizing/desensitizing capacity of orally applied allergens in diagnosed food allergic patients started with several clinical trials in the 1980s. These studies showed promising results (135) although in some cases serious gastrointestinal adverse events were reported. In the last decade the interest in non-invasive routes for specific immunotherapy increased again. Currently this approach undergoes the most intensive research. Meglio *et al* showed that from 21 cow's milk allergic children above 5 years of age 71% tolerated 200 ml of cow's milk after 6 months of OIT and were still tolerant in a 4-years follow-up. However, the weakness of this study was that no control group was included to study the natural course of cow's milk allergy (136-137). The safety and efficacy of cow's milk OIT was confirmed in children with severe cow's milk allergy (138). After 1 year the threshold dose was increased in 54% of the children and 36% of the children became tolerant whereas in the control group all children were still cow's milk allergic. Side effects occurred but were controllable with medication. Also for hen's egg and peanut allergy the efficacy of OIT was studied and confirmed (139-142) but more research is needed to optimize treatment protocols (i.e. rush versus semi-rush) and to study the underlying mechanism. It is still not known whether persistent immune modulation or a transient desensitization is induced by OIT (143). However, even if desensitization is induced, clinical tolerance due to regular intake of the offended food has the advantage of increasing the threshold dose for allergic reactions which can improve the quality of life substantially for the allergic patient. However, it can not be excluded that diseases (i.e. infections) affect the increased threshold dose. OIT with peanut is currently studied in patients with atopic dermatitis. In the Learning Early About Peanut Allergy study 480 children aged 4 to 10 months with eczema and egg allergy (as a predictor for peanut allergy) are assigned to either avoid consumption of peanuts or to be fed peanut snacks three times a week. After five years the development of peanut allergy will be compared. This study can give important insight in the capacity of OIT to diminish new sensitizations and ultimately to pause the atopic march.

Summary

Prevention of food allergy induced by the three major food allergens, hen's egg, cow's milk and peanut is considered important and might prevent related diseases like atopic dermatitis, allergic rhinitis and allergic asthma later in life. Breastfeeding is still considered the best way of preventing food sensitization. Prebiotic oligosaccharides and cytokines like IL-10, TGF_{β} which are abundantly present in human milk, might provide an immunological milieu that favors the induction of oral tolerance in the Th2 prone infant. The early introduction of food proteins or peptides (i.e. hydrolysed formulae) seems to be the most promising approach to induce oral tolerance and prevent sensitization to harmless food antigens. In addition, food proteins seem to be involved in stimulating maturation of the immature gut. In the allergic child, allergen specific immune therapies are important strategies to induce hypo-responsiveness to the offending food either by restoring tolerance or by transient desensitization. They include subcutaneous immunotherapy, sublingual immunotherapy and oral immunotherapy. Although allergen specific immunotherapy seems very promising and might prevent secondary sensitizations and thereby even diminishing or stopping the atopic march, still much research is needed to further optimize the protocols and to study the underlying mechanisms.

References

[1] Asher, M. I., S. Montefort, B. Bjorksten, C. K. Lai, D. P. Strachan, S. K. Weiland, and H. Williams. 2006. Worldwide time trends in the prevalence of symptoms of asthma, allergic rhinoconjunctivitis, and eczema in childhood: ISAAC Phases One and Three repeat multicountry cross-sectional surveys. *Lancet* 368:733-743.

[2] Sly, R. M. 1999. Changing prevalence of allergic rhinitis and asthma. *Ann Allergy Asthma Immunol* 82:233-248; quiz 248-252.

[3] Williams, H., C. Robertson, A. Stewart, N. Ait-Khaled, G. Anabwani, R. Anderson, I. Asher, R. Beasley, B. Bjorksten, M. Burr, T. Clayton, J. Crane, P. Ellwood, U. Keil, C. Lai, J. Mallol, F. Martinez, E. Mitchell, S. Montefort, N. Pearce, J. Shah, B. Sibbald, D. Strachan, E. von Mutius, and S. K. Weiland. 1999. Worldwide variations in the prevalence of symptoms of atopic eczema in the International Study of Asthma and Allergies in Childhood. *J Allergy Clin Immunol* 103:125-138.

[4] Hill, D. J., R. G. Heine, C. S. Hosking, J. Brown, L. Thiele, K. J. Allen, J. Su, G. Varigos, and J. B. Carlin. 2007. IgE food sensitization in infants with eczema attending a dermatology department. *J Pediatr* 151:359-363.

[5] Hauk, P. J. 2008. The role of food allergy in atopic dermatitis. *Curr Allergy Asthma Rep* 8:188-194.

[6] Werfel, T., and K. Breuer. 2004. Role of food allergy in atopic dermatitis. *Curr Opin Allergy Clin Immunol* 4:379-385.

[7] Lack, G. 2008. Epidemiologic risks for food allergy. *J Allergy Clin Immunol* 121:1331-1336.

[8] Levy, Y., A. Broides, N. Segal, and Y. L. Danon. 2003. Peanut and tree nut allergy in children: role of peanut snacks in Israel? *Allergy* 58:1206-1207.

[9] Hourihane, J. O., R. Aiken, R. Briggs, L. A. Gudgeon, K. E. Grimshaw, A. DunnGalvin, and S. R. Roberts. 2007. The impact of government advice to pregnant mothers regarding peanut avoidance on the prevalence of peanut allergy in United Kingdom children at school entry. *J Allergy Clin Immunol* 119:1197-1202.

[10] Wennergren, G. 2009. What if it is the other way around? Early introduction of peanut and fish seems to be better than avoidance. *Acta Paediatr* 98:1085-1087.

[11] Branum, A. M., and S. L. Lukacs. 2008. Food allergy among U.S. children: trends in prevalence and hospitalizations. *NCHS Data Brief*:1-8.

[12] Strobel, S. 2001. Immunity induced after a feed of antigen during early life: oral tolerance v. sensitisation. *Proc Nutr Soc* 60:437-442.

[13] Sicherer, S. H., and H. A. Sampson. 2009. 10. Food allergy. *J Allergy Clin Immunol.*

[14] Skripak, J. M., E. C. Matsui, K. Mudd, and R. A. Wood. 2007. The natural history of IgE-mediated cow's milk allergy. *J Allergy Clin Immunol* 120:1172-1177.

[15] Savage, J. H., E. C. Matsui, J. M. Skripak, and R. A. Wood. 2007. The natural history of egg allergy. *J Allergy Clin Immunol* 120:1413-1417.

[16] Spergel, J. M., and A. S. Paller. 2003. Atopic dermatitis and the atopic march. *J Allergy Clin Immunol* 112:S118-127.

[17] Rhodes, H. L., R. Sporik, P. Thomas, S. T. Holgate, and J. J. Cogswell. 2001. Early life risk factors for adult asthma: a birth cohort study of subjects at risk. *J Allergy Clin Immunol* 108:720-725.

[18] Carroll, N. G., S. Mutavdzic, and A. L. James. 2002. Increased mast cells and neutrophils in submucosal mucous glands and mucus plugging in patients with asthma. *Thorax* 57:677-682.

[19] Peterson, C. G., T. Hansson, A. Skott, U. Bengtsson, S. Ahlstedt, and J. Magnussons. 2007. Detection of local mast-cell activity in patients with food hypersensitivity. *J Investig Allergol Clin Immunol* 17:314-320.

[20] Shek, L. P., L. Bardina, R. Castro, H. A. Sampson, and K. Beyer. 2005. Humoral and cellular responses to cow milk proteins in patients with milk-induced IgE-mediated and non-IgE-mediated disorders. *Allergy* 60:912-919.

[21] Kraneveld, A. D., M. Kool, A. H. van Houwelingen, P. Roholl, A. Solomon, D. S. Postma, F. P. Nijkamp, and F. A. Redegeld. 2005. Elicitation of allergic asthma by immunoglobulin free light chains. *Proc Natl Acad Sci U S A* 102:1578-1583.

[22] Redegeld, F. A., M. W. van der Heijden, M. Kool, B. M. Heijdra, J. Garssen, A. D. Kraneveld, H. Van Loveren, P. Roholl, T. Saito, J. S. Verbeek, J. Claassens, A. S. Koster, and F. P. Nijkamp. 2002. Immunoglobulin-free light chains elicit immediate hypersensitivity-like responses. *Nat Med* 8:694-701.

[23] Paliwal, V., R. F. Tsuji, M. Szczepanik, I. Kawikova, R. A. Campos, M. Kneilling, M. Rocken, J. Schuurman, F. A. Redegeld, F. P. Nijkamp, and P. W. Askenase. 2002. Subunits of IgM reconstitute defective contact sensitivity in B-1 cell-deficient xid mice: kappa light chains recruit T cells independent of complement. *J Immunol* 169:4113-4123.

[24] van Houwelingen, A. H., K. Kaczynska, A. D. Kraneveld, M. Kool, F. P. Nijkamp, and F. A. Redegeld. 2007. Topical application of F991, an immunoglobulin free light chain antagonist, prevents development of contact sensitivity in mice. *Clin Exp Allergy* 37:270-275.

[25] van Esch, B. C., B. Schouten, B. R. Blokhuis, G. A. Hofman, L. Boon, J. Garssen, L. M. Knippels, L. E. Willemsen, and F. A. Redegeld. 2010. Depletion of CD4(+)CD25(+) T cells switches the whey-allergic response from immunoglobulin E- to immunoglobulin free light chain-dependent. *Clin Exp Allergy* 40(9):1414-21. Epub 2010 Apr 19

[26] Schouten, B., B. C. van Esch, A. O. van Thuijl, B. R. Blokhuis, T. Groot Kormelink, G. A. Hofman, G. E. Moro, G. Boehm, S. Arslanoglu, A. B. Sprikkelman, L. E. Willemsen, L. M. Knippels, F. A. Redegeld, and J. Garssen 2010. Contribution of IgE and immunoglobulin free light chain in the allergic reaction to cow's milk proteins. *J Allergy Clin Immunol* 125:1308-1314.

[27] Powe, D. G., T. G. Kormelink, M. Sisson, B. J. Blokhuis, M. F. Kramer, N. S. Jones, and F. A. Redegeld. 2010. Evidence for the involvement of free light chain immunoglobulins in allergic and nonallergic rhinitis. *J Allergy Clin Immunol* 125(1):139-45.e1-3. Epub 2009 Oct 8

[28] Flinterman, A. E., A. C. Knulst, Y. Meijer, C. A. Bruijnzeel-Koomen, and S. G. Pasmans. 2006. Acute allergic reactions in children with AEDS after prolonged cow's milk elimination diets. *Allergy* 61:370-374.

[29] Leung, D. Y. 2000. Atopic dermatitis: new insights and opportunities for therapeutic intervention. *J Allergy Clin Immunol* 105:860-876.

[30] Jakasa, I., M. M. Verberk, M. Esposito, J. D. Bos, and S. Kezic. 2007. Altered penetration of polyethylene glycols into uninvolved skin of atopic dermatitis patients. *J Invest Dermatol* 127:129-134.

[31] McGrath, J. A., and J. Uitto. 2008. The filaggrin story: novel insights into skin-barrier function and disease. *Trends Mol Med* 14:20-27.

[32] Palmer, C. N., A. D. Irvine, A. Terron-Kwiatkowski, Y. Zhao, H. Liao, S. P. Lee, D. R. Goudie, A. Sandilands, L. E. Campbell, F. J. Smith, G. M. O'Regan, R. M. Watson, J. E. Cecil, S. J. Bale, J. G. Compton, J. J. DiGiovanna, P. Fleckman, S. Lewis-Jones, G. Arseculeratne, A. Sergeant, C. S. Munro, B. El Houate, K. McElreavey, L. B. Halkjaer, H. Bisgaard, S. Mukhopadhyay, and W. H. McLean. 2006. Common loss-of-function variants of the epidermal barrier protein filaggrin are a major predisposing factor for atopic dermatitis. *Nat Genet* 38:441-446.

[33] Seguchi, T., C. Y. Cui, S. Kusuda, M. Takahashi, K. Aisu, and T. Tezuka. 1996. Decreased expression of filaggrin in atopic skin. *Arch Dermatol Res* 288:442-446.

[34] Cookson, W. O., B. Ubhi, R. Lawrence, G. R. Abecasis, A. J. Walley, H. E. Cox, R. Coleman, N. I. Leaves, R. C. Trembath, M. F. Moffatt, and J. I. Harper. 2001. Genetic linkage of childhood atopic dermatitis to psoriasis susceptibility loci. *Nat Genet* 27:372-373.

[35] Compton, J. G., J. J. DiGiovanna, K. A. Johnston, P. Fleckman, and S. J. Bale. 2002. Mapping of the associated phenotype of an absent granular layer in ichthyosis vulgaris to the epidermal differentiation complex on chromosome 1. *Exp Dermatol* 11:518-526.

[36] Smith, F. J., A. D. Irvine, A. Terron-Kwiatkowski, A. Sandilands, L. E. Campbell, Y. Zhao, H. Liao, A. T. Evans, D. R. Goudie, S. Lewis-Jones, G. Arseculeratne, C. S. Munro, A. Sergeant, G. O'Regan, S. J. Bale, J. G. Compton, J. J. DiGiovanna, R. B. Presland, P. Fleckman, and W. H. McLean. 2006. Loss-of-function mutations in the gene encoding filaggrin cause ichthyosis vulgaris. *Nat Genet* 38:337-342.

[37] Lowe, A. J., C. S. Hosking, C. M. Bennett, J. B. Carlin, M. J. Abramson, D. J. Hill, and S. C. Dharmage. 2007. Skin prick test can identify eczematous infants at risk of asthma and allergic rhinitis. *Clin Exp Allergy* 37:1624-1631.

[38] Strid, J., J. Hourihane, I. Kimber, R. Callard, and S. Strobel. 2004. Disruption of the stratum corneum allows potent epicutaneous immunization with protein antigens resulting in a dominant systemic Th2 response. *Eur J Immunol* 34:2100-2109.

[39] Spergel, J. M., E. Mizoguchi, J. P. Brewer, T. R. Martin, A. K. Bhan, and R. S. Geha. 1998. Epicutaneous sensitization with protein antigen induces localized allergic dermatitis and hyperresponsiveness to methacholine after single exposure to aerosolized antigen in mice. *J Clin Invest* 101:1614-1622.

[40] Lack, G., D. Fox, K. Northstone, and J. Golding. 2003. Factors associated with the development of peanut allergy in childhood. *N Engl J Med* 348:977-985.

[41] Kissling, S., and B. Wuthrich. 1993. [Follow-up of atopic dermatitis after early childhood]. *Hautarzt* 44:569-573.

[42] Wuthrich, B., and P. Schudel. 1983. [Atopic neurodermatitis after childhood stage; follow-up study of 121 cases]. *Z Hautkr* 58:1013-1023.

[43] Burgess, J. A., A. J. Lowe, M. C. Matheson, G. Varigos, M. J. Abramson, and S. C. Dharmage. 2009. Does eczema lead to asthma? *J Asthma* 46:429-436.

[44] van der Hulst, A. E., H. Klip, and P. L. Brand. 2007. Risk of developing asthma in young children with atopic eczema: a systematic review. *J Allergy Clin Immunol* 120:565-569.

[45] Lowe, A. J., J. B. Carlin, C. M. Bennett, C. S. Hosking, M. J. Abramson, D. J. Hill, and S. C. Dharmage. 2008. Do boys do the atopic march while girls dawdle? *J Allergy Clin Immunol* 121:1190-1195.

[46] Illi, S., E. von Mutius, S. Lau, R. Nickel, C. Gruber, B. Niggemann, and U. Wahn. 2004. The natural course of atopic dermatitis from birth to age 7 years and the association with asthma. *J Allergy Clin Immunol* 113:925-931.

[47] Brockow, I., A. Zutavern, U. Hoffmann, A. Grubl, A. von Berg, S. Koletzko, B. Filipiak, C. P. Bauer, H. E. Wichmann, D. Reinhardt, D. Berdel, U. Kramer, and J. Heinrich. 2009. Early allergic sensitizations and their relevance to atopic diseases in children aged 6 years: results of the GINI study. *J Investig Allergol Clin Immunol* 19:180-187.

[48] Host, A. 2002. Frequency of cow's milk allergy in childhood. *Ann Allergy Asthma Immunol* 89:33-37.

[49] Field, C. J. 2005. The immunological components of human milk and their effect on immune development in infants. *J Nutr* 135:1-4.

[50] Hoppu, U., M. Kalliomaki, K. Laiho, and E. Isolauri. 2001. Breast milk--immunomodulatory signals against allergic diseases. *Allergy* 56 Suppl 67:23-26.

[51] Lara-Villoslada, F., M. Olivares, S. Sierra, J. M. Rodriguez, J. Boza, and J. Xaus. 2007. Beneficial effects of probiotic bacteria isolated from breast milk. *Br J Nutr* 98 Suppl 1:S96-100.

[52] Ando, T., K. Hatsushika, M. Wako, T. Ohba, K. Koyama, Y. Ohnuma, R. Katoh, H. Ogawa, K. Okumura, J. Luo, T. Wyss-Coray, and A. Nakao. 2007. Orally administered TGF-beta is biologically active in the intestinal mucosa and enhances oral tolerance. *J Allergy Clin Immunol* 120:916-923.

[53] Vos, A. P., L. M'Rabet, B. Stahl, G. Boehm, and J. Garssen. 2007. Immune-modulatory effects and potential working mechanisms of orally applied nondigestible carbohydrates. *Crit Rev Immunol* 27:97-140.

[54] Palmer, D. J., M. S. Gold, and M. Makrides. 2008. Effect of maternal egg consumption on breast milk ovalbumin concentration. *Clin Exp Allergy* 38:1186-1191.

[55] Vadas, P., Y. Wai, W. Burks, and B. Perelman. 2001. Detection of peanut allergens in breast milk of lactating women. *Jama* 285:1746-1748.

[56] Lifschitz, C. H., H. K. Hawkins, C. Guerra, and N. Byrd. 1988. Anaphylactic shock due to cow's milk protein hypersensitivity in a breast-fed infant. *J Pediatr Gastroenterol Nutr* 7:141-144.

[57] Gibson, G. R., and M. B. Roberfroid. 1995. Dietary modulation of the human colonic microbiota: introducing the concept of prebiotics. *J Nutr* 125:1401-1412.

[58] van Hoffen, E., B. Ruiter, J. Faber, L. M'Rabet, E. F. Knol, B. Stahl, S. Arslanoglu, G. Moro, G. Boehm, and J. Garssen. 2009. A specific mixture of short-chain galacto-oligosaccharides and long-chain fructo-oligosaccharides induces a beneficial immunoglobulin profile in infants at high risk for allergy. *Allergy* 64:484-487.

[59] Moro, G., S. Arslanoglu, B. Stahl, J. Jelinek, U. Wahn, and G. Boehm. 2006. A mixture of prebiotic oligosaccharides reduces the incidence of atopic dermatitis during the first six months of age. *Arch Dis Child* 91:814-819.

[60] Schouten, B., B. C. van Esch, G. A. Hofman, S. A. van Doorn, J. Knol, A. J. Nauta, J. Garssen, L. E. Willemsen, and L. M. Knippels. 2009. Cow milk allergy symptoms are reduced in mice fed dietary synbiotics during oral sensitization with whey. *J Nutr* 139:1398-1403.

[61] Vos, A. P., B. C. van Esch, B. Stahl, L. M'Rabet, G. Folkerts, F. P. Nijkamp, and J. Garssen. 2007. Dietary supplementation with specific oligosaccharide mixtures decreases parameters of allergic asthma in mice. *Int Immunopharmacol* 7:1582-1587.

[62] Arshad, S. H., B. Bateman, A. Sadeghnejad, C. Gant, and S. M. Matthews. 2007. Prevention of allergic disease during childhood by allergen avoidance: the Isle of Wight prevention study. *J Allergy Clin Immunol* 119:307-313.

[63] Strid, J., M. Thomson, J. Hourihane, I. Kimber, and S. Strobel. 2004. A novel model of sensitization and oral tolerance to peanut protein. *Immunology* 113:293-303.

[64] Palmer, D. J., and M. Makrides. 2006. Diet of lactating women and allergic reactions in their infants. *Curr Opin Clin Nutr Metab Care* 9:284-288.

[65] Du Toit, G., Y. Katz, P. Sasieni, D. Mesher, S. J. Maleki, H. R. Fisher, A. T. Fox, V. Turcanu, T. Amir, G. Zadik-Mnuhin, A. Cohen, I. Livne, and G. Lack. 2008. Early consumption of peanuts in infancy is associated with a low prevalence of peanut allergy. *J Allergy Clin Immunol* 122:984-991.

[66] Kull, I., A. Bergstrom, G. Lilja, G. Pershagen, and M. Wickman. 2006. Fish consumption during the first year of life and development of allergic diseases during childhood. *Allergy* 61:1009-1015.

[67] Kraehenbuhl, J. P., and M. R. Neutra. 1992. Transepithelial transport and mucosal defence II: secretion of IgA. *Trends Cell Biol* 2:170-174.

[68] Menezes, J. S., D. S. Mucida, D. C. Cara, J. I. Alvarez-Leite, M. Russo, N. M. Vaz, and A. M. de Faria. 2003. Stimulation by food proteins plays a critical role in the maturation of the immune system. *Int Immunol* 15:447-455.

[69] Chehade, M., and L. Mayer. 2005. Oral tolerance and its relation to food hypersensitivities. *J Allergy Clin Immunol* 115:3-12; quiz 13.

[70] 70. Jang, M. H., N. Sougawa, T. Tanaka, T. Hirata, T. Hiroi, K. Tohya, Z. Guo, E. Umemoto, Y. Ebisuno, B. G. Yang, J. Y. Seoh, M. Lipp, H. Kiyono, and M. Miyasaka. 2006. CCR7 is critically important for migration of dendritic cells in intestinal lamina propria to mesenteric lymph nodes. *J Immunol* 176:803-810.

[71] Worbs, T., U. Bode, S. Yan, M. W. Hoffmann, G. Hintzen, G. Bernhardt, R. Forster, and O. Pabst. 2006. Oral tolerance originates in the intestinal immune system and relies on antigen carriage by dendritic cells. *J Exp Med* 203:519-527.

[72] Viney, J. L., A. M. Mowat, J. M. O'Malley, E. Williamson, and N. A. Fanger. 1998. Expanding dendritic cells in vivo enhances the induction of oral tolerance. *J Immunol* 160:5815-5825.

[73] Goubier, A., B. Dubois, H. Gheit, G. Joubert, F. Villard-Truc, C. Asselin-Paturel, G. Trinchieri, and D. Kaiserlian. 2008. Plasmacytoid dendritic cells mediate oral tolerance. *Immunity* 29:464-475.

[74] Min, S. Y., K. S. Park, M. L. Cho, J. W. Kang, Y. G. Cho, S. Y. Hwang, M. J. Park, C. H. Yoon, J. K. Min, S. H. Lee, S. H. Park, and H. Y. Kim. 2006. Antigen-induced, tolerogenic CD11c+,CD11b+ dendritic cells are abundant in Peyer's patches during the induction of oral tolerance to type II collagen and suppress experimental collagen-induced arthritis. *Arthritis Rheum* 54:887-898.

[75] de Heer, H. J., H. Hammad, T. Soullie, D. Hijdra, N. Vos, M. A. Willart, H. C. Hoogsteden, and B. N. Lambrecht. 2004. Essential role of lung plasmacytoid dendritic cells in preventing asthmatic reactions to harmless inhaled antigen. *J Exp Med* 200:89-98.

[76] Bilsborough, J., T. C. George, A. Norment, and J. L. Viney. 2003. Mucosal CD8alpha+ DC, with a plasmacytoid phenotype, induce differentiation and support function of T cells with regulatory properties. *Immunology* 108:481-492.

[77] Martin, P., G. M. Del Hoyo, F. Anjuere, C. F. Arias, H. H. Vargas, L. A. Fernandez, V. Parrillas, and C. Ardavin. 2002. Characterization of a new subpopulation of mouse CD8alpha+ B220+ dendritic cells endowed with type 1 interferon production capacity and tolerogenic potential. *Blood* 100:383-390.

[78] Iwasaki, A., and B. L. Kelsall. 2001. Unique functions of CD11b+, CD8 alpha+, and double-negative Peyer's patch dendritic cells. *J Immunol* 166:4884-4890.

[79] Mowat, A. M. 2003. Anatomical basis of tolerance and immunity to intestinal antigens. *Nat Rev Immunol* 3:331-341.

[80] Jaensson, E., H. Uronen-Hansson, O. Pabst, B. Eksteen, J. Tian, J. L. Coombes, P. L. Berg, T. Davidsson, F. Powrie, B. Johansson-Lindbom, and W. W. Agace. 2008. Small intestinal CD103+ dendritic cells display unique functional properties that are conserved between mice and humans. *J Exp Med* 205:2139-2149.

[81] Pabst, O., G. Bernhardt, and R. Forster. 2007. The impact of cell-bound antigen transport on mucosal tolerance induction. *J Leukoc Biol* 82:795-800.

[82] Spahn, T. W., H. L. Weiner, P. D. Rennert, N. Lugering, A. Fontana, W. Domschke, and T. Kucharzik. 2002. Mesenteric lymph nodes are critical for the induction of high-dose oral tolerance in the absence of Peyer's patches. *Eur J Immunol* 32:1109-1113.

[83] Coombes, J. L., K. R. Siddiqui, C. V. Arancibia-Carcamo, J. Hall, C. M. Sun, Y. Belkaid, and F. Powrie. 2007. A functionally specialized population of mucosal

CD103+ DCs induces Foxp3+ regulatory T cells via a TGF-beta and retinoic acid-dependent mechanism. *J Exp Med* 204:1757-1764.

[84] Takayama, N., O. Igarashi, M. N. Kweon, and H. Kiyono. 2007. Regulatory role of Peyer's patches for the inhibition of OVA-induced allergic diarrhea. *Clin Immunol* 123:199-208.

[85] Sato, A., and A. Iwasaki. 2005. Peyer's patch dendritic cells as regulators of mucosal adaptive immunity. *Cell Mol Life Sci* 62:1333-1338.

[86] Tsuji, N. M., K. Mizumachi, and J. Kurisaki. 2003. Antigen-specific, CD4+CD25+ regulatory T cell clones induced in Peyer's patches. *Int Immunol* 15:525-534.

[87] Tsuji, N. M., K. Mizumachi, and J. Kurisaki. 2001. Interleukin-10-secreting Peyer's patch cells are responsible for active suppression in low-dose oral tolerance. *Immunology* 103:458-464.

[88] Frossard, C. P., L. Tropia, C. Hauser, and P. A. Eigenmann. 2004. Lymphocytes in Peyer patches regulate clinical tolerance in a murine model of food allergy. *J Allergy Clin Immunol* 113:958-964.

[89] Kunkel, D., D. Kirchhoff, S. Nishikawa, A. Radbruch, and A. Scheffold. 2003. Visualization of peptide presentation following oral application of antigen in normal and Peyer's patches-deficient mice. *Eur J Immunol* 33:1292-1301.

[90] Cantor, H. M., and A. E. Dumont. 1967. Hepatic suppression of sensitization to antigen absorbed into the portal system. *Nature* 215:744-745.

[91] Yang, R., Q. Liu, J. L. Grosfeld, and M. D. Pescovitz. 1994. Intestinal venous drainage through the liver is a prerequisite for oral tolerance induction. *J Pediatr Surg* 29:1145-1148.

[92] Mucida, D., N. Kutchukhidze, A. Erazo, M. Russo, J. J. Lafaille, and M. A. Curotto de Lafaille. 2005. Oral tolerance in the absence of naturally occurring Tregs. *J Clin Invest* 115:1923-1933.

[93] Saurer, L., and C. Mueller. 2009. T cell-mediated immunoregulation in the gastrointestinal tract. *Allergy* 64:505-519.

[94] Shreffler, W. G., N. Wanich, M. Moloney, A. Nowak-Wegrzyn, and H. A. Sampson. 2009. Association of allergen-specific regulatory T cells with the onset of clinical tolerance to milk protein. *J Allergy Clin Immunol* 123:43-52 e47.

[95] Winkler, B., K. Hufnagl, A. Spittler, M. Ploder, E. Kallay, S. Vrtala, R. Valenta, M. Kundi, H. Renz, and U. Wiedermann. 2006. The role of Foxp3+ T cells in long-term efficacy of prophylactic and therapeutic mucosal tolerance induction in mice. *Allergy* 61:173-180.

[96] Nagatani, K., K. Sagawa, Y. Komagata, and K. Yamamoto. 2004. Peyer's patch dendritic cells capturing oral antigen interact with antigen-specific T cells and induce gut-homing CD4(+)CD25(+) regulatory T cells in Peyer's patches. *Ann N Y Acad Sci* 1029:366-370.

[97] Zhang, X., L. Izikson, L. Liu, and H. L. Weiner. 2001. Activation of CD25(+)CD4(+) regulatory T cells by oral antigen administration. *J Immunol* 167:4245-4253.

[98] Hays, T., and R. A. Wood. 2005. A systematic review of the role of hydrolyzed infant formulas in allergy prevention. *Arch Pediatr Adolesc Med* 159:810-816.

[99] Osborn, D. A., and J. Sinn. 2006. Formulas containing hydrolysed protein for prevention of allergy and food intolerance in infants. *Cochrane Database Syst Rev*:CD003664.

[100] Zeiger, R. S., and S. Heller. 1995. The development and prediction of atopy in high-risk children: follow-up at age seven years in a prospective randomized study of combined maternal and infant food allergen avoidance. *J Allergy Clin Immunol* 95:1179-1190.

[101] Halken, S., K. S. Hansen, H. P. Jacobsen, A. Estmann, A. E. Faelling, L. G. Hansen, S. R. Kier, K. Lassen, M. Lintrup, S. Mortensen, K. K. Ibsen, O. Osterballe, and A. Host. 2000. Comparison of a partially hydrolyzed infant formula with two extensively hydrolyzed formulas for allergy prevention: a prospective, randomized study. *Pediatr Allergy Immunol* 11:149-161.

[102] Chan, Y. H., L. P. Shek, M. Aw, S. H. Quak, and B. W. Lee. 2002. Use of hypoallergenic formula in the prevention of atopic disease among Asian children. *J Paediatr Child Health* 38:84-88.

[103] von Berg, A., S. Koletzko, A. Grubl, B. Filipiak-Pittroff, H. E. Wichmann, C. P. Bauer, D. Reinhardt, and D. Berdel. 2003. The effect of hydrolyzed cow's milk formula for allergy prevention in the first year of life: the German Infant Nutritional Intervention Study, a randomized double-blind trial. *J Allergy Clin Immunol* 111:533-540.

[104] Vandenplas, Y., B. Hauser, C. Van den Borre, C. Clybouw, T. Mahler, S. Hachimi-Idrissi, L. Deraeve, A. Malfroot, and I. Dab. 1995. The long-term effect of a partial whey hydrolysate formula on the prophylaxis of atopic disease. *Eur J Pediatr* 154:488-494.

[105] Peng, H. J., S. N. Su, J. J. Tsai, L. C. Tsai, H. L. Kuo, and S. W. Kuo. 2004. Effect of ingestion of cow's milk hydrolysed formulas on whey protein-specific Th2 immune responses in naive and sensitized mice. *Clin Exp Allergy* 34:663-670.

[106] Fritsche, R., J. J. Pahud, S. Pecquet, and A. Pfeifer. 1997. Induction of systemic immunologic tolerance to beta-lactoglobulin by oral administration of a whey protein hydrolysate. *J Allergy Clin Immunol* 100:266-273.

[107] Pecquet, S., L. Bovetto, F. Maynard, and R. Fritsche. 2000. Peptides obtained by tryptic hydrolysis of bovine beta-lactoglobulin induce specific oral tolerance in mice. *J Allergy Clin Immunol* 105:514-521.

[108] van Esch, B. C., B. Schouten, G. A. Hofman, T. van Baalen, F. P. Nijkamp, L. M. Knippels, L. E. Willemsen, and J. Garssen. 2010.. Acute allergic skin response as a new tool to evaluate the allergenicity of whey hydrolysates in a mouse model of orally induced cow's milk allergy. *Pediatr Allergy Immunol* 21(4 Pt 2):e780-6. Epub 2009 Jun 26.

[109] Cantani, A. 1999. Hidden presence of cow's milk proteins in foods. *J Investig Allergol Clin Immunol* 9:141-145.

[110] Knippels, L. M., and A. H. Penninks. 2005. Recent advances using rodent models for predicting human allergenicity. *Toxicol Appl Pharmacol* 207:157-160.

[111] Burks, A. W., S. Laubach, and S. M. Jones. 2008. Oral tolerance, food allergy, and immunotherapy: implications for future treatment. *J Allergy Clin Immunol* 121:1344-1350.

[112] Vissers, J. L., B. C. van Esch, G. A. Hofman, M. L. Kapsenberg, F. R. Weller, and A. J. van Oosterhout. 2004. Allergen immunotherapy induces a suppressive memory response mediated by IL-10 in a mouse asthma model. *J Allergy Clin Immunol* 113:1204-1210.

[113] Taher, Y. A., B. J. Piavaux, R. Gras, B. C. van Esch, G. A. Hofman, N. Bloksma, P. A. Henricks, and A. J. van Oosterhout. 2008. Indoleamine 2,3-dioxygenase-dependent tryptophan metabolites contribute to tolerance induction during allergen immunotherapy in a mouse model. *J Allergy Clin Immunol* 121:983-991 e982.

[114] Taher, Y. A., B. C. van Esch, G. A. Hofman, P. A. Henricks, and A. J. van Oosterhout. 2008. 1alpha,25-dihydroxyvitamin D3 potentiates the beneficial effects of allergen immunotherapy in a mouse model of allergic asthma: role for IL-10 and TGF-beta. *J Immunol* 180:5211-5221.

[115] Cox, L., D. Larenas-Linnemann, R. F. Lockey, and G. Passalacqua. Speaking the same language: The World Allergy Organization Subcutaneous Immunotherapy Systemic Reaction Grading System. *J Allergy Clin Immunol* 125:569-574, 574 e561-574 e567.

[116] Nelson, H. S., J. Lahr, R. Rule, A. Bock, and D. Leung. 1997. Treatment of anaphylactic sensitivity to peanuts by immunotherapy with injections of aqueous peanut extract. *J Allergy Clin Immunol* 99:744-751.

[117] Knol, E. F. 2006. Requirements for effective IgE cross-linking on mast cells and basophils. *Mol Nutr Food Res* 50:620-624.

[118] Lerch, E., and U. R. Muller. 1998. Long-term protection after stopping venom immunotherapy: results of re-stings in 200 patients. *J Allergy Clin Immunol* 101:606-612.

[119] Larche, M. 2005. Peptide therapy for allergic diseases: basic mechanisms and new clinical approaches. *Pharmacol Ther* 108:353-361.

[120] Larche, M. 2007. Peptide immunotherapy for allergic diseases. *Allergy* 62:325-331.

[121] Yang, M., C. Yang, and Y. Mine. Multiple T cell epitope peptides suppress allergic responses in an egg allergy mouse model by the elicitation of forkhead box transcription factor 3- and transforming growth factor-beta-associated mechanisms. *Clin Exp Allergy*.

[122] Pajno, G. B., L. Caminiti, D. Vita, G. Barberio, G. Salzano, F. Lombardo, G. W. Canonica, and G. Passalacqua. 2007. Sublingual immunotherapy in mite-sensitized children with atopic dermatitis: a randomized, double-blind, placebo-controlled study. *J Allergy Clin Immunol* 120:164-170.

[123] Passalacqua, G., and G. W. Canonica. 2006. Sublingual immunotherapy: update 2006. *Curr Opin Allergy Clin Immunol* 6:449-454.

[124] Wahn, U., A. Tabar, P. Kuna, S. Halken, A. Montagut, O. de Beaumont, and M. Le Gall. 2009. Efficacy and safety of 5-grass-pollen sublingual immunotherapy tablets in pediatric allergic rhinoconjunctivitis. *J Allergy Clin Immunol* 123:160-166 e163.

[125] Bufe, A., P. Eberle, E. Franke-Beckmann, J. Funck, M. Kimmig, L. Klimek, R. Knecht, V. Stephan, B. Tholstrup, C. Weisshaar, and F. Kaiser. 2009. Safety and efficacy in children of an SQ-standardized grass allergen tablet for sublingual immunotherapy. *J Allergy Clin Immunol* 123:167-173 e167.

[126] Cox, L. 2008. Allergen immunotherapy and asthma: efficacy, safety, and other considerations. *Allergy Asthma Proc* 29:580-589.

[127] Mascarell, L., V. Lombardi, A. Louise, N. Saint-Lu, H. Chabre, H. Moussu, D. Betbeder, A. M. Balazuc, L. Van Overtvelt, and P. Moingeon. 2008. Oral dendritic cells mediate antigen-specific tolerance by stimulating TH1 and regulatory CD4+ T cells. *J Allergy Clin Immunol* 122:603-609 e605.

[128] Rask, C., J. Brimnes, and K. Lund. Shorter dosing intervals of sublingual immunotherapy lead to more efficacious treatment in a mouse model of allergic inflammation. *Scand J Immunol* 71:403-412.

[129] Van Overtvelt, L., V. Lombardi, A. Razafindratsita, N. Saint-Lu, S. Horiot, H. Moussu, L. Mascarell, and P. Moingeon. 2008. IL-10-inducing adjuvants enhance sublingual immunotherapy efficacy in a murine asthma model. *Int Arch Allergy Immunol* 145:152-162.

[130] Lombardi, V., L. Van Overtvelt, S. Horiot, H. Moussu, H. Chabre, A. Louise, A. M. Balazuc, L. Mascarell, and P. Moingeon. 2008. Toll-like receptor 2 agonist Pam3CSK4 enhances the induction of antigen-specific tolerance via the sublingual route. *Clin Exp Allergy* 38:1819-1829.

[131] Calamita, Z., H. Saconato, A. B. Pela, and A. N. Atallah. 2006. Efficacy of sublingual immunotherapy in asthma: systematic review of randomized-clinical trials using the Cochrane Collaboration method. *Allergy* 61:1162-1172.

[132] Penagos, M., E. Compalati, F. Tarantini, R. Baena-Cagnani, J. Huerta, G. Passalacqua, and G. W. Canonica. 2006. Efficacy of sublingual immunotherapy in the treatment of allergic rhinitis in pediatric patients 3 to 18 years of age: a meta-analysis of randomized, placebo-controlled, double-blind trials. *Ann Allergy Asthma Immunol* 97:141-148.

[133] Wilson, D. R., M. T. Lima, and S. R. Durham. 2005. Sublingual immunotherapy for allergic rhinitis: systematic review and meta-analysis. *Allergy* 60:4-12.

[134] Enrique, E., F. Pineda, T. Malek, J. Bartra, M. Basagana, R. Tella, J. V. Castello, R. Alonso, J. A. de Mateo, T. Cerda-Trias, M. San Miguel-Moncin Mdel, S. Monzon, M. Garcia, R. Palacios, and A. Cistero-Bahima. 2005. Sublingual immunotherapy for hazelnut food allergy: a randomized, double-blind, placebo-controlled study with a standardized hazelnut extract. *J Allergy Clin Immunol* 116:1073-1079.

[135] Patriarca, C., A. Romano, A. Venuti, D. Schiavino, V. Di Rienzo, E. Nucera, and S. Pellegrino. 1984. Oral specific hyposensitization in the management of patients allergic to food. *Allergol Immunopathol (Madr)* 12:275-281.

[136] Meglio, P., E. Bartone, M. Plantamura, E. Arabito, and P. G. Giampietro. 2004. A protocol for oral desensitization in children with IgE-mediated cow's milk allergy. *Allergy* 59:980-987.

[137] Meglio, P., P. G. Giampietro, S. Gianni, and E. Galli. 2008. Oral desensitization in children with immunoglobulin E-mediated cow's milk allergy--follow-up at 4 yr and 8 months. *Pediatr Allergy Immunol* 19:412-419.

[138] Longo, G., E. Barbi, I. Berti, R. Meneghetti, A. Pittalis, L. Ronfani, and A. Ventura. 2008. Specific oral tolerance induction in children with very severe cow's milk-induced reactions. *J Allergy Clin Immunol* 121:343-347.

[139] Buchanan, A. D., T. D. Green, S. M. Jones, A. M. Scurlock, L. Christie, K. A. Althage, P. H. Steele, L. Pons, R. M. Helm, L. A. Lee, and A. W. Burks. 2007. Egg oral immunotherapy in nonanaphylactic children with egg allergy. *J Allergy Clin Immunol* 119:199-205.

[140] Jones, S. M., L. Pons, J. L. Roberts, A. M. Scurlock, T. T. Perry, M. Kulis, W. G. Shreffler, P. Steele, K. A. Henry, M. Adair, J. M. Francis, S. Durham, B. P. Vickery, X. Zhong, and A. W. Burks. 2009. Clinical efficacy and immune regulation with peanut oral immunotherapy. *J Allergy Clin Immunol* 124:292-300, 300 e291-297.

[141] Hofmann, A. M., A. M. Scurlock, S. M. Jones, K. P. Palmer, Y. Lokhnygina, P. H. Steele, J. Kamilaris, and A. W. Burks. 2009. Safety of a peanut oral immunotherapy protocol in children with peanut allergy. *J Allergy Clin Immunol* 124:286-291, 291 e281-286.

[142] Clark, A. T., S. Islam, Y. King, J. Deighton, K. Anagnostou, and P. W. Ewan. 2009. Successful oral tolerance induction in severe peanut allergy. *Allergy* 64:1218-1220.

[143] Staden, U., C. Rolinck-Werninghaus, F. Brewe, U. Wahn, B. Niggemann, and K. Beyer. 2007. Specific oral tolerance induction in food allergy in children: efficacy and clinical patterns of reaction. *Allergy* 62:1261-1269.

In: Food Allergies: Symptoms, Diagnosis, and Treatment
Editor: Patricia M. Rodgers
ISBN: 978-1-61728-748-0

Chapter 10

MANAGEMENT OF THE CHILD WITH FOOD ALLERGY*

Alexander K.C. Leung[1,**] and Kam-lun Ellis Hon[2]
[1] University of Calgary, Alberta Children's Hospital, Calgary, Alberta, Canada
[2] Chinese University of Hong Kong, Prince of Wales Hospital, Shatin, Hong Kong.

ABSTRACT

The definitive treatment of food allergy is strict elimination of the offending food from the diet. Symptomatic reactivity to food allergens is generally very specific, and patients rarely react to more than one food in a botanical or animal species. If elimination diets are prescribed, care must be taken to ensure that they are palatable and nutritionally adequate. Patients must have a good knowledge of food containing the allergen and must be taught to scrutinize the labels of all packaged food carefully.

Formula-fed infants with cow's milk allergy should be fed an elemental or extensively hydrolysed hypoallergenic formula. Soy formulas are inappropriate alternatives as a significant number of infants who are allergic to cow's milk are also allergic to soy. Most children outgrow their food hypersensitivity. As such, rechallenge testing for food allergy should be performed; the interval between rechallenges should be dictated by the specific food allergen in question, the age of the child, and the degree of difficulty in avoiding the food in question

Emergency treatment of food-induced anaphylaxis should follow the basic life support ABC principles, with the simultaneous intramuscular injection of adrenaline. A fast-acting H_1 antihistamine should be considered for the child with progressive or generalized urticaria or disturbing pruritus. Pharmacological therapies such as mast cell stabilizers have very little role to play in the treatment of gastrointestinal manifestations of food allergy.

---

[*] A version of this chapter was also published in *Food Allergies: New Research*, edited by Carrie M. Chesterton, published by Nova Science Publishers. It was submitted for appropriate modifications in an effort to encourage wider dissemination of research.

[**] Correspondence to: Dr. Alexander K.C. Leung, MBBS, FRCPC, FRCP(UK&Irel), FRCPCH, FAAP, Clinical Professor of Pediatrics, The University of Calgary, #200, 233 – 16th Avenue NW, Calgary, Alberta, Canada T2M 0H5; Telefax: (403) 230-3322, e-mail: aleung@ucalgary.ca

In high-risk infants, exclusive breastfeeding with introduction of solid foods not earlier than 6 months of age may delay or possibly prevent the onset of food allergy in some children. Avoidance of allergenic foods by lactating mothers is often recommended. When breastfeeding is not possible, the use of a partially or extensively hydrolysed hypoallergenic formula is desirable. Prophylactic medications have not been shown to be consistently effective in the prevention of life-threatening reactions to food. Their use may mask a less severe reaction to a culprit food, knowledge of which might prevent a more severe reaction to that food in the future.

Keywords: allergen avoidance, breastfeeding, hydrolysed hypoallergenic formula

INTRODUCTION

Food allergy affects approximately 4 to 8% of young children and 1 to 4% of adults [1-4]. The key to the management of food allergy is avoidance of foods known to or suspected of having caused a reaction [5]. Other approaches include pharmacotherapy, education of patients, and dietary manipulations for the prevention of food allergy in high-risk individuals. Currently, there is no effective and safe immunotherapy in the management of patients with food allergy.

AVOIDANCE OF FOOD ALLERGENS

The definitive treatment of food allergy is strict elimination of the offending food from the diet [6,7]. It is unusual for a child to be allergic to more than one food. Bock studied 480 children with probable food hypersensitivity and found that allergic reaction to more than two foods occurred in only 10 (2.1%) of the 480 children [8]. Crespo et al. studied 355 children with food allergy and found that 222 (62.5%) had allergic reactions to only one food, 86 (24.2%) had allergic reactions to two foods, and 47 (13.2%) had allergy to three or more foods [9]. Symptomatic reactivity to food allergens is generally very specific, and patients rarely react to more than one food in a botanical or animal species [7,10-12]. However, in pollen-related food allergy, cross-reactions can occur between phylogenetically distantly related species such as birch and kiwi or soy [2].

The avoidance of the offending food antigen sounds simple but in reality it is not, especially if the offending food is ubiquitous and thus difficult to avoid. Avoidance can be difficult because of cross-contamination of food which may lead to inadvertent ingestion of the offending food [13]. Accidents most frequently happen in daycare centers, schools, and restaurants [13,14]. Approximately 50% of affected individuals experience accidental exposure and reactions every 3 to 5 years [15]. Of the 32 food-related fatalities reported by Bock et al, at least 87% of patients had a previous history of reaction to the responsible food allergen [16]. Avoidance of skin contact and inhalation of offending food allergen is also necessary [17-19]. The importance of education about allergen avoidance cannot be over-emphasized.

On the other hand, the indiscriminate use of elimination diets without a firm diagnosis is a widespread malpractice and may lead to psychological dependence on an unsound diet, as well as vitamin deficiencies, malnutrition, and failure to thrive if multiple foods are inadvertently avoided [7,20-23]. The diagnosis of food allergens should be based on placebo-controlled food challenges. Venter et al followed a birth cohort of 966 infants on the Island of Wight, United Kingdom born between September 2001 and August 2002 to the age of one year [24]. Cumulative incidence of parentally reported food hypersensitivity was 25.8%. Open or double-blind, placebo-controlled food challenges were used to confirm suspected reactions. Only 2.2% of those tested were confirmed to have food allergy, indicating the need to evaluate suspected food allergy to avoid needless dietary restriction.

Oral allergy syndrome generally occurs in patients with inhalant allergy to birch, mugwort, or ragweed pollen and is associated with the ingestion of various fresh fruits (e.g., bananas, melons, citrus fruits) and raw vegetables (e.g. carrots, tomatoes, celery) [13,25]. It is interesting to note that if the offending fruit or vegetable is cooked, then the patient does not usually experience any symptom as the food allergens are generally destroyed by heating [26]. Thus, avoiding the offending fruit or vegetable which has been cooked may not always be necessary.

In some children ingesting ludicrous elimination diets, eating disorders may develop. If elimination diets are prescribed, care must be taken to ensure that they are palatable and nutritionally adequate. Patients should be provided with information on what alternative foods are available so that good variety in the diet can be maintained [27]. A formal dietetic evaluation is recommended.

Patients and/or their caregivers must have a good knowledge of foods containing the allergen and must be taught to scrutinize the labels of all packaged food carefully [28]. Careful label reading is the cornerstone of food allergy management [29]. In one study, only 4 (7%) of 60 parents were able to identify milk protein in 14 sample labels [30]. Incorrect or ambiguous labeling of foods may result in accidental ingestion of the offending food [13]. Also, some of the terms used do not clearly indicate the presence of a food allergen. The United States Food and Drug Administration (FDA) now requires food manufacturers to declare and clear label all functional ingredients on food labels [31]. The Food Allergen Labeling and Consumer Protection Act (FALCPA) effective in January 2006 requires simple terms to indicate the presence of major food allergens [4]. FALCPA requires food manufacturers to state explicitly the presence of eight major food allergens, namely, milk, egg, wheat, soybean, peanut, tree nuts, fish, and shellfish. New EU labeling laws require the presence of the following food allergens at any level to be stated on the label: celery, cereals containing gluten (wheat, barley, rye and oats), crustaceans, eggs, fish, milk, mustard, tree nuts, peanuts, sesame seeds, soybeans, SO_2 and sulfites (at level >10 mg/kg or >10 mg/L) [32]. It is mandatory to list all subgredients and specify the source of ingredients previously listed as "natural flavor". However, foods that are not prepacked are not covered by this legislation [27]. Patients and/or their caregivers should be cautioned about the presence of the offending food as a "hidden" ingredient in processed foods [33,34]. The importance of communicating with restaurant staff about ingredients when one is dining out cannot be over-emphasized [35].

Cow's milk allergy affects 0.3 to 7.5% of infants [36]. The incidence of self-diagnosed cow's milk allergy is substantially higher than that reported in randomized, controlled, food challenge trials [37]. Infants with cow's milk protein allergy should not be fed either whole cow's milk or formulas containing intact whole cow's milk proteins [36]. It has been estimated that 15 to 25% of infants who have IgE-mediated cow's milk allergy are also allergic to soy, but the rate of tolerance is only 50% for those with non-IgE-mediated cow's milk allergy [4,38,39]. A Cochrane analysis of studies comparing soy to hydrolysed cow's milk formulas found a significant increase in infant and childhood allergy cumulative incidence in infants fed soy formulas [40]. As such, soy formula is not a suitable alternative [37]. Goat's milk is not recommended in infants with cow's milk allergy as goat's milk also shares some allergenic protein fractions with cow's milk [37,41,42]. Infants with cow's milk or soy hypersensitivity should be fed a hypoallergenic formula [43]. Extensively hydrolysed casein formulas such as Nutramigen, Pregestimil, and Alimentum have also been used successfully in this regard [43,44]. These formulas are hypoallergenic and well tolerated by children [45]. These formulas, however, are expensive and unpalatable. The partially hydrolyzed whey hydrolysate Good Start is less expensive and has a better taste [46]. However, it contains slightly larger peptides and significantly more immunologically identifiable cow's milk protein, and therefore not suitable for the treatment of cow's milk allergy [1,39,47]. Formulas whose protein source is free amino acids (e.g., Vivonex, Ele Care, and Neocate) are available and are considered as nonallergenic [1,42]. These formulas should be tried in infants who are very sensitive to cow's milk protein and cannot tolerate even extensively hydrolysed formulas [14]. Amino acid-based formulas are also useful in the treatment of allergic eosinophilic esophagitis and allergic eosinophilic gastroenteropathy [48-51].

Breastfed infants who develop symptoms of food allergy may benefit from maternal restriction of cow's milk, egg, fish, peanuts, and tree nuts [52]. Approximately 50% of infants who have food protein-induced proctocolitis while nursing improve with elimination of cow's milk from the maternal diet [53]. If maternal restriction of food allergens is not successful, an extensively hydrolysed formula should be tried [52]. If allergic symptoms persist, a free amino acid-based formula should be considered [52].

Most children outgrow their food hypersensitivity [46]. In contrast, the prognosis for adults with food allergy is less favorable [2]. It has been shown that approximately 30 to 40% of children lose their food hypersensitivity after 1 to 2 years of allergen avoidance, even though the results of skin tests and radioallergosorbent tests may not change [54]. The loss of hypersensitivity is especially likely to occur in infants and young children, although older children and adults may also lose their hypersensitivity [55]. The degree of compliance with allergen avoidance and the allergen responsible may influence the outcome [46]. The majority of children outgrow cow's milk allergy by 4 years of age [42]. Hypersensitivity to peanuts, nuts, egg, fish, and shellfish tends to be more persistent [27,42,54,56]. Consequently, rechallenge testing for food allergy should be performed; the interval between rechallenges should be dictated by the specific food allergen in question, the age of the child, and the degree of difficulty in avoiding the food in question [12,47].

PHARMACOTHERAPY

Symptomatic treatment of complications resulting from the inadvertent ingestion of food is essentially the same as that for the specific complication resulting from any other cause [57]. Patients with a history of anaphylactic reaction over the age of seven years as well as caregivers should be taught how to self-administer epinephrine and should have an epinephrine auto-injector such as Anapen/Anapen Jr, EpiPen/EpiPen Jr, or Twinjet/Twinjet Jr and antihistamine available at all times [2,58]. The physician should take appropriate steps to ensure that the patients and their caregivers understand the indications and use of the device thoroughly. These individuals should also be provided with a written anaphylaxis action plan. The instructions should be clear, simple, and age appropriate. Rehearsal of the procedure is important.

Epinephrine helps to block severe allergic reactions and anaphylaxis by suppressing leukotriene and histamine release [59,60]. Epinephrine reverses vasodilatation, increases blood pressure, dilates airways, reduces laryngeal edema and angioedema, and increases myocardial contractility [59,60]. For the treatment of anaphylaxis, the recommended dose of epinephrine 1:1000 (1mg/ml) is 0.01 mg/kg intramuscularly, up to a maximum of 0.3 mg (0.3 ml) in children and 0.5 mg (0.5 ml) in adults [14,59,61]. Peak concentrations are reached within 10 minutes of intramuscular administration [60,62]. As Anapen Jr, EpiPen Jr, and Twinjet Jr contain 0.15 mg of epinephrine and Anapen, EpiPen, and Twinjet contain 0.3 mg of epinephrine, it would be desirable to have a wider range of auto-injector doses [13,59]. The subcutaneous route is no longer recommended as the systemic levels of epinephrine are highly unpredictable from this mode of administration [59]. It has been shown that intramuscular injections into the thigh result in more rapid absorption and higher plasma epinephrine levels than intramuscular injections into the arm [28,61,63-65]. Epinephrine works best when given early [13,59].

After the first aid treatment, the patient should be transferred to the nearest emergency department for monitoring and additional treatment as required [14]. If necessary, the dose of epinephrine may be repeated at 5 minutes intervals according to cardiorespiratory function [59,64]. In one study, 16% of patients presenting to the emergency department with food-induced anaphylaxis required two doses of epinephrine [64]. In patients with severe anaphylaxis unresponsive to intramuscular epinephrine or with cardiovascular collapse, epinephrine should be given intravenously with blood pressure and continuous cardiac monitoring [60,61]. Some of these patients may require volume support, oxygen, nebulized bronchodilators, parenteral diphenhydramine, ranitidine, and glucocorticosteroids [28,66]. Should this be the case, the patient should be placed in a recumbent position with lower limbs elevated, as tolerated symptomatically [28,61,63]. This may prevent orthostatic hypotension. Because of the possibility of a biphasic response, all patients with anaphylaxis should be observed for at least four hours before discharge.

Patients and/or their caregivers must be educated about early recognition of allergic symptoms and early management of an anaphylactic reaction [67]. Schools should be equipped to treat anaphylaxis in allergic students and physicians should help instruct school personnel about these issues [2]. The Food Allergy & Anaphylaxis Network (FAAN) (10,400 Easton Place, Fairfax, VA 22030-5647; tel.800-929-4040; or www.foodallergy.org) has excellent educational material for patients, schools, and physicians dealing with food allergy in addition to a written emergency plan for treatment of an accidental ingestion [12]. It is suggested that patients at risk for anaphylaxis should always carry two doses of self-injectable epinephrine [64,68]. An identification necklace or bracelet such as MedicAlert or Medi-Tag stating the patient's sensitivity is also advised [1,34]. Referral to an allergist is also recommended [69].

For the child with progressive or generalized urticaria or distressing pruritus, the administration of a fast-acting oral H_1 antihistamine such as hydroxyzine or diphenhydramine should be considered [10,59,61,70]. H_2 receptor blockers such as ranitidine are less helpful as only a small number of H_2 receptors are found in the skin [70]. Although antihistamines do not block systemic reactions, they do relieve the itchiness [67].

The use of drugs such as disodium cromoglycate, ketotifen, and prostaglandin synthetase inhibitors in the treatment of food allergy has generally been disappointing, either because of minimal efficacy or unacceptable adverse effects [7,12]. Systemic corticosteroids are rarely used in the treatment of food allergy, except in severe anaphylaxis, allergic eosinophilic esophagitis, allergic eosinophilic gastroenteropathy, and dietary-induced enteropathy [67,71]. The side effects of long-term systemic corticosteroid therapy are unacceptable.

Currently, oral administration of activated charcoal is not considered a practical first-aid treatment for food anaphylaxis [14]. Prophylactic medications have not been shown to be consistently effective in the prevention of severe life-threatening reactions to foods [5]. Their use may mask a less severe allergic reaction to a culprit food, the knowledge of which might prevent a more severe allergic reaction to that food in the future [5]. The use of prophylactic medications is therefore discouraged.

PROBIOTICS AND PREBIOTICS

The use of probiotics and prebiotics in the management of food allergy is controversial [72]. It has been hypothesized that the increased sensitization to food allergens might result from reduced infection or exposure to microbial products such as endotoxin in early childhood [73]. Prospective studies have found that infants who are prone to develop atopic dermatitis have lower numbers of *Bifidobacterium* in their intestinal microflora [74-76]. It has been shown that probiotics might reverse the increased intestinal permeability characteristic of children with food allergy and enhance specific IgA responses frequently defective in children with food allergy [77]. *In vitro* studies show that allergic patients induce less IL-10 production and more proinflammatory cytokine production than those nonallergic individuals [78,79]. Presumably, probiotics act on the intestinal mucosa and stimulate T-cell differentiation in favor of Th1 over Th2, with resultant decreased production of IgE and increased production of IgA [1,78,80]. Probiotics might also correct aberrations in gut permeability [81,82]. Prebiotics work by selectively stimulating the growth or activity of a limited number of bacterial strains in the intestinal flora.

Much work has been done on the use of probiotics and, to a lesser extent, prebiotics in the management of atopic dermatitis. Several randomized controlled trials failed to show the beneficial effects of probiotics in the prevention of atopic dermatitis [83]. Other studies yielded different results [83-88]. Kalliomäki et al. randomized 159 mothers and their respective infants with a family history of atopy to receive either a placebo or 10^{10} CFU of *Lactoobacillus* GG for 2 to 4 weeks before delivery and for 6 months after delivery, respectively [84]. Twenty three percent of the children in the probiotic group versus 46% of children in the control group were found to have atopic dermatitis at two years of age (RR: 0.51; 95% confidence interval: 0.32-0.84) [84]. The effect was still observed two years later: 26% of children in the treatment group versus 46% of children in the placebo group had atopic dermatitis (RR: 0.57; 95% confidence interval: 0.33-0.97) [85].

Viljanen et al. randomized 230 infants who had suspected cow's milk allergy in a double-blinded study to receive *L. rhamnosus* GG (n=80), a mixture of four probiotic strains (n=76), or a placebo (n=74), given twice daily with food for four weeks [88]. The authors found that *L. rhamnosus* GG was an effective therapy for atopic dermatitis in IgE-sensitized infants but not in non-IgE-sensitized infants.

In a double-blind, placebo-controlled trial, Tamura et al. randomized 109 adult patients with allergic rhinitis to drink fermented milk containing *Lactobacilli casei* strain Shirota (n=55) or placebo (n=54) for 8 weeks [89]. The authors found no significant difference between the two groups during the ingestion period. In the subgroup of patients with moderate to severe nasal symptom scores before starting ingestion of test samples, supplementation with the probiotic tended to reduce nasal symptom-medication scores.

In a double-blind placebo-controlled trial, Taylor et al randomized 226 newborn infants of atopic mothers to receive either 3×10^9 CFU of *Lactobacillus acidophilus* (n=115) or placebo (n=111) daily for 6 months [90]. A total of 178 infants (89 in each group) completed the study. The authors found that the rates of atopic dermatitis were similar in the two groups at 6 months and 12 months of follow-up. At 12 months, the rate of sensitization was significantly higher in the probiotic group (p=0.03). These findings challenge the use of probiotics in the prevention of allergy.

Kukkonen et al. randomized 1,223 pregnant women carrying high risk infants at increased risk for allergy to receive a probiotic (n=610) or a placebo (n=613) for 2 to 4 weeks before delivery [91]. Their infants received the same probiotic plus galacto-oligosaccharides (n=461) or a placebo (n=464) for 6 months. These children were evaluated at 2 years of age for cumulative incidence of allergic diseases (food allergy, eczema, asthma, and allergic rhinitis) and IgE sensitization (positive skin prick test response or serum antigen-specific IgE level). The authors found that probiotic and prebiotic treatment, compared with placebo, had no effect on the cumulative incidence of allergic diseases but tended to reduce IgE-associated atopic diseases (odds ratio: 0.71; 95% confidence interval: 0.5 to 1; p=0.052). Probiotic and prebiotic treatment did reduce eczema (odds ratio: 0.74; 95% confidence interval: 0.55 to 0.98; p=0.35) and atopic eczema (odds ratio: 0.66; 95% confidence interval: 0.46 to 0.95; p=0.025).

In a double-blind placebo-controlled trial, Weston et al. randomized 56 children aged 6 to 18 months who had moderate to severe atopic dermatitis to receive *L. fementum* VRI-033 PCC (n=28) or placebo (n=28) twice daily for eight weeks [92]. Fifty children completed the study. The authors found that the reduction in the SCORAD index was significant in the probiotic group (p=0.03) but not in the placebo group. In a double-blind study, Passeron et al. randomized 48 children to receive either *L. rhamnosus* Lcr 35 plus a prebiotic preparation (n=28) or an identically appearing probiotic preparation alone three times a day for three months [93]. In the symbiotic group, the mean total SCORAD score was 39.1 before treatment versus 20.7 after three months of treatment (p< 0.0001). In the probiotic group, the mean SCORAD score was 39.3 before treatment versus 24 after three months of treatment (p<0.0001). The authors concluded that symbiotics and prebiotics used alone were effective in the treatment of atopic dermatitis.

Probiotics and prebiotics are included in some infant formulas with the aim of inducing the development of a *Bifidobacterium*-dominated intestinal flora [37]. At present, probiotics or prebiotics are not established treatment modalities for atopic dermatitis [72,78]. They are ineffective in the prevention and treatment of reactive airway disease [78]. The routine use of probiotics and prebiotics in food allergy management requires further study.

Dietary Manipulations in the Prevention of Food Allergy in High-Risk Individuals

Breastfeeding has a protective effect on the incidence of atopic disease in children who have a genetic predisposition for atopy [53,94-97], especially so for the prevention of asthma [95]. Gdalevich et al. performed a systematic review and meta-analysis of 12 prospective studies (n=8,183) that evaluated the association between exclusive breastfeeding in the first three months of life and asthma [95]. The mean follow-up was 4.1 years. The pooled odds ratio for the protective effect of breastfeeding was 0.7 (95% confidence interval: 0.6 to 0.81). The protective effect was more pronounced in the subset of studies that assessed children with a family history of atopy (odds ratio: 0.52; 95% confidence interval: 0.35 to 0.79) compared to studies with an unstratified population, and to studies that included children without atopic first-degree relatives (odds ratio: 0.73; 95% confidence interval: 0.62 to 0.86).

The protective effects of breastfeeding on atopic dermatitis are controversial. The American Academy of Dermatology Guidelines Task Force reviewed the subject in 2004 and found no conclusive evidence that exclusive breastfeeding influences the development of atopic dermatitis [98]. The American Academy of Dermatology Guidelines Task Force did find suggestive evidence that prolonged breastfeeding might delay the onset of atopic dermatitis [98]. The Section of Pediatrics of the European Academy of Allergology and Clinical Immunology critically reviewed the existing literature and concluded that exclusive breastfeeding for at least 4 to 6 months in infants with a family history of atopy results in a lower incidence of atopic dermatitis [99]. A recent study reported that breastfeeding for 4 months or more reduces the risk of atopic dermatitis and the onset of the allergy to 4 years of age [100]. Kull et al followed a birth cohort of 4,089 children [100]. Data on breastfeeding, allergic symptoms, and potential confounding factors were obtained from questionnaires that were answered by parents when the children were 2 months, and 1, 2, and 4 years of age. The authors found that exclusive breastfeeding for 4 months or more reduced the risk of atopic dermatitis at 4 years of age (odds ratio: 0.78; 95% confidence interval: 0.63 to 0.96). The decreased risk was most evident for children who had atopic dermatitis with an onset during the first 2 years of life and that persisted to 4 years (odds ratio: 0.59; 95% confidence interval: 0.45 to 0.77). A protective effect of breastfeeding was also noted among children with early onset atopic dermatitis, regardless of whether it was persistent, and among children who developed early or late onset asthma which was followed by late onset atopic dermatitis (odds ratio: 0.48; 95% confidence interval: 0.3 to 0.76).

Breastfeeding might have a protective effect on the development of allergic rhinitis, although not to the same extent as that reported for asthma and atopic dermatitis [95,100,101]. Minouni Bloch et al. performed a meta-analysis of six prospective studies (n=3,303) that examined the effect of exclusive breastfeeding in the first 3 months of life on the development of allergic rhinitis [101]. The overall odds ratio was 0.74 (95% confidence interval: 0.54 to 1.01). The protective association was considered substantial notwithstanding borderline statistical significance. More recently, Siltanen et al. prospectively followed 456

Finnish children from an unselected birth cohort of 4,674 infants for 4 years [102]. The authors found in children with a family history of atopy, exclusive breastfeeding for 3 months protected against allergic rhinoconjunctivitis and sensitization to pets [102].

In high-risk infants who are exclusively breastfeed and in whom solids are not introduced until six months of age, breastfeeding might delay, or possibly prevent, the onset of food allergy [6,23,39,103,104]. Infants with elevated cord serum IgE and a positive family history of atopy are at risk for the development of atopic disease [105-107]. Breastfeeding protects against the development of allergy by several potential mechanisms. Colostrum provides a protective coating to the gut that prevents the entrance of large foreign proteins and minimizes the possibility of an allergic response. Colostrum also prevents the adherence of pathogens. Breastfeeding reduces the amount of foreign protein in the gastrointestinal tract and passively transfers maternal IgA to the infant, which minimizes the risk for absorption of antigens from the gastrointestinal tract [6,108]. Transfer of cell-mediated immunity from mother to infant stimulates IgA synthesis in the infant [109]. Epidermal growth factor present in human milk hastens maturation of intestinal mucosa and epithelium, and strengthens the mucosal barrier to antigen [108]. Several studies have shown that respiratory and gastrointestinal infections can predispose to the development of allergic diseases [109]. The allergy-preventive effect of breastfeeding might be secondary to a reduction in the number of infections in the infant.

Because small amounts of food antigens ingested by the mother are excreted in breast milk [55], avoidance of allergenic foods by lactating mothers is often recommended [6,33,36,110,111]. A meta-analysis of two studies [112,113] concludes that avoidance of allergenic foods by lactating mothers may transiently reduce the development of atopic dermatitis in early childhood [111]. Several studies suggest that a strict food allergen avoidance regimen followed by mothers during pregnancy may result in a significant reduction in the infants of food-related allergic disorders [06,114,115]. Other authors disagree [105,116,117]. Studies that have demonstrated a beneficial effect of a strict food allergen avoidance regimen followed by mothers during pregnancy and lactation on the prevalence and severity of atopic disease in high-risk, breast-fed infants probably reflect only the influence of maternal dietary restriction during lactation [105]. The present consensus is that dietary intervention in utero is potentially harmful and is not indicated unless future studies prove otherwise [11,37,111,118].

Marini et al. prospectively studied 279 infants with high atopic risk who were put on an allergy prevention program and 80 infants with similar atopic risk but no intervention [119]. The intervention program included dietary measures (exclusive and prolonged milk feeding followed by a hypoallergenic weaning diet) and environmental measures such as avoidance of parental smoking in the presence of the babies. The incidence of allergic manifestations was much lower in the intervention group than in the nonintervention group at 1 year (11.5% vs. 54.4%), 2 years (14.9% vs. 65.6%), and 3 years (20.6% vs. 74.1%). Atopic dermatitis and recurrent wheezing were found in both the intervention group and the nonintervention group from birth to the second year of life, whereas urticaria and gastrointestinal disorders were only present in the nonintervention group in the first year of life. Halken et al. studied 105 "high-risk" infants who were breast-fed and/or receiving a hypoallergenic formula combined with avoidance of solid foods during the first 6 months of life [120]. This prevention group was compared with a control group consisting of 54 identically defined "high-risk" infants who were on an unrestricted diet. The cumulative prevalence of atopic symptoms was significantly lower at 18 months in the prevention group (32%) than in the control group (74%) ($p < 0.01$) because of a reduced prevalence of recurrent wheezing (13% vs. 37%; $p < 0.01$), atopic dermatitis (14% vs. 31%; $p < 0.01$), vomiting/diarrhea (5% vs. 28%; $p < 0.01$), and infantile colic (9% vs. 24%; $p < 0.01$). The cumulative prevalence of food allergy was significantly lower in the prevention group (6% vs. 17%; $p < 0.05$). The authors concluded that feeding high-risk infants with breast milk and/or hypoallergenic formula, combined with the avoidance of solid foods during the first 6 months of life, has a protective effect on the risk of atopic symptoms developing during the first 18 months of life. The American Academy of Pediatrics recommends that mothers of high-risk infants should avoid allergens, such as peanuts and nuts, during lactation [52].

When breastfeeding is not possible, the use of a partially or completely hydrolyzed hypoallergenic formula is desirable for infants at risk [37,52,117,118,121]. A meta-analysis of studies that compared prolonged feeding with hydrolysed formulas versus cow's milk formulas in high risk infants found a significant reduction in infant allergy (seven studies, 2514 infants; typical risk ratio: 0.79; 95% CI: 0.66 to 0.94), but not in the incidence of childhood allergy (two studies, 950 infants; typical risk ratio: 0.85; 95% CI: 0.69 to 1.05 [122].

Partially hydrolysed formulas are often used for the prevention of atopy when breastfeeding is not possible in infants with a strong family history of allergy or elevated cord IgE levels to reduce possible food allergy symptoms [6,14,121]. These formulas have been developed with the aim of minimizing the number of sensitizing epitopes within milk proteins, while at the same time retaining peptides of sufficient size and immunogenicity to stimulate the induction of oral tolerance [37]. Compared with extensively hydrolysed formulas, partially hydrolysed formulas are less expensive and more palatable [46]. Prospective controlled trials examining the use of extensively hydrolysed formulas and partially hydrolysed formulas for allergy prevention among high-risk infants show significant reductions in the cumulative incidence of atopic disease through the first five years of life compared with those fed with cow's milk formulas [121]. In the meta-analysis performed by Osborn et al, infants fed extensively hydrolysed formulas versus partially hydrolysed formulas had a significant reduction in food allergy (two studies, 341 infants; typical risk ratio: 0.43; 95%confidence interval: 0.19 to 0.99), but there was no significant difference in all allergy or any other specific allergy incidence [122].

Soy protein is immunogenic and allergenic, although less than cow's milk [118]. A meta-analysis of two studies (n=283) found no significant differences in childhood allergy cumulative incidence from the use of a soy formula compared to a cow's milk formula (typical risk ratio: 0.67; 95% confidence interval: 0.18 to 2.46) [40]. As there is no evidence of benefit, the use of a soy formula for prevention of food allergy cannot be recommended [40,52].

Early introduction of solid food may increase the risk of food allergy [52,53,102, 123,124]. The existing literature suggests that the optimal time for the introduction of selected supplemental food should be six months. For infants at risk, dairy products should not be introduced before 12 months, eggs 24 months, and peanut, tree nuts, fish, and seafood at least 36 months of age [125]. It is recommended that foods should be introduced one at a time and gradually [125]. Cooked, homogenized foods should be preferred to their fresh counterparts when a reduction of allergenicity has been clinically demonstrated for that processed food [125].

It has been suggested that supplementation with long-chain polyunsaturated fatty acids might reduce the incidence of atopic diseases [126-128]. A Cochrane systematic review showed no consistent beneficial effect on marine fatty acids (fish oil) supplementation in asthma prevention [129]. A meta-analysis showed that supplementation with fish oil did not improve the severity of atopic dermatitis [130].

MISCELLANEOUS ASPECTS

Patients with food-dependent exercise-induced anaphylaxis should refrain from exercise within 2 to 3 hours after ingesting the triggering food [66]. Affected patients should exercise with their friends and should stop exercise and seek help immediately if symptoms develop [66].

High-risk environments have to be avoided if the patient is highly allergic and particularly if the patient is allergic to airborne food allergens [5]. High-risk areas include common eating places such as childcare centers, school cafeterias, restaurants, and ice cream shops [5]. School and childcare centers should have policies facilitating food allergen avoidance such as prohibition of sharing of food or utensil and increased staff supervision during meal times [5].

It has been demonstrated that vapors containing proteins emitted from cooking food (e.g. steaming fish) can induce asthmatic attacks [18,67]. Inhalational exposures to foods, particular in the workplace, account for approximately 1% of asthmatic attacks in the adult population [67,131]. Baker's asthma caused by inhalation of flour or mold-derived enzymes used as flour additives is a good example [5]. Affected individuals have asthmatic attacks in association with exposure to aerosolized wheat proteins and have positive skin prick tests or serum specific IgE to wheat proteins [131]. Likewise, peanut dust in airplanes can provoke allergic reactions in susceptible individuals [132]. Allergenic proteins may also reach the respiratory tract via the circulation or they may act via inflammatory mediators released from the skin or gastrointestinal tract [131]. Exposure to known food allergens via inhalation (e.g. flour, peanut dust, steaming fish), skin (e.g. peanut oil in moisturizers), and mucous membrane (e.g. kissing), should be avoided [133].

FUTURE THERAPEUTIC OPTIONS

Currently, there is no effective and safe specific immunotherapy for food allergens. The study of injectable specific immune therapy using peanuts was suspended because of the high rate of adverse reactions [134]. Traditional injection immunotherapy for other food allergies is not recommended either because of the risk of serious systemic reactions associated with such therapy [135]. Sublingual immunotherapy to food allergens is better tolerated and preliminary results are encouraging [48,136,137]. Long-term efficiency of sublingual immunotherapy, however, remains to be determined.

Vaccines for immunotherapy specially for food-induced anaphylaxis that are being developed include humanized anti-IgE monoclonal antibody therapy, sublingual immunotherapy, peptide immunotherapy, mutated protein immunotherapy, plasmid DNA immunotherapy, engineered recombinant protein immunotherapy, immunostimulatory sequence-modulated immunotherapy, cytokine-modulated immunotherapy, bacterial-encapsulated allergen immunotherapy, and homologous protein immunotherapy [2,7,13,137-140]. Allergen-specific immunotherapy should be considered for patients who have specific IgE antibodies to clinically relevant allergens and whose allergic symptoms are severe enough to warrant the time and risk of allergen immunotherapy [137].

Preliminary studies showed the potential use of humanized monoclonal anti-IgE antibody in food-allergic subjects [141,142]. Humanized monoclonal anti-IgE antibody binds to the third domain of the Fc region of the IgE molecule and prevents its binding to the high affinity receptor on mast cells and basophils [143]. The anti-IgE also downregulates the expression of the high affinity receptor on mast cells and decreases the release of histamine from basophils [144]. In a randomized, double-blind, placebo-controlled trial in 84 patients with a history of peanut allergy, Leung et al showed an increased threshold of tolerance in patients with severe peanut allergy on oral food challenge after being given every 4 weeks subcutaneous injection of TNX-901 for four doses [138]. TNX-901 is a humanized IgG_1 monoclonal antibody against IgE that binds with high affinity to an epitope in the CH_3 domain [138]. The effect was highly significant at the 450 mg dose level. However, even at the highest dose of TNX-901, approximately 25% of patients were not protected. The treatment was well tolerated with no systemic adverse events. Unfortunately, anti-IgE therapy is expensive and such therapy has to be administered on a regular basis so as to maintain its protective effect [35,67]. Currently, another anti-IgE humanized IgG_1 antibody (omalizumab) is being tested in subjects older than 6 years of age with peanut anaphylaxis [19]. Stern et al. treated four adults with eosinophilic esophagitis with a human monoclonal IgG_1 antibody against interleukin-5 (mepolizumab) given by infusion on a monthly basis [145]. After three months of treatment (750 mg monthly), the mean and maximal esophageal eosinophilic count fell from 46 to 6 and from 153 to 28 per high-power field, respectively. The patients also reported improvement of clinical symptoms and quality of life.

Oral immunotherapy seems to represent an interesting and promising approach for the management of food allergy [137,146]. Enrique et al. randomized in a double-blind, placebo-controlled fashion 23 patients with hazelnut allergy to receive either a standardized hazelnut extract or placebo using a sublingual-spit rush protocol over four days [147]. They then received maintenance sublingual immunotherapy for approximately three months. On repeat double-blind, placebo-controlled food challenge, patients in the treatment group had a mean quantity of hazelnut provoking objective symptoms and increased tolerance to hazelnuts from 2.29 gm to 11.59 gm ($p=0.02$) while patients in the placebo group had a non-significant increase from 3.49 gm to 4.14 gm.

Peptide immunotherapy utilizes peptide fragments containing T-cell-reactive epitopes rather complete protein molecules [135]. Apparently, this kind of therapy would induce T-cell unresponsiveness and production of interferon-γ in a concentration-dependent manner [19]. Peptide immunotherapy allows for formulation of vaccines against any target in which major allergenic proteins are known because IgE binding sites for each major allergen do not have to be mapped [19]. It is hoped that such therapy would render T-cells unresponsive to subsequent allergen exposure. Peptide immunotherapy might play a role in the future therapy of food allergy.

Mutated protein immunotherapy is based on the modification of the primary amino acid sequences of IgE-binding allergenic epitopes of the major allergens present in food, with the aim of reducing allergen potential thereby eliminating activation of mast cells and basophils [19,135]. Mutation of the IgE-binding sites leaves the T-cell response unaffected [148]. Such therapy is hampered by the large numbers of allergens present in each food.

Plasmid DNA immunotherapy results in transcription and translation of encoded genes and elicits an antibody response in the host, thereby preferentially induces a Th1 immune response and suppression of IgE [15,149] Plasmid DNA requires immunostimulatory sequences for optimal immunogenicity [149].

Engineered recombinant protein technology makes room for the development of hypoallergenic derivatives of natural allergens, which would minimize the adverse effect of immunotherapy. Such allergens should not be able to activate cells via cross-linking of IgE antibodies, but should preserve T-cell epitopes and activate B-cells to induce blocking IgG antibodies [15].

Immunostimulatory sequence-modulated immunotherapy using CpG has been shown to be effective in reversing IgE-mediated sensitization in patients with ragweed allergy [150,151]. Likewise, immunostimulatory sequence-conjugated Ara h 2 has been shown to be beneficial in the treatment allergy in a murine model [67].

In animal studies, various Chinese herbs have been shown to block anaphylactic reactions resulting from food allergy [152-154]. The therapeutic effect was associated with immunoregulatory effects on Th1-Th-2 responses and reductions in IgE levels [153]. The exact mechanism is not known and further studies are required.

Vaccinations and Food Allergies

Although measles-German measles-mumps (MMR) vaccine is cultured from chick embryos, MMR vaccination is not contraindicated in children allergic to eggs [59,155]. The vaccination should, however, be administered in a supervised setting [59,156]. On the other hand, the vaccine is contraindicated in children with known systemic allergic reaction to neomycin or gelatin [157]. Patients with egg allergy should be tested before getting influenza or yellow fever vaccines, which contain egg protein [158].

Conclusion

Currently, strict avoidance of the allergenic food and ready access to self-injectable epinephrine are the standards of care. Recent advances in our understanding of the immunological processes involved in the pathogenesis of food allergy have opened the door to the investigation and development of novel therapeutic and prophylactic therapies against food allergy. It is hoped that safe and effective vaccines for immunotherapy will be available in the future for the prevention and treatment of food allergy. In particular, anti-IgE therapy may eventually turn out to be a useful adjunct to allergen avoidance.

REFERENCES

[1] Bangash, SA; Bahna, SL. Pediatric food allergy update. *Curr. Allergy Asthma Rep.* 2005;5:437-444.

[2] Burks, AW; Ballmer-Weber, BK. Food allergies. *Mol. Nutr. Food Res.* 2006;50:595-603.

[3] Chehade, M. IgE and non-IgE-mediated food allergy: treatment in 2007. *Curr. Opin. Allergy Clin. Immunol.* 2007;7:264-268.

[4] Sicherer, SH; Sampson, HA. Food allergy. *J. Allergy Clin. Immunol.* 2006;117:S470-S475.

[5] American College of Allergy, Asthma, & Immunology. Food allergy: a practice parameter. *Ann. Allergy Asthma Immunol.* 2006;96(Suppl 2):S1-S68.

[6] Leung, AK. Food allergy: a clinical approach. *Adv. Pediatr.* 1998;45:145-177.

[7] Scurlock, AM; Lee, LA; Burks, AW. Food allergy in children. *Immunol. Allergy Clin. North Am.* 2005;25:369-388.

[8] Bock, SA. Prospective appraisal of complaints of adverse reactions to foods in children during the first 3 years of life. *Pediatrics.* 1987;79:683-688.

[9] Crespo, JF; Pascual, C; Burks, AW; et al. Frequency of food allergy in a pediatric population from Spain. *Pediatr. Allergy Immunol.* 1995;6:39-43.

[10] Bock, SA; Sampson, HA. Food allergy in infancy. *Pediatr. Clin. North Am.* 1994;41:1047-1067.

[11] Hoffman, KM; Sampson, HA. Evaluation and management of patients with adverse food reactions. In: Bierman, CW; Pearlman, DS; Shapiro, GG; et al. (eds). *Allergy, Asthma, and Immunology from Infancy to Adulthood.* Philadelphia: WB Saunders. 1996; pp.665-686.

[12] Sampson, HA. Food allergies. In: McMillan, JA; Feigin, RD; DeAngelis, C; et al. (eds). *Oski's Pediatrics: Principles & Practice*. Philadelphia: Lippincott Williams & Wilkins. 2006; pp.2417-2423.

[13] Lee, LA; Burks, AW. Food allergies: prevalence, molecular characterization, and treatment/prevention strategies. *Annu. Rev. Nutr.* 2006;26;539-565.

[14] Anderson, JA. Food allergy and intolerance. In: Lieberman, P; Anderson, JA. (ed). *Current Clinical Practice: Allergic Diseases: Diagnosis and Treatment.* 3rd edition. Totowa: Humana Press, 2007, pp. 271-294.

[15] Nieuwenhuizen, N; Lopata, A. Fighting food allergy: current approaches. *Ann. N. Y. Acad. Sci.* 2005;1056:30-45.

[16] Bock, SA; Munoz-Furlong, A; Sampson, HA. Fatalities due to anaphylactic reactions to foods. *J. Allergy Clin. Immunol.* 2001;107:191-193.

[17] Fiocchi, A; Martelli, A. Dietary management of food allergy. *Pediatr. Ann.* 2006;35:755-763.

[18] James, JM; Crespo, JF. Allergic reactions to foods by inhalation. *Curr. Allergy Asthma Rep.* 2007;7:167-174.

[19] Nowak-Wegrzyn, A. Immunotherapy for food allergy. *Inflamm. Allergy Drug Targets.* 2006;5:23-34.

[20] Altman, DR; Chiaramonte, LT. Public perception of food allergy. *J. Allergy Clin. Immunol.* 1996;97:1247-1251.

[21] Opper, PH; Burakoff, R. Food allergy and intolerance. *Gastroenterologist.* 1993;1:211-220.

[22] Sicherer, SH; Leung, DY. Advances in allergic skin disease, anaphylaxis, and hypersensitivity reactions to foods, drugs, and insects. *J. Allergy Clin. Immunol.* 2007;119:1462-1469.

[23] Stern, M. Gastrointestinal allergy. In: Walker, WA; Durie, PR; Hamilton, JR; et al. (eds). *Pediatric Gastrointestinal Disease.* St. Louis: Mosby. 1991; pp.557-574.

[24] Venter, C; Pereira, B; Grundy, J; et al. Incidence of parentally reported and clinically diagnosed food hypersensitivity in the first year of life. *J. Allergy Clin. Immunol.* 2006;117:1118-1124.

[25] Leung AK, Kamat D. Clinical manifestations of food allergy. In: Columbus F, ed. Food Allergies: New Research. New York: Nova Science Publishers, Inc. (in press).

[26] Nash, S; Burks, AW. Oral allergy syndrome. *Curr. Allergy Asthma Rep.* 2007;7:1-2.

[27] Grimshaw, KE. Dietary management of food allergy in children. *Proc. Nutr. Soc.* 2006;65:412-417.

[28] Joint Task Force on Practice Parameters; American Academy of Allergy, Asthma and Immunology; American College of Allergy, Asthma and Immunology; Joint Council of Allergy, Asthma and Immunology. The diagnosis and management of anaphylaxis: an updated practice parameter. *J. Allergy Clin. Immunol.* 2005;115:S483-S523.

[29] Muňoz-Furlong, A. Daily coping strategies for patients and their families. *Pediatrics.* 2003;111:1654-1661.

[30] Joshi, P; Mofidi, S; Sicherer, SH. Interpretation of commercial food ingredient labels by parents of food-allergic children. *J. Allergy Clin. Immunol.* 2002;109:1019-1021.

[31] Taylor, SL; Hefle, SL. Food allergen labeling in the USA and Europe. *Curr. Opin. Allergy Clin. Immunol.* 2006;6:186-190.

[32] European Commission. Directive 2003/89/EC of the European Parliament and of the Council of 10 November 2003 amending Directive 2000/13/EC as regards indication of the ingredients present in foodstuffs. *Official J. Euro. Comminities.* 2003;L308:15-18.

[33] Lee, BW. Food and allergy. *Ann. Acad. Med. Singapore.* 1995;24:238-241.

[34] Steinman, HA. "Hidden" allergens in foods. *J. Allergy Clin. Immunol.* 1996;98:241-250.

[35] Keet, CA; Wood RA. Food allergy and anaphylaxis. *Immunol. Allergy Clin. North Am.* 2007;27:193-212.

[36] Leung, AK; Sauve, RS. Whole cow's milk in infancy. *Paediatr. Child. Health.* 2003;8:419-421.

[37] Crittenden, RG; Bennett, LE. Cow's milk allergy: a complex disorder. *J. Am. Coll. Nutr.* 2005;24:S582-S591.

[38] Garcia-Careaga, M; Kerner, JA, Jr. Gastrointestinal manifestations of food allergies in pediatric patients. *Nutr. Clin. Pract.* 2005;20:526-535.

[39] Duggan, C; Walker, WA. Protein intolerance. In: Oski, FA; DeAngelis, CD; Feigin, RD. (eds). *Principles and Practice of Pediatrics.* Philadelphia: JB Lippincott. 1994; pp.1887-1890.

[40] Osborn, DA; Sinn, J. Soy formula for prevention of allergy and food intolerance in infants (review). *Cochrane Database Syst. Rev.* 2006 Oct 18;(4):CD003741.

[41] Bellioni-Businco, B; Paganelli, R; Lucenti, P; et al. Allergenicity of goat's milk in children with cow's milk allergy. *J. Allergy Clin. Immunol.* 1999;103:1191-1194.

[42] Beyer, K. Hypoallergenicity: a principle for the treatment of food allergy. *Nestlé Nutr. Workshop Ser. Pediatr. Program.* 2007;59:37-47.

[43] Committee on Nutrition, American Academy of Pediatrics. Food hypersensitivity. In: Barness, LA .(ed). *Pediatric Nutrition Handbook.* Elk Grove Village, Ill: American Academy of Pediatrics. 1993; pp.274-285.

[44] Sampson, HA; Bernhisel-Broadbent, J; Yang, E; et al. Safety of casein hydrolysate formula in children with cow milk allergy. *J. Pediatr.* 1991;118:520-525.

[45] Sampson, HA; James, JM; Bernhisel-Broadbent, J. Safety of an amino acid-derived infant formula in children allergic to cow's milk. *Pediatrics.* 1992;90:463-465.

[46] Leung, AK; Bowen, TJ. Seasonal allergic rhinitis and food allergy. In: Bergman, AB. (ed). *Twenty Common Problems in Pediatrics.* New York: McGraw-Hill. 2001, pp. 219-233.

[47] Stern, M. Allergic enteropathy. In: Walker, WA; Durie, PR; Hamilton, JR; et al. (eds). *Pediatric Gastrointestinal Disease.* St. Louis: Mosby. 1996; pp.677-692.

[48] Chehade, M; Magid, MS; Mofidi, S; et al. Allergic eosinophilic gastroenteritis with protein-losing enteropathy: intestinal pathology, clinical course, and long-term follow-up. *J. Pediatr. Gastroenterol. Nutr.* 2006;42:516-521.

[49] Kagalwalla, AF; Sentongo, TA; Ritz, S; et al. Effect of six-food elimination diet on clinical and histologic outcomes in eosinophilic esophagitis. *Clin. Gastroenterol. Hepatol.* 2006;4:1097-1102.

[50] Liacouras, CA. Eosinophilic esophagitis: treatment in 2005. *Curr. Opin. Gastroenterol.* 2006;22:147-142.

[51] Miller TP, Leung AK. Eosinophilic gastrointestinal disorders. In: Columbus F, ed. Food Allergies: New Research. New York: Nova Science Publishers, Inc. (in press).

[52] American Academy of Pediatrics, Committee on Nutrition. Hypoallergenic infant formulas. *Pediatrics.* 2000;106:346-349.

[53] Hyams, JS. Food allergy (food hypersensitivity). In: Kliegman, RM; Behrman, RE; Jenson, HB; et al. *Nelson Textbook of Pediatrics.* Philadelphia: Saunders Elsevier. 2007, pp.1585-1587.

[54] Burks, AW; Sampson, H. Food allergies in children. *Curr. Probl. Pediatr.* 1993;23:230-252.

[55] Dannaeus, A. Food allergy in infancy and children. *Ann. Allergy.* 1987;59:124-126.

[56] Tariq, SM; Stevens, M; Matthew, S; et al. Cohort study of peanut and tree nut sensitisation by age of 4 years. *BMJ.* 1996;313:514-517.

[57] Golbert, TM. Food allergy and immunological diseases of the gastrointestinal tract. In: Patterson, R; Zeiss, CR; Grammer, LC. (eds). *Allergic Diseases - Diagnosis and Management.* Philadelphia: JB Lippincott. 1993; pp.353-394.

[58] Metcalfe, DD. Allergic reactions to foods. In: Frank, MM; Austen, KF; Claman, HN; et al.(eds). *Samter's Immunological Diseases.* Boston: Little, Brown. 1995; pp.1357-1366.

[59] Baral, VR; Hourihane, JO. Food allergy in children. *Postgrad. Med. J.* 2005;81:693-701.

[60] Muraro, A; Roberts, G; Clark, A; et al. The management of anaphylaxis in childhood: position paper of the European Academy of Allergology and Clinical Immunology. *Allergy.* 2007;62:857-871.

[61] Wang, J; Sampson, HA. Food anaphylaxis. *Clin. Exp. Allergy.* 2007;37:651-660.

[62] Simons, FE; Roberts, JR; Gu, X; et al. Epinephrine absorption in children with a history of anaphylaxis. *J. Allergy Clin. Immunol.* 1998;101:33-37.

[63] Brown, SG. Cardiovascular aspects of anaphylaxis: implications for treatment and diagnosis. *Curr. Opin. Allergy Clin. Immunol.* 2005;5:359-364.

[64] Oren, E; Banerji, A; Clark, S; et al. Food-induced anaphylaxis and repeated epinephrine treatments. *Ann. Allergy Asthma Immunol.* 2007;99:429-432.

[65] Simons, FE. First-aid treatment of anaphylaxis to food: focus on epinephrine. *J. Allergy Clin. Immunol.* 2004;113:837-844.

[66] Sampson, HA; Leung, DY. Anaphylaxis. In: Kliegman, RM; Behrman, RE; Jenson, HB; et al. (eds). *Nelson Textbook of Pediatrics*. Philadelphia: Saunders Elsevier. 2007, pp.983-985.

[67] Sampson, HA. Update on food allergy. *J. Allergy Clin. Immunol.* 2004;113:805-819.

[68] Kelso, JM. A second dose of epinephrine for anaphylaxis: how often needed and how to carry. *J. Allergy Clin. Immunol.* 2006;117:464-465.

[69] Clark, S; Camargo, CA, Jr. Emergency management of food allergy: systems perspective. *Curr. Opin. Allergy Clin. Immunol.* 2005;5:293-298.

[70] Du Toit, G; Fox, A; Morris, A. Managing food allergy in children. *Practitioner.* 2006;250:45-46, 49-52.

[71] Metcalfe, DD. Food hypersensitivity. *J. Allergy Clin. Immunol.* 1984;73:749-762.

[72] Leung, AK; Hon, KL; Robson, WL. Atopic dermatitis. *Adv. Pediatr.* 2007;54:241-273.

[73] Bailey, M; Haverson, K; Inman, C; et al. The development of the mucosal immune system pre- and post-weaning: balancing regulatory and effector function. *Proc. Nutr. Soc.* 2005;64:451-457.

[74] Kalliomäki, M; Kirjavainen, P; Eerola, E; et al. Distinct patterns of neonatal gut microflora in infants in whom atopy was and was not developing. *J. Allergy Clin. Immunol.* 2001;107:129-134.

[75] Watanabe, S; Narisawa, Y; Arase, S; et al. Differences in fecal microflora between patients with atopic dermatitis and healthy control subjects. *J. Allergy Clin. Immunol.* 2003;111:587-591.

[76] Björkstén, B; Sepp, E; Julge,K; et al. Allergy development and the intestinal microflora during the first year of life. *J. Allergy Clin. Immunol.* 2001;108:516-520.

[77] Laitenen, K; Isolauri, E. Management of food allergy: vitamins, fatty acids or probiotics? *Eur. J. Gastroenterol. Hepatol.* 2005;17:1305-1311.

[78] Boyle, RJ; Tang, ML. The role of probiotics in the management of allergic disease. *Clin. Exp. Allergy*. 2006;36:568-576.

[79] He, F; Morita, H; Hashimoto, H; et al. Intestinal *Bifidobacterium* species induce varying cytokine production. *J. Allergy Clin. Immunol.* 2002;109:1035-1036.

[80] Kirjavainen, PV; Apostolou, E; Salminen, SJ, et al. New aspects of probiotics – a novel approach in the management of food allergy. *Allergy.* 1999;54:909-915.

[81] O'Sullivan, GC; Kelly, P; O'Halloran, S; et al. Probiotics: an emerging therapy. *Curr. Pharm. Des.* 2005;11:3-10.

[82] Rosenfeld, V; Benfeldt, E; Valerius, NH; et al. Effect of probiotics on gastrointestinal symptoms and small intestinal permeability in children with atopic dermatitis. *J. Pediatr.* 2004;145:612-616.

[83] Williams, HC. Two "positive" studies of probiotics for atopic dermatitis – or are they? *Arch. Dermatol.* 2006;142:1201-1203.

[84] Kalliomäki, M; Salminen, S; Arvilommi, H; et al. Probiotics in primary prevention of atopic disease: a randomized placebo-controlled trial. *Lancet.* 2001b;357:1076-1079.
[85] Kalliomäki, M; Salminen, S; Poussa, T; et al. Probiotics and prevention of atopic disease: 4-year follow-up of a randomized placebo-controlled trial. *Lancet.* 2003;361:1869-1871.
[86] Lodinová-Zádníková, R; Cukrowska, B; Tlaskalova-Hogenova, H. Oral administration of probiotic *Escherichia coli* after birth reduces frequency of allergies and repeated infections later in life (after 10 and 20 years). *Int. Arch. Allergy Immunol.* 2003;131:209-211.
[87] Rosenfeld, V; Benfeldt, E; Nielsen, SD; et al. Effect of probiotic *lactobacilli* strains in children with atopic dermatitis. *J. Allergy Clin. Immunol.* 2003;111:389-395.
[88] Viljanen, M; Savilahti, E; Haahtela, T; et al. Probiotics in the treatment of atopic eczema/dermatitis syndrome in infants: a double-blind placebo-controlled trial. *Allergy.* 2005;60:494-500.
[89] Tamura, M; Shikina, T; Morihana, T; et al. Effects of probiotics on allergic rhinitis induced by Japanese cedar pollen: randomized double-blind, placebo-controlled clinical trial. *Int. Arch. Allergy Immunol.* 2007;143:75-82.
[90] Taylor, AL; Dunstan, JA; Prescott, SL, et al. Probiotic supplementation for the first 6 months of life fails to reduce the risk of atopic dermatitis and increases the risk of allergen sensitization in high-risk children: a randomized controlled trial. *J. Allergy Clin. Immunol.* 2007;119:184-191.
[91] Kukkonen, K; Savilahti, E; Haahtela, T; et al. Probiotic and prebiotic galacto-oligosaccharides in the prevention of allergic diseases: a randomized, double-blind, placebo-controlled trial. *J. Allergy Clin. Immunol.* 2007;119:192-198.
[92] Weston, S; Halbert, A; Richmond, P; et al. Effects of probiotics on atopic dermatitis: a randomized controlled trial. *Arch. Dis. Child.* 2005;90:892-897.
[93] Passeron, T; Lacour, JP; Fontas, E; et al. Prebiotics and synbiotics: two promising approaches for the treatment of atopic dermatitis in children above 2 years. *Allergy.* 2006;61:431-437.
[94] Chulada, PC; Arbes, SJ Jr; Dunson, D; et al. Breast-feeding and the prevalence of asthma and wheeze in children: analyses from the Third National Health and Nutrition Examination Survey, 1988-1994. *J. Allergy Clin. Immunol.* 2003;111:328-336.
[95] Gdalevich, M; Mimouni, D; Mimouni, M. Breast-feeding and the risk of bronchial asthma in childhood: a systematic review with meta-analysis of prospective studies. *J. Pediatr.* 2001;139:261-266.
[96] Leung, AK; Barber, KA. Managing childhood atopic dermatitis. *Adv. Ther.* 2003;20:120-137.
[97] Leung, AK; Sauve, RS. Breast is best for babies. *J. Natl. Med. Assoc.* 2005;97:1010-1019.
[98] Hanifin, JM; Cooper, KD; Ho, VC; et al. Guidelines for care of atopic dermatitis. *J. Am. Acad. Dermatol.* 2004;50:391-404.
[99] Muraro, A; Dreborg, S; Halken, S; et al. Dietary prevention of allergic diseases in infants and children. Part III: critical review of published peer-reviewed observational and interventional studies and final recommendations. *Pediatr. Allergy Immunol.* 2004;15:291-307.
[100] Kull, I; Böhme, M; Wahlgren, CF; et al. Breast-feeding reduces the risk for childhood

eczema. *J. Allergy Clin. Immunol.* 2006;116:657-661.

[101] Mimouni Bloch, AM; Mimouni, D; Mimouni, M; et al. Does breastfeeding protect against allergic rhinitis during childhood? A meta-analysis of prospective studies. *Acta Paediatr.* 2002;91:275-279.

[102] Siltanen, M; Kajosaari, M; Poussa, T; et al. A dual long-term effect of breastfeeding on atopy in relation to heredity in children at 4 years of age. *Allergy.* 2003;58:524-530.

[103] Host, A; Halken, S. Primary prevention of food allergy in infants who are at risk. *Curr. Opin. Allergy Clin. Immunol.* 2005;5:255-259.

[104] Schmitz, J. Prevention of food allergy during late infancy and early childhood. *Nestle Nutr. Workshop Ser. Pediatr. Program.* 2005;56:15-25.

[105] Sampson, HA; Fomon, SJ. Antigen-antibody interactions and adverse reactions to food. In: Fomon, SJ. (ed). *Nutrition of Normal Infants.* St. Louis: Mosby. 1993; pp.395-408.

[106] Zeiger, RS; Heller, S; Mellon, MH; et al. Effect of combined maternal and infant food-allergen avoidance on development of atopy in early infancy: a randomized study. *J. Allergy Clin. Immunol.* 1989;84:72-89.

[107] Brostoff, J; Hawk, LJ. Food allergy in children. *Eur. J. Clin. Nutr.* 1991;45:S11-S15.

[108] Leung, AK; Robson, WL. Breastfeeding. In: Carter, LV. (ed). *Child Nutrition Research Advances.* New York: Nova Science Publishers, Inc. (in press).

[109] Björkstén, B; Kjellman, NI. Does breast-feeding prevent food allergy? Allergy Proc. 1991;12:233-237.

[110] Bahna, SL. Management of food allergies. *Ann. Allergy.* 1984;53:678-682.

[111] Kramer, MS; Kakuma, R. Maternal dietary antigen avoidance during pregnancy and/or lactation for preventing or treating atopic disease in the child. *Cochrane Database Syst. Rev.* 2003(4):CD000133.

[112] Chandra, RK; Puri, S; Hamed, A. Influence of maternal diet during lactation and use of formula feeds on development of atopic eczema in high risk infants. *BMJ.* 1989;299:228-230.

[113] Hattevig, G; Sigurs, N; Kjellman, B. Maternal food antigen avoidance during lactation and allergy during the first 10 years of age. *J. Allergy Clin. Immunol.* 1996;97:241.

[114] Chandra, RK; Puri, S; Suraiya, C; et al. Influence of maternal food antigen avoidance during pregnancy and lactation on incidence of atopic eczema in infants. *Clin. Allergy.* 1986;16:563-571.

[115] Hattevig, G; Sigurs, N; Kjellman, B. Effects of maternal dietary avoidance during lactation on allergy in children at 10 years of age. *Acta Paediatr.* 1999;88:7-12.

[116] Falth-Magnusson, K; Kjellman, NIM. Development of atopic disease in babies whose mothers were receiving exclusion diet during pregnancy: a randomized study. *J. Allergy Clin. Immunol.* 1987;80:868-875.

[117] von Berg, A. The concept of hypoallergenicity for atopy prevention. *Nestlé Nutr. Workshop Ser. Pediatr. Program.* 2007;59:49-62.

[118] Zeiger, RS. Food allergen avoidance in the prevention of food allergy in infancy and children. *Pediatrics.* 2003;111:1662-1671.

[119] Marini, A; Agosti, M; Motta, G; et al. Effects of a dietary and environmental prevention programme on the incidence of allergic symptoms in high atopic risk infants: three years follow-up. *Acta Paediatr.* 1996;414:S1-S22.

[120] Halken, S; Host, A; Hansen, LG; et al. Effect of an allergy prevention programme on incidence of atopic symptoms in infancy: a prospective study of 159 "high-risk" infants.

Allergy. 1992;47:545-553.

[121] Hays, T; Wood, RA. A systematic review of the role of hydrolysed infant formulas in allergy prevention. *Arch. Pediatr. Adolesc. Med.* 2005;159:810-816.

[122] Osborn, DA; Sinn, J. Formulas containing hydrolysed protein for prevention of allergy and food intolerance in infants (review). *Cochrane Database Syst. Rev.* 2006 Oct 18;(4):CD003664.

[123] Kajosaari, M; Saarinen, UM. Prophylaxis of atopic disease by six months' total solid foods elimination. *Acta Paediatr. Scand.* 1983;72:411-421.

[124] Morgan, J; Williams, P; Norris, F; et al. Eczema and early solid feeding in preterm infants. *Arch. Dis. Child.* 2004;89:309-314.

[125] Fiocchi, A; Assa'ad, A; Bahna, S; et al. Food allergy and the introduction of solid foods to infants: a consensus document. *Ann. Allergy Asthma Immunol.* 2006;97:10-21.

[126] [126] Hodge, L; Salome, CM; Peat, JK; et al. Consumption of oily fish and childhood asthma risk. *Med. J. Aust.* 1998;164:137-140.

[127] Mayser, P; Mayer, K; Mahloudjian, M; et al. A double-blind, randomized, placebo-controlled trial of n-3 versus n-6 fatty acid-based lipid infusion in atopic dermatitis. *J. Parent. Enter. Nutr.* 2002;26:151-158.

[128] Nafstad, P; Nystad, W; Magnus, P; et al. Asthma and allergic rhinitis at 4 years of age in relation to fish consumption in infancy. *J. Asthma*. 2003;40:343-348.

[129] Thien, FCK; Woods, R; de Lucas S; et al. Dietary marine fatty acids (fish oil) for asthma in adults and children. *Cochrane Database Sys. Rev.* 2002;3:CD001283.

[130] Gool, CJ; Zeegers, MP; Thijs, C. Oral essential fatty acid supplementation in atopic dermatitis – a meta-analysis of placebo-controlled trials. *Br. J. Dermatol.* 2004;150:728-740.

[131] Roberts, G; Lack, G. Relevance of inhalational exposure to food allergens. *Curr. Opin. Allergy Clin. Immunol.* 2003;3:211-215.

[132] Sicherer, SH; Furlong, TJ; DeSimone, J; et al. Self-reported allergic reactions to peanuts on commercial airlines. *J. Allergy Clin. Immunol.* 1999;104:186-189.

[133] Nowak-Wegrzyn, A. Food allergy to proteins. *Nestlé Nutr. Workshop Ser. Pediatr. Program*. 2007;59:17-35.

[134] Nelson, HS; Lahr, J; Rule, R, et al. Treatment of anaphylactic sensitivity to peanuts by immunotherapy with injections of aqueous peanuts extract. *J. Allergy Clin. Immunol.* 1997;99:744-751.

[135] Pons, L; Burks, W. Novel treatments for food allergy. *Expert Opin. Investig. Drugs*. 2005;14:829-834.

[136] Allen, KJ; Hill, DJ, Heine, RG. 4. Food allergy in childhood. *MJA*. 2006;185:394-400.

[137] Enrique, E; Cisteró-Bahíma, A. Specific immunotherapy for food allergy: basic principles and clinical aspects. *Curr. Opin. Allergy Clin. Immunol.* 2006;6:466-469.

[138] Leung, DY; Sampson, HA; Yunginger, JW; et al. Effect of anti-IgE therapy in patients with peanut allergy. *N. Engl. J. Med.* 2003;348:986-993.

[139] Li, XM; Zhang, TF; Huang, CK; et al. Food Allergy Herbal Formula-1 (FAHF-1) blocks peanut-induced anaphylaxis in a murine model. *J. Allergy Clin. Immunol.* 2001;108:639-646.

[140] Li, XM; Srivastava, K; Grishin, A; et al. Persistent protective effect of heat-killed *Escherichia coli* producing "engineered," recombinant peanut proteins in a murine model of peanut allergy. *J. Allergy Clin. Immunol.* 2003;112:159-167.

[141] Mankad, VS; Burks, AW. Omalizumab: other indications and unanswered questions. *Clin. Rev. Allergy Immunol.* 2005;29:17-30.

[142] Okubo, K; Ogino, S; Nagakura, T; et al. Omalizumab is effective and safe in the treatment of Japanese cedar pollen-induced seasonal allergic rhinitis. *Allergol. Int.* 2006;55:379-386.

[143] Crespo, JF; James, JM; Rodriguez J. Diagnosis and therapy of food allergy. *Mol. Nutr. Food Res.* 2004;48:347-355.

[144] MacGlashan, DW; Bochner, BS; Adelman, DC, et al. Down-regulation of Fc (epsilon) RI expression on human basophils during vivo treatment of atopic patients with anti-IgE antibody. *J. Immunol.* 1997;158:1438-1445.

[145] Stein, ML; Collins, MH; Villanueva, JM; et al. Anti-IL-5 (mepolizumab) therapy for eosinophilic esophagitis. *J. Allergy Clin. Immunol.* 2006;118:1312-1319.

[146] Bieber, T. Allergen-specific sublingual immunotherapy: less mystic, more scientific. *Allergy.* 2006;61:149-150.

[147] Enrique, E; Pineda, F; Malek, T; et al. Sublingual immunotherapy for hazelnut food allergy: a randomized double-blind placebo-controlled study with a standardized hazelnut extract. *J. Allergy Clin. Immunol.* 2005;116:1073-1079.

[148] King, N; Helm, R; Stanley, JS; et al. Allergenic characteristics of a modified peanut allergen. *Mol. Nutr. Food Res.* 2005;49:963-971.

[149] Peng, HJ; Su, SN; Chang, ZN; et al. Induction of specific Th1 responses and suppression of IgE antibody formation by vaccination with plasmid DNA encoding Der f 11. *Vaccine.* 2002;20:1761-1768.

[150] Horn, AA; Raz, E. Immunostimulatory sequence oligodeoxynucleotide-based vaccination and immunomodulation: two unique but complementary strategies for the treatment of allergic diseases. *J. Allergy Clin. Immunol.* 2002;110:706-712.

[151] Marshall, JD; Abtahi, S; Eiden, JJ; et al. Immunostimulatory sequence DNA linked to the Amb a 1 allergen promotes T(H)1 cytokine expression while downregulating T(H)2 cytokine expression in PBMCs from human patients with ragweed allergy. *J. Allergy Clin. Immunol.* 2001;108:191-197.

[152] Hsieh, KY; Hus, CI; Lim JY; et al. Oral administration of an edible-mushroom-derived protein inhibits the development of food-allergic reactions in mice. *Clin. Exp. Allergy.* 2003;33:1595-1602.

[153] Li, XM; Srivastava, K; Huleatt, JW; et al. Engineered recombinant peanut proteins and heat-killed *Listeria monocytogenes* coadministration protects against peanut-induced anaphylaxis in a murine model. *J. Immunol.* 2003;170:3289-3295.

[154] Srivastava, KD; Kattan, JD; Zou, ZM; et al. The Chinese herbal medicine formula FAHF-2 completely blocks anaphylactic reactions in a murine model of peanut allergy. *J. Allergy Clin. Immunol.* 2005;115:171-178.

[155] James, JM; Burks, AW; Robertson, PK; et al. Safe administration of the measles vaccine to children allergic to eggs. *N. Engl. J. Med.* 1995;332:1262-1266.

[156] Khakoo, GA; Lack, G. Recommendations for using MMR vaccine in children allergic to eggs. *BMJ.* 2000;320:929-932.

[157] Lacksman, R; Finn, A. MMR vaccine and allergy. *Arch. Dis. Child.* 2000;82:93-95.

[158] Sampson, HA; Leung, DY. Adverse reactions to food. In: Kliegman, RM; Behrman, RE; Jenson, HB; et al. (eds). *Nelson Textbook of Pediatrics.* Philadelphia: Saunders Elsevier. 2007, pp.986-990.

Index

A

B

C

D

E

F

G

H

I

J

K

L

M

N

Q

R

S

T

U

V

W

X

Y